Health Care Ethics

A Theological Analysis

Benedict M. Ashley, O.P., Ph.D., S.T. M.

Kevin D. O'Rourke, O.P., J.C.D., S.T. Lr.

The Catholic Hospital Association
St. Louis, Missouri 63104

Nihil Obstat:
    Dennis R. Zusy, O.P.

Imprimatur:
    + James J. Byrne, S.T.D.
        Archbishop of Dubuque

November 23, 1977

To our brothers in the Dominican Province of St. Albert the Great, in thanksgiving for their fraternal charity.

Library of Congress Catalog Card No. 77-088355
ISBN 0-87125-044-6

1) Medical ethics
2) Medicine- Religious aspects- Catholic Church
3) Christian Ethics- Catholic authors
4) Pastoral medicine- Catholic Church

PREFACE

In the course of writing this book, we have called upon several people for help and received support and encouragement from many others. Though it will not be possible to name all those who have been instrumental in bringing this work to fulfillment, we do wish to express publicly our thanks to those who were more directly involved. First of all, to our colleagues at The Catholic Hospital Association, the Institute of Religion, and Aquinas Institute of Theology, we wish to express our thanks for the fraternal support and intellectual stimulation which led us to undertake this project. To the many readers of our manuscript, we also wish to express our thanks: especially, to John Doyle, Ph.D., Richard Fox, Ph.D., William May, S.T.D., Rev. Donald McCarthy, Ph.D., Edward Spillane, Ph.D., Edmund Pellegrino, M.D., Sister Maria Rieckelman, M.M., M.D., and Thomas Hilgers, M.D., for their comments, observations and corrections.

After the manuscript was completed Bea Rockstroh labored long and diligently to prepare it for publication and Fathers Thomas O'Meara, O.P., S.T.D., and Dennis Zusy, O.P., Ph.D., read it as theological advisors. The help of all three improved and strengthened the text. Through the whole process, June Granville cheerfully coordinated the compilation of the manuscript and also typed the manuscript too many times to mention. Others who aided through competence and advice were Lynnette Sodha, Mary Krieger, Ed Pollock and Tom Callahan. Lastly, we would like to thank Sister Mary Maurita Sengelaub, R.S.M., under whose presidency at CHA this book was begun, and Sister Helen Kelley, D.C., under whose presidency it has been published.

Naturally, we take responsibility for all mistakes, over or understatements that might be contained in this book. But we also acknowledge wholeheartedly that the book would never have been produced without the help and support of the above-mentioned people.

ABOUT THE AUTHORS

Rev. Benedict M. Ashley, O.P., was reared in Oklahoma, received his undergraduate training at the University of Chicago, and a PhD from the University of Notre Dame in Political Science. After joining the Dominican Order, he earned degrees in philosophy and theology and was ordained in 1948. His numerous books and articles on ethical issues, as well as his dedication to teaching, resulted in the recent conferral of the prestigious Master of Sacred Theology (STM) by the Dominican Order.

Father Ashley's interest in medical ethics was stimulated by his experience at the Texas Medical Center as a professor at the Institute of Religion and Human Development. At present he serves as a member of the Medical Moral Commission, Archdiocese of Dubuque, and Professor of Moral Theology, Aquinas Institute of Theology, Dubuque, Iowa.

* * * *

Rev. Kevin D. O'Rourke, O.P., was reared in the Chicago area, attended the University of Notre Dame as an undergraduate and received advanced degrees in theology (STL) and canon law (JCD) at the Angelicum in Rome after joining the Dominican Order. Ordained in 1954, he served as professor of canon law and moral theology at Aquinas Institute of Theology in Dubuque, Iowa, and also as president of the Institute from 1968-72. Since 1973 he has served as director of Medical-Moral Affairs, The Catholic Hospital Association, and was recently named a vice president of the Association. In this position he helps Catholic health care facilities. face the practical ethical questions that arise in contemporary health care and also has written several articles on ethical issues arising as a result of medical progress and human need.

CONTENTS

INTRODUCTION

Purpose of Book

Modern medicine gives us unprecedented power to heal human beings of physical and mental disease, to keep them healthy, and even to improve our human race for the future. This power can be used to humanize life or to dehumanize and destroy it. It can be used justly to benefit all, or it can be used to benefit the few at the expense of the many. How to use such power is a question of values and, therefore, of individual and group decisions which are not merely technical but ethical.

Hence, recently there has been a deluge of publications on medicoethical and bioethical topics (Boné, 1973). Two reasons have induced us to add to this flood. First, we think too much of this literature focuses on a few controversial but sometimes minor topics, while neglecting the broader and major issues affecting human health and the health care professions. Second, we want to be of assistance to Christian, and especially Catholic, health care professionals and health care facilities faced with the difficult and often puzzling responsibility to give witness to a long tradition of humanistic health care, while working with other professionals and government agencies committed to diverse value systems.

Outline and Method

We believe each person bears primary responsibility for personal health and the right to retain ultimate control over personal health. We also believe each person has the right to the help and care of the community in achieving personal health as well as the reciprocal obligation to assist other members of the community in the same search. Hence, in Part I we deal with the dignity of the human person in community and his or her right to health and the responsibility for it.

In Part II we deal with the responsibilities of the community, of the government, and of the health care profession in particular to assist persons in the search for health. As members of the clerical profession, we do not presume to pass judgment on our brothers and sisters of the health care profession with whom we have been associated as theological consultants in recent

1

years. All professions today are struggling under heavy public criticism for betraying the values which the learned professions have always been thought to exemplify for society. As clergy, we confess the truth of some of these allegations against our own profession and are in no mood to accuse members of other professions. We do believe, however, that all the professions must give each other mutual friendly criticism and support, so that it is not presumptious for us to join in the ethical debate now going on within the health care profession itself.

We use the broad term *health care* rather than *medical* profession because we address this book not only to physicians but also to all those engaged in serving others in their search for health. If sometimes we devote more attention to physicians than to other members of the health team, it is only because physicians are more visible and their responsibilities more clearly defined by professional traditions. What we say of them, the reader should apply *mutatis mutandis* to other health team members.

Because of our emphasis on the individual's primary responsibility for health, we believe this book can also be helpful to the general public in understanding their own rights and responsibilities in relation to the health care profession which exists only to serve them.

After dealing with the mutual relation between the health seeker and the health care professional, we turn in Parts III and IV to the process of ethical decision making in which both health seeker and professional are involved.

Too often today, bioethical controversies are confused and frustrating because the participants do not make explicit the value systems to which they are committed. Scientifically educated health care professionals know how to deal with facts, but often are untrained in any method of dealing with values. Consequently, in Part III we deal with the logic of ethical decision making, showing that currently there are many such logics which are not necessarily in contradiction with one another, but which are often very one-sided.

Two pioneers of medical ethics in the United States, Paul Ramsey (1970b) and Joseph Fletcher (1954), oppose each other on most issues because Ramsey works from a deontological ethics (duty ethics) of abstract, universal, rational rules of moral obligation, while Fletcher works from a teleological (means-ends utilitarian, consequentialist, situationist) ethics which emphasizes pragmatic decisions in unique contexts. In order to escape this stultifying polarization of ethical debate, we propose what we call Prudential Personalism. Like teleological ethics, it is "prudential" because it is an effort to make intelligent practical decisions about the means to be chosen to meet concrete human needs, but like deontological ethics it rejects a merely pragmatic, utilitarian calculation of consequences as an adequate method of moral decision by human persons. However, it is not a deontology but a personalism, because it does not base ethical decisions on axiomatic rules but on principles derived from our experience of the needs of human persons as they share in the historically developing human community.

It is not enough, however, to choose a logic or formal procedure for ethical decision making; we must also make our decisions in the context of some specific value system. Many assume today that the theological value systems of the various religions, Catholic, Protestant, Jewish and so forth will always remain pitted against each other in polemics that have no rational solution, and that if there is to be any public debate and consensus, it must be in terms of a neutral, philosophical, secular, and humanistic value system.

We take a different view and in Part III propose a system of values or ethical principles frankly Christian and Roman Catholic (not denying room for pluralism even here). We believe that every human being has a value system of some sort which is either religious or equivalent to a religion. To label one of these as neutral or humanistic is from the outset to give it a privileged position which can only frustrate honest debate and any effort to achieve some measure of sincere cooperation in a pluralistic society. For a long time in this country, the Protestant value system was taken somehow as self-evident, and all efforts of Jews and Catholics to speak in behalf of their own value systems was rejected as an intrusion of a private religion on public civil debate. Today it is assumed in the academy and the media that Humanism is self-evident (just as is Marxism in some countries) and any effort to speak up in the name of a "religious" value system is decried as an imposition.

Catholics reason ethically in terms of a value system rooted in a view of reality given by the Christian Gospel, interpreted by the Church in its life of faith, and authoritatively formulated by the pope and the bishops. Catholics believe this Gospel with the commitment of faith, and they accept its ordinary formulation and application by the pope and bishops with "religious assent" (Vatican II, 1965c) even when this lacks the final authority of solemn definition. However, this commitment to authoritative teaching, as well as our respect for a long tradition of Catholic theological reflection, cannot exempt the educated Catholic from listening honestly to other systems of belief, nor from comparing our beliefs with the discoveries of science and history and with our personal experience of life.

Such testing of belief leads Catholics to a development in the way we understand and apply our fundamental convictions. The same must be said of those who adhere to other beliefs and value systems and who also have an obligation to be open to dialogue undertaken in a truth-seeking spirit. None of us has the right to say to another, "You are biased because you are committed to your belief system, while I am not biased because I am only committed to the truth." Each of us seeks the truth through a belief and value system in which we think and which, if we are honest, we seek to deepen, broaden, and make more adequate to reality. Since the Second Vatican Council, Catholics have had the experience of how fruitful such an ecumenical approach can be, not for *conversion* of others so much as for a *convergence* of insight. In this book we attempt to follow that method, which requires both an openness to the options of others and a deepening of our own Christian and Catholic identity.

In Part IV we apply this method of seeking truth to the major issues now under controversy ranging from birth to death. This requires us to engage to a degree in a kind of ecumenism internal to the Catholic community which the events of the Second Vatican Council also opened up for us, namely, the problem of theological pluralism within Catholic thinking. Today we see our Catholic ethical system not as something complete and absolutely fixed, but as essentially historical and dynamic in character. At any given historical moment there exists in the Catholic community an authoritative moral teaching which provides a firm basis for any ethical discussion. In the medicoethical field, this teaching developed remarkably even before the Second Vatican Council (1963-1965) in the writings of Pope Pius XII (d. 1958) who was keenly aware of the emergence of such issues in our times. The United States Catholic Conference has collected some of these teachings in the *Ethical and Religious Directives for Catholic Health Facilities* (1971). Because we hope that our book will be useful for those working in such facilities, in our own ethical reasoning we give due recognition to the pastoral guidance of the Second Vatican Council and to the teaching of the popes and bishops, especially as expressed in the *Ethical and Religious Directives*.

Nevertheless, at any given moment in the history of the Catholic Church, a development of moral understanding goes on in response to current problems. We cannot assume that this development is always well balanced or even healthy. In the efforts of Catholics to live in a world of competing value systems, we may learn from the value systems of others, but we may also lose a good deal in the process. A frequently cited example of this is the distortion suffered by Christian sexual ethics from the influence of Stoicism when it was the popular value system of the Roman Empire (Noonan, 1965).

We do not pretend that in this process of development there is any easy way to distinguish progress from retrogression; neither conservatives nor liberals have any guarantee that they are automatically in the right. Consequently, along with an exposition of the authoritative position of the pastors of the Roman Catholic Church, we have included considerable discussion of different interpretations of such positions and of proposals for their refinement, revision, and even correction being made by committed Catholics theologians. Sometimes we opt for a liberal position, sometimes for a conservative one, as best we can see the truth at this moment. We hope that in so doing we are in line with the intellectual independence, combined with respect for authority and tradition, which seems to us one of the chief features of a Catholic and Christian value system.

Because we present our ethical discussion of concrete issues within the Catholic value system, we have subtitled this book "A Theological Analysis." By "analysis" we understand an effort to solve concrete ethical problems in terms of principles which are themselves formulations of human needs and values. We believe these values are most adequately discovered when we employ every kind of insight available to us: historical and personal experience, scientific discovery, philosophical reflection, and the Gospel light shining in Scripture and in the living tradition of the Christian community.

Such an analysis leads us to complete the book with Part V devoted to health care precisely as it is a Christian ministry.

Outcome

In this final Part V, we attempt to show that in a health care team which aims at healing the total human person, spiritual ministry must necessarily play an integral and integrating part. The chaplain in any health care facility or its pastoral care department has the essential function of assisting health care to take on a fully human and Christian vitality. This cannot be achieved if the chaplain and the department monopolize this ministry, but only if they are able to help all members of the health care team to recognize that as Christian professionals they are also engaged in a Christian ministry. Physicians, nurses, administrators, and all the variety of auxiliaries in a Catholic health care facility are gifted with talents and professional competence by which they truly minister the healing power of Jesus Christ present through them in our suffering and hoping world.

PART I

THE HEALTH SEEKER

CHAPTER 1 THE RIGHT TO BE FULLY HUMAN

1.1   HEALTH IS FOR PERSONS

Overview

In medical ethics, our first concern should be the persons who seek health rather than the professionals or institutions which exist only to serve the need of persons for health. Hence, Part I of this book deals with *The Health Seeker*.

In this chapter, we will discuss the right to be fully human, because the search for health is but one aspect of that search for complete humanness with which all ethics is concerned. In the next chapter, we will develop the notion of the right to health which is rooted in this right to be fully human. In chapter 3, we will present the conclusion that while each person has the primary responsibility for his or her own health this can be achieved only with the help and care of the community.

In the present chapter, we will argue that the basic principle of health ethics is the dignity of the human person (1.1). However, the human person can be healthy and whole only in a human community because to be a person is to be capable of interpersonal relations (1.2). An important implication of this fact is that an ethics of health must also be a politics of health, that is, it must consider how a community can arrive at consensus on the values, norms, and standards by which the community can work together to help all its members achieve health. However, in the United States and in the world there are many competing ethical systems.   For many, this seems to make a workable medical ethics impossible. We will argue, however, that even in pluralistic societies progress can be made toward ethical consensus (1.3).   Finally, we will argue that the chief problem in forming such a consensus is not disagreement about the human values to be sought, but about priorities. Hence, as we strive to resolve some of the ethical conflicts in the field of health care, our attention must be focused sharply on the issue of the hierarchy of values (1.4). This chapter is summed up by formulation of the basic ethical *Principle of Human Dignity in Community* on which the argument of this whole book rests (1.5).

8

Personhood

Every one of us is concerned about his or her health. Nothing is more human, more personal. Health, in fact, is and always has been one of the main preoccupations of the human community. We express our human fellowship by saying, "How are you this morning?" and "How-do-you-do?"

Our concern is about physical well-being, but it goes beyond that. In 1958 the World Health Organization declared: "Health is a state of complete physical, mental and social well-being and not merely the absence of disease or infirmity." That definition has been widely accepted and widely criticized (Callahan, 1973c), but at least it has made us aware that human health cannot be limited to the parameters of veterinary medicine. Animals need health care. Yet for us human beings, *need, care,* and *health* mean something different than they do for animals precisely because we are human.

Today, it is no longer easy to explain what *human* means. We live in a technological age in an artificial environment, and we view our world through scientific eyes. We need to recover the sense of our own humanity, our difference from the machine and even from the world of nature which has become so subject to scientific probing and technological manipulation (Nasr, 1968). In trying to define what makes us human beings different from animals, plants, and the dust of the earth and stars, we need not isolate or alienate human beings from the natural world of physics or biology (I. Ramsey, 1965). Rather, we must try to locate ourselves in the universe of things to which we are related in countless ways and yet in which we feel sometimes so alone both as a human being and as *this* individual human being who asks, Who am I?

Perhaps the best way to approximate a working definition of the human person in the ethical context of this book is to begin with the notion of human need (Handy, 1970). The human being is not definable as a static entity, but as a dynamic system of needs (Maslow, 1970). We humans need many of the same things plants and animals need, but we need even these common necessities in a special human way. Animals experience need when they hunger, thirst, gasp for air, or pursue a mate; we humans not only feel such needs, but we also have at least some understanding of *why* we need what we need. We also devise alternative ways of satisfying these needs, puzzle over what we need most, and even create needs never felt by human beings who came before us.

However, it is not easy to determine what human needs and capacities are genetically determined and common to the whole human species and which have been created by human culture. Of course the evolutionary continuity of our species with its primate ancestors guarantees some kind of biological origin of human values (Pugh, 1977). Nevertheless, biologists (Dobzhansky, 1956; Alcock, 1975) recognize that the evolution of our remarkable human brain has given us the capacity to break through the largely fixed and genetically determined kinds of behavior characteristic of even our closest primate relatives. Human beings have the need and the capacity to use symbols, invent tools, communicate by speech with its variety of invented languages, and to create and modify social and political systems in a manner only faintly foreshadowed in the behavior of other animals (Premack, 1976).

Yet this need and capacity to develop a diversity of cultural patterns masks the genetically inherent and common needs and capacities which might serve to define human nature. Anthropology and history have found it difficult to verify cross-cultural universals (Edel, 1968). Nor can we have recourse to the behavior of so-called primitive peoples, because their cultural history is as long as ours. Even the study of infant behavior yields only equivocal results, because infants behave only in response to the culture into which they are born.

Nevertheless, this very difficulty we experience in trying to separate human nature from human culture gives us our clue. What defines us as human beings is precisely this limited but real transcendence of rigid biological determinism (Adler, 1967). We are indeed bodily, biological animal beings with inherent needs for food, shelter, and reproduction, but we also have the kinds of brains and intelligence which make it possible and necessary for us to choose from a vast range of possible ways to satisfy these inherent needs. Culture is only the expression of our nature, which is to be intelligently free. This embodied intelligent freedom defines us as human and gives unity and continuity to the human family across time and space.

Personal Development

To have this need and capacity for intelligent freedom is to be a *person*. The reason ordinary language does not apply the term *person* to an animal, even a pet, is because we human beings, do not experience animals as self-conscious autonomous beings. Animals don't talk back. This is why some philosophers today want to add to the defining characteristics of person, not only "intelligence," and "freedom," but also "ability to communicate," and "to care," and "to be called forth" (Mounier, 1952; Tournier, 1957; Walgrave, 1965; Johann, 1968; Bertocci, 1970; Benjamin, 1971). We should note, however, that in ordinary usage the terms *person* and *personality* are not identical. We say that a person "has a personality," that is, that persons are the kinds of beings that understand and feel for each other in a human, freely intelligent manner. It is this *expression* of personhood which is personality (Lavely, 1967; Allport, 1937; Hall and Lindzey, 1970).

Medical ethics is confronted by the obvious fact that there are a good many human beings who hardly seem to be persons as we have just defined that term: the infant, the seriously defective, the senile, and the unconscious human being, and, yes, even ourselves when we are asleep! Certainly such human beings exhibit little that can be called personality, since their behavior seems to be only at the animal or even the plant level. We sometimes say of a comatose, brain-damaged victim of an accident, "He is now nothing more than a vegetable."

The fact is that in the human organism intelligent freedom is intimately linked to the central nervous system and more precisely to the frontal lobes of the cerebral cortex. When this relatively small but extremely complex part of a human being is inhibited in this normal functioning, that person ceases to be actively, intelligently free. He or she sinks back into the deterministic reflexes or physiological reactions of the animal or vegetative level of functioning. Yet as long as these higher brain centers function, a human being manifests a personality even when the rest of the body is largely destroyed. Such a person seems to need little from the rest of the body except a supply of oxygenated and nutritive blood to bring energy to the brain and carry away its wastes. Theoretically, at least, someday we may be able to maintain a living and conscious brain without a body at all. Will the human person in his or her own unique individuality still be present, be actively self-aware and posses intelligent freedom?

Does this mean that a human person exists only when that person is actually functioning in self-awareness and freedom? This conception would be altogether too static. The human person is not a pure intelligence, but a bodily being, sharing with the natural world, emerging through evolution out of that world, yet never being separated from it. Consequently, our human self-awareness and freedom emerge only at high points of a very complex process, much of which is subconscious and part of the determination of nature. When a unique human organism comes into existence at conception, his or her uniqueness is already genetically determined by a novel combination and fusion of different traits never previously combined. At this moment a unique human body comes into being and is continuously identifiable. In refutation of idealistic conceptions of the human person as a "self-conscious mind," recent philosophy insists that bodily identity is necessary to the notion of the human person (Strawson, 1959; Penelham, 1967; Danto, 1967). Even the medieval scholastics who argued for the survival of the human soul did not consider the soul a complete human person and believed that it received its identity from its relation to the body it would receive again at the resurrection (Thomas Aquinas, 1976 ed.). The whole life process that follows involves a development of this unique body-person in constant interaction with its environment.

Every individual has a *biography* that leads toward mature actualization of intelligent freedom and the manifestation of a unique personality. This life story passes through many phases of fetal and infant life before the higher functioning of the brain becomes possible. Even during adult life persons function with intelligent freedom only at certain times and in certain relations to their environment. Much of the adult's life is taken up with sleep, with routine, with times of feeding and relaxation when intelligence is working at a level below that of creative freedom. Yet this same, identical person carries on the total process of living in all its phases. Getting sick and getting well are both parts of this continuous, struggling process of living development. Thus by defining human person-hood as "embodied intelligent freedom" we are defining a life process which goes on at many levels of activity, but which is more clearly manifest and definable by its maximum, its high point of integration. Medical ethics must always keep in mind that the person who needs help in a particular crisis of illness is a being who exists not merely here and now but with a history and a future.

The term *personality* as commonly used also emphasizes this unique individuality of each of us within the human race. Because the essence of human nature is embodied intelligent freedom, each human being transcends the common determinations of this nature and attains a unique biography of personal choices. To be truly human I must also be truly *myself*. I must live out my life, taking responsibility for its ultimate direction. Such is a reasonable interpretation of the paradoxical view of some existentialist philosophers who say, "Man has no nature, but only a history." Individual differences between one human being and another are immense, resulting in a vast range of varied personalities (Allport, 1937). Even identical twins, who have great genetic similarity, are still able to live personal lives and to have distinct biographies (Stern, 1973). Twins can disagree, can each go separate ways. No doubt if someday science produces human clones, a test-tube production of many individuals of the same species (Francoeur, 1970; Watson, 1971), these human beings would each still have a life to live and would live it in a unique way.

With this account of what it is to be a human person, we can now come to a conclusion about what it is that makes human health care truly human by proposing a *preliminary* formulation of the goal of health care:

> The goal of health care is to contribute to the full development of human persons, that is, *to help human beings live in intelligent freedom*. Health care fails whenever it tends to depersonalize its clients by reducing this freedom.

1.2 PERSONAL HEALTH IN COMMUNITY

We have argued that every ethical problem about health care ultimately reduces to our conception of what it is to be a human person and to actualize that personhood in its fullness. However, this must not lead us into the error of individualism, so influential in American culture, which conceives the person in isolation, continually defending himself or herself against the encroachments of society. What then is the relation of human person to human community?

The classical definition "man is a rational animal" makes sense only if the terms *animal* and *rational* are understood as tags for a vast, ever-increasing array of information gathered by the behavioral sciences and the humanistic disciplines. *Animal* refers to our evolutionary origin and our complex physiochemicobiological structure. *Rational* does not mean that we are *only* rational, but that our very complex human behavior rises at peak moments to a freedom that transcends the instinctive life of animals. To say "man is a rational animal" is to say we men and women of every race belong to a single, interacting human community that is not only able to eat, drink, and procreate, but also to think scientifically and creatively, to debate and make political decisions, and to make love personally. Aristotle indicated this by saying "man is a *political* animal" (*Politics* I, 1253a).

Thus the notion of person is correlative to the notion of society or community and like any such term cannot be satisfactorily defined except in relation to its correlative. John Walgrave (1965), speaking in phenomenological terms, has written:

> That which is proper to a person and finds its fulfillment in personality cannot be defined exclusively as "self-possession." A complete definition should read "self-possession with an objectively directed project of life." The closedness of self-possession has meaning only through openness to objective life. That to which the activities of the objective project of life are directed is ultimately the personal world in which being-real finds its proper realization. In this way we ultimately arrive at "personal community" as the unitary formula which defines the objective of the activity making a person. This activity itself can be summed up in the word "love." Love then, which creates the personal community, is the proper perfection of personality. (pp. 114-115)

In fact, no human person can exist apart from a human community. Each of us comes into existence from parents, and no one of us can develop either physically or psychologically without constant interhuman relationships. The human brain cannot develop its full function without language, and language is a cultural, social creation. Even if in the future persons are produced in a test tube, they will be the product of a technological community and will be able to develop only within it.

The correlation of person and community is not merely superficial. We need a community not merely because the community supplies us with certain instrumental needs (food, housing, clothing, defense), but because the fulfillment of our personalities is to be found only in the act of communication and sharing with each other. If personhood is embodied intelligent freedom, it is then fulfilled in the free act of knowing and loving. Yet in the whole universe the most complex, varied, integrated, and beautiful beings are persons, and it is only in them that our desire to know and love can find full play. All the striving of science to understand the universe comes to its culmination in exploring the mystery of human persons who are the highest outcome of the evolutionary process, summing it all up in their complexity and emerging freedom and intercommunication (Mounier, 1952; MacMurray, 1961; Ligneuel, 1968).

Our knowledge of each other, however, cannot be achieved by simple observation in the way we can study a rock, a tree, or a dog. To know *you* I must pass beyond the relation of mere observer. To understand you intimately I must form a specifically human relation with you, whether as an enemy, a master, a slave, or better, a co-worker, a lover, or a friend. Such knowledge also involves feeling, even love. I must freely reveal myself to you if you are freely to reveal yourself to me. This means that a health care professional cannot really understand a patient or diagnose his ailment as if he were a thing, because the patient is a person whose whole mode of existence in his health or sickness is *relational*.

For Christians this correlation of person and community takes on a still deeper significance for two reasons (Kress, 1976). (1) The Christian God is a personal God, a Trinity of Persons who live in the total sharing of one single being, life, knowledge, and love. Thus the ultimate reality is a Community of Persons which sets the pattern for all other realities including our human reality. (2) The Christian God has created each unique human person *for* Himself, that is, with the intention of drawing each of us to share in his own eternal, trinitarian life. "This fellowship of ours is with the Father and His Son, Jesus Christ" (I John 1:3). Consequently, the Christian health care professional in his or her effort to heal another human being is a minister of God helping that patient to share more fully in the everlasting community of the Father, Son, and Holy Spirit.

This emphasis on the intimate relation of person to community should not, however, lead us into the exaggeration of those who argue that personhood is *conferred* on the individual by the community not by reason of some inherent right, but on the basis of conditions set by the community. Thus the philosopher Ronald M. Green (1974), making use of a "social contract" theory similar to that of John Rawls (1971), argues, "The issue of abortion . . . comes down to the question of whether rational agents could find it rational in the circumstances of moral choice to confer rights on the fetus, and if so, the nature and extent of these rights" (p. 62). The geneticist Joshua Lederberg (1967) locates human personhood as beginning around the first year of life, because "at this point only does [a person] enter into a cultural tradition which has been the special attribute of man by which he is set apart from the rest of the species." More moderately, the philosopher and medical ethicist H. T. Engelhardt, Jr. (1973b) argues:

> Though human biological life has value, it does not have an intrinsic value as persons possess in virtue of being self-conscious moral agents, and,

therefore, possessors of moral worth . . .

> Although a newborn infant is not yet a person, its promise of becoming
> a person allows entry into the role of person. The value of potential
> personhood is expressed in the "as if" social interactions of the infant
> which point to a future when the "as if" will be an "is" . . . The role of
> the child allows some biological human life to be appreciated as if it were
> a person. This appreciation and imputation of personhood, though, re-
> quires the minimal amount of interaction of which the infant is capable.
> (p. 24)

The significance of this theory of imputed personhood for the abortion
debate will be discussed in chapter 9. As an explanation of the relation
of person to community, it fails to take into account that, as we have
seen, the human person is essentially a capacity and openness to knowledge and love of other persons. Consequently, human personhood is
never completely actualized in this earthly life, but is always in the
process of growth, a growth which consists primarily in the extension
and deepening of communal relations.

Community, in its turn, exists to assist each of its member-persons
in this process of growth. Thus, as soon as a person comes into bodily
existence as a unique human organism, it enters into this actualizing
process and has a right to help from the human community to complete
this process. In other words, to *be* a person is to be in the process of
actualizing personhood (Eller, 1975). The community, therefore, does
not confer on or impute personhood to the sleeping, unself-conscious
infant or fetus but responds to its silent demand to live and grow.

This point becomes clear when we think of a hospital as a human
community dedicated to the care of the health of human persons. The
hospital does not confer the power to get well on the patients; it is inherent in their capacity for personal life. These patients include not only
the self-conscious, but also the comatose, the senile, the child, the infant,
and the unborn. Each is a human organism in the process of living out a
human life. Each has an ethical claim on the hospital community to give
such help as it can (and this has limits) to help this human being in its
growth, its struggle to actualize its inherent capacity for knowledge, love,
and human relationship which depend so intimately on its physical health.
The very purpose and meaning of the hospital community, as of every
human community, is to help its members grow in personhood.

Similar to the theories of imputation as a source of personhood
is the attempt of Joseph Fletcher (1972, 1974c) to enumerate "indicators
of humanhood," because along with the biological criterion of
"neocortical function," he selects "self-awareness," "euphoria" (as
found in a retarded but happy child), and "human relationships." Such
signs certainly indicate stages in the process of the actualization of a
person, but they do not necessarily mark the beginning of that process.
Nor do they indicate when a person with rights first exists and demands
the care of the community.

1.3   POLITICS OF PERSONHOOD

Christian Ethical Consensus

The intrinsic relation of persons to community implies that there is a *political* aspect to all human events. Therefore, an ethics of the human person in community must also be a *politics*, that is it must take into account the ways by which human persons develop value systems socially — sometimes through debate and often through social conflict. If we do not realistically face up to this political aspect of ethics, we will find ourselves each defending his or her own subjective ethical stance in endless and fruitless polemics. Today it has become all too apparent that health because it is human is a profoundly political issue, not merely in terms of the argument over "socialized medicine," but in the sense that the problems of poverty, food, population, and pollution are central both to national and international political struggles. There is discussion today about whether the medical profession has become a political weapon for thought control (Szasz, 1970, 1977) or genocide (Frankel, 1974).

In the face of this fact, many Christians are tempted to despair and withdraw from ethical controversy. In the pluralistic world of today, how is ethical debate even possible, let alone practical consensus? Warring value systems appear to be irreconcilable. Only political power will prevail, but today Christians form a minority often bitterly opposed by their fellow Christians and accused of politicizing religious differences and imposing sectarian morality on the public. In the health field, this disagreement among Chrisitians has become very evident in matters such as contraception, sterilization, abortion, and euthanasia.

Nevertheless, an attitude of withdrawal by Christians from ethical debate was not countenanced by the Second Vatican Council (1964b, 1965a, 1965b), which recognized the fact of pluralism, renounced any policy of religious imperialism, and proposed an ecumenical approach to differences in faith and value systems. First of all, Catholics must be convinced that they form a single faith community with all others who acknowledge Jesus as Lord, ordinarily signified by baptism. Within this community, of course, are great differences of opinion on certain ethical questions as a result of the historical divergence and isolation of one church from another. Such differences should not, however, overshadow the profound agreement among Christians that they all look toward Jesus Christ, portrayed for them in the Scriptures and the living history of his faithful followers, for the norm of ethical personhood and communal life.

Thus it is possible for Christians to move toward ethical consensus by turning together to Jesus in prayer, meditation, fraternal dialogue, and cooperation (Slater, 1963; Tavard, 1973). To lose hope in this possibility is to lose hope in him. Care for the sick was one of Jesus' first concerns. He healed before he preached, and he went out to the lepers, the most neglected members of the community. If Christians begin with this concern for the bodily needs of the alienated, the experience of charity will sweep away many of the one-sided views that divide us. It was no accident that the source of the recent upsurge in the ecumenical spirit was the common experience of Christians of every denomination who found themselves together in opposition to the tyranny of totalitarian governments in the days of Hitler, Mussolini, and Stalin.

A Wide Consensus

The Second Vatican Council (1965a) insisted that this spirit of dialogue must extend beyond the Christian family to other religions. Judaism and Islam believe in the same personal God as do Christians and also share the same fundamental convictions as to the dignity of the human person in relation to God (Smart, 1976). In the history of health care, Jews and Muslims made fundamental contributions which have become part of the tradition of Christian health care (Guthrie, 1946; Munter, 1971).

The Eastern religions of India and China are beginning to be influential in American life, but at first sight their outlook might appear to be incompatible with the Christian emphasis on the dignity of the human person in relation to a personal God, since they teach that the individual, after a series of reincarnations, is destined to be absorbed into the unity of the Absolute. (Tachibana, 1926; C. A. Moore, 1967). Closer study, however, reveals that this Absolute is not subpersonal, nor impersonal, but superpersonal. Thus it becomes possible for monotheists to join with believers in these Eastern religions in a common search for authentic spiritual self-hood (Zaehner, 1970; Merton, 1973). We are beginning to appreciate how much these religions, with their meditative disciplines, can contribute to our efforts to achieve personal integration and total health.

Nor should we forget the contributions of the *nature religions* of our native Americans and of other native peoples to a more profound appreciation of our relation to nature in its mysterious wisdom and cosmic rhythm. Modern medicine is beginning to learn from the ecological experience of such peoples. We cannot return to Eden, but woe to us if we forget it (Dubos, 1959)!

Thus, in other world religions, Christians will find much that can form a basis for ethical dialogue and much they can learn in the pursuit of true health for persons in a world community (Hocking, 1956; Tillich, 1963). Today, however, these religious systems of values seem to be receding before the worldwide advance of secularization which dominates both the First World of the democracies and the Second World of the Marxists, both competing for the domination of the Third World of underdeveloped peoples. Moreover this secularized view of man seems more congenial to the science and technology upon which modern medicine is based than do the older religions which often seem to substitute prayer for scientific health care. Yet the Second Vatican Council (1965a) has also indicated how dialogue between believers and non-believers is a practical hope.

The Christian is inclined to look at the agnostic world view of Humanism which prevails in the democratic countries and the atheistic world view of the Marxists as absolutely contradictory to Christianity. However, if we trace the origin of these new world philosophies we see that they are sociologically equivalent to the older world religions (Stark, 1966). The religious wars which resulted from the breakdown of Christian unity in the sixteenth and seventeenth centuries and the shock of discovering other ethically admirable religions of the New World and Asia led to a religious vacuum in Europe. Out of this arose the new philosophy of secular Humanism (the Enlightenment) which enthusiastically accepted the rise of science and technology as more efficient means to solve human problems than prayer, ritual, and traditional dogmas.

Thus in the well-known *Humanist Manifesto* (1933), signed by a group of distinguished American thinkers under the leadership of our most famous American philosopher, John Dewey, we read:

> Religion consists of those actions, purposes, and experiences which are humanly significant. Nothing human is alien to religion. It includes labor, art, science, philosophy, love, friendship, recreation — all that is in its degree expressive of intelligently satisfying human living . . . Religious Humanism considers the complete realization of human personality to be the end of man's life and seeks its fulfillment and development in the here and now. This is the explanation of the humanist's social passion. (p. 13)

Thus, Humanism rejects the notion of an afterlife for man and his dependence on a God or an Absolute, but it does so precisely in the interest of human dignity. Believing that the older religions tend to excuse man from full responsibility to create a good society here and now, this humanist position has been reaffirmed by an international group in the *Paris Statement* of 1966 (Kurtz and Dondeyne, 1972) and in this country in the *Humanist Manifesto II* (1973).

Where Humanism is not dominant, Marxism has become the contemporary equivalent of a religious system of values. While Marxism shares many common values with Humanism, it insists more emphatically on a materialistic conception of humanity, according to which we human beings emerge from nature by our struggle to control and refashion nature (even our own nature) to suit our own purposes. Historically, the human community has employed much of its energies in an internal class struggle of man against man.   Today, Marxists believe, we are on the threshold of an age when this class struggle will be overcome by the rise to power of the productive members of society, so that all humankind will at last be free to apply all its energies to the conquest of nature through the use of scientific technology (Fromm, 1974).

The humanistic Marxist Milan Prucha (1965) writes:

> Man is not the universal purpose of the world which religious illusion believes him to be.   Man came into existence in a certain part of the universe, under certain favorable conditions, as a partial product of the development of matter.   He must, therefore, assert himself through his practical activity against the world as a whole; rooted in the world, he must carry into it a meaning given by human existential needs. (p. 140)

> Marx comprehends the essence of man as the result of specific human activity, in accordance with his concept of practical materialism.   Man as a natural being creates social reality.   This is a new reality, in which the being of each individual achieves its content only in relation to other individuals, in relation to the social entity. (p. 144)

Many Catholics are under the impression that the Catholic Church opposes Communism and favors Capitalism.   They are unacquainted with the fully developed social teaching of recent popes (Mainelli, 1975; Gremillion, 1976) which must be taken into consideration in any Catholic approach to today's ethical problems, including those in the medical field.   This Catholic teaching attempts to transcend the Capitalist-Communist impasse based in both camps on a materialistic conception of society.   The popes urge us to work for a world community based on spiritual goals and economic cooperation.   They link the problem of human health with the problem of world poverty as the most fundamental ethical problems of our time, problems which in the United States are often ignored by bioethics, while much is made over esoteric problems such as eugenics and heart transplants (Illich, 1976b).

The Second Vatican Council has made clear that Christians have much to learn from the Humanist's emphasis on man's responsibility to use reason, science, and technology to solve human problems.   The other worldly view of religion rightly deserves the accusation that religion is often an "opiate of the people" when it should be a challenge to use the talents given us by God to overcome poverty, disease, and injustice.   For this reason, Catholic health care professionals should strive to heal any schizoid dualism in their own thinking between their religious view of life and an enlightened scientific view of the world.   Christians cannot accept the agnostic and sometimes mechanistic and materialistic interpretation which some scientists give the findings of science, but we can and should join enthusiastically in the advance of scientific research and its application to the solution of human problems of health.

Catholic liberation theologians (Gutierrez, 1973) have taken a further step by arguing that Catholics also need to learn from the Marxist criticism of Capitalism.   They point out that when Jesus announced the coming of the Kingdom of God he was not talking merely about a temporal reality, but was declaring the realization of the Old Testament prophetic demands for justice to the poor and oppressed. The Kingdom of God *begins* here on earth with social justice (Paul VI, 1971a, 1971b), and no one will gain its heavenly fulfillment who has neglected to work for social justice on earth. Jesus himself declared this in the parables of the sheep and goats (Matt. 25:31-46) and of Lazarus and the rich man (Luke 16:19-31). Consequently, a genuine Christian ethics cannot be written from the viewpoint of the status quo which in a sinful world tends to reflect the materialistic spirit of domination and possessiveness. It must view the world from the side of the oppressed whose needs have been ignored and neglected. Thus Jesus pointed to his preaching of the Gospel to the poor as the best sign of the authenticity of his own mission (Matt. 11:5). Therefore, can we not conclude that a Christian politics of health care must be based on advocacy for the rights of the neglected?

Why is the conflict between the individualism of Capitalism and the collectivism of Communism so unresolvable? Christian theology thinks of this conflict as the result of a profound misunderstanding of the relation of person to community (DeKoninck, 1943). We often confuse the notion of personal with the notion of private. Hence, it appears that to favor the community is to *sacrifice* the person to the collective. This is true if the community is based on a sharing of material goods. Such goods can be shared among individuals only by dividing them up and giving to each his private share. What I get, you lose, and vice versa. This is the way it works in modern societies based primarily on the sharing of material goods such as economic production and military power. Consequently, those who oppose selfish individualism sometimes turn to Communism wherein the person is sacrificed to the society.

Christian politics, however, aims at the sharing of *spiritual* goods: truth and love. Material goods should be distributed in such a way as to promote spiritual sharing, but they are not the primary basis of community. When spiritual goods are shared, no one loses, but each gains. The more I share such spiritual goods as truth and friendship, the more perfectly I possess them for myself. Only in such spiritual sharing is profound community between human persons possible. Thus the common good is not something opposed to the personal good. Rather it is the deepest heart of the personal good of each person. While private goods are actually *less* personal than this common good.

This theory may sound tempting, but impractical, until we realize that scientific truth is such a spiritual good. Is it not true that today scientists all over the world are able to come close to each other in the common advancement and sharing of scientific research, although they are deeply divided by the politics of their country based on economic and military power?

Therefore, a Christian politics today will aim at overcoming world conflict by constantly witnessing to a community based on spiritual values and subordinating material values as instruments to spiritual community. This is why dialogue in an ecumenical spirit has to be the great political strategy of the Christian. Health care is directed to the body, but as a process of healing it is directed to a spiritual goal, the appreciation of persons in their intelligent freedom.

Individualism and Human Rights

Now it should be clear why Catholic theology perceives as the greatest danger to the development of an ethical consensus in a pluralistic society that extreme form of Humanism which is sometimes called radical individualism. Typical Humanism has a strong concern for social justice, but radical individualism rejects the belief that community as such is a moral value. This ethic, proposed by Hobbes in the seventeenth century, supported in more moderate form by Locke, and given a new form by Nietzsche in the nineteenth century, has had a profound effect in American society from Emerson to its diverse advocates among the young counter-culturalists and psychotherapists (Szasz, 1961) on the left and libertarians like Ayn Rand (1964) and Robert Nozick (1974) on the right.

The ethic of radical individualism is summed up in the principle "I have a right to live my own life as long as I don't hurt anybody else," meaning by "hurt" direct harm by bodily injury or damage or theft of private property. According to this ethic, society exists only as a means to protect one individual from another, so as to leave each to pursue his or her private purposes. Moreover, any claim of one human being on another which is not contractual goes beyond the right to be let alone and is therefore unethical. Ethical behavior becomes the consistent pursuit of self-interest within a minimal code of law and contract enforcement. Proponents of this ethic often argue (1) that in fact people really act this way and other ethics are therefore hypocritical and (2) that this system of laissez faire is actually more productive of economic prosperity and human progress than are collectivist and altruistic ethics.

However, in reply we can point out that for laissez faire capitalists to argue they have a right to amass a fortune because it is "good for society" is itself hypocritical, because their real belief is that they have a right to their own lives no matter what the social consequences as long as they do not provoke those more powerful than themselves to destroy them.

This extreme form of individualism is perhaps best labeled privatism, and it was also the ethic of some of the counterculturists of the 1960s. Although they were in revolt against the aggressive money-making privatism of their parents, they had learned its basic attitudes which they reinterpreted in terms of freedom and love, that is, as an individualistic search for selfish pleasure and irresponsibility.

Privatism seems to be growing in American society in the 1970s. It is the most difficult value system to deal with, even for a Christian who has the will to try to find some point of contact. Yet even here we should give the individualists their due. When Ayn Rand (1964) attacks altruism and proposes the new selfishness, she obviously supposes that Christians teach an alturistic ethics in which the person is called upon to sacrifice his or her self-fulfillment to the community. Rightly she sees this as unreal and sentimental. What she does not realize is that Catholic ethics insists that the command "Love thy neighbor as thyself" (Mark 12:31) implies that we must *love ourselves* before we can love anyone else. Selfishness is not repudiated because it seeks the good of the self, but because it *closes* the self to those goods which can be achieved only by sharing with other persons. Thus Catholics can agree with radical individualists that each of us has as his or her first moral duty to seek genuine self-fulfillment. This is not sinful selfishness, but a duty to the God who made us to make good use of his gifts.

Furthermore, as Christians we should take up the challenge to show by hardheaded, realistic, and rational arguments that this self-fulfillment demands that we should not close ourselves off in sinful selfishness, but open ourselves to community in which alone we can find this self-fulfillment. In this way, we also learn something from privatism about good health care, namely, that (as we will argue in detail in chapter 2) each person has the primary responsibility for the care of his own health, a responsibility which he cannot pass on to the health care profession or to society.

This ecumenical search for ethical consensus has its solid legal and political foundations in the United Nations' *Universal Declaration of Human Rights* (1948) signed by almost all the countries of the world and supported by all the major religions, as well as by Humanists and Marxists. Catholics have been urged by the Pontifical Commission on Peace and Justice (1973) and by Pope Paul VI (1973) to support this *Declaration* as a sound (although not complete) basis for modern ethics. It begins with the fundamental statement which formulates the very notion of person and community for which we have just argued:

Article 1: All human beings are born free and equal in dignity and rights.
They are endowed with reason and conscience and should
act towards one another in a spirit of brotherhood.

Here "reason and conscience" is equivalent to the "intelligent freedom" and "brotherhood" to "community" in terms of which we have defined the human person. The *Declaration* then effectively concretizes this abstract principle by enumerating twenty-nine basic human rights. Among these are the following which should serve as the Magna Charta for a modern health care ethics:

Article 3: Everyone has the right to life, liberty and security of person.
Article 22: Everyone, as a member of society, has the right to social
security and is entitled to realization, through national effort

and international cooperation and in accordance with the organization and resources of each state, of the economic, social and cultural rights indispensable for his dignity and the free development of his personality.

Article 25: (1) Everyone has the right to a standard of living adequate for the health and well-being of himself and of his family, including food, clothing, housing and medical care and necessary social services, and the right to security in the event of unemployment, sickness, disability, widowhood, old age or other lack of livelihood in circumstances beyond his control . . . (3) Motherhood and childhood are entitled to special care and assistance. All children, whether born in or out of wedlock, shall enjoy the same social protection.

According to Article 2 all these rights apply to all human beings "without distinction of any kind, such as race, color, sex, language, religion, political or other opinion, national or social origin, property, birth or other status." Moreover, Article 29 (1) asserts, "Everyone has duties to the community in which alone the free and full development of his personality is possible."

Of course, we are far from having fulfilled our obligations under this *Declaration* in our own country, let alone in the whole world. Nevertheless, it stands as a proof that in the twentieth century there is already a basic consensus on the fundamental ethical values on which world community must be based (De La Chapelle, 1969; Cassin, 1969; Leclercq, 1969; Downie and Telfer, 1970). The aim of this book is to take that ethic very seriously.

1.4   PRIORITIES IN NEEDS AND VALUES

The fact that the nations of the world are at least nominally agreed on a list of human rights or values is an important step toward increasing ethical consensus, but it is only a first step. Sad experience since the adoption of the *Universal Declaration* has shown how diverse are the interpretations of many of these rights. When carefully examined, this diversity reveals ethics must not only list agreed-upon values, but must also deal with the question of priorities. What is the "hierarchy of values"? Some will reply that this question of emphases and priorities is a wholly subjective matter about which rational discussion is impossible. Whether this is the case can be decided only if we examine more closely the concept of value and its relation to objective facts.

We have already argued that ethics has to do with the satisfaction of the *needs* of human persons in their lives as intelligently free social beings. We have now to ask more precisely: What are these needs? Are some needs more basic than others? The general answer is that human needs are satisfied by human values, and the most basic needs by the most basic values, but the term *value* is vague. It was originally used in economics, but has been extended in usage to cover a spectrum of analogical meanings (Rescher, 1969). However, a given human value is always correlative to a human need, that is, it is desired to satisfy the need. In contrast are the negative value, which is inimical to the need, and the valueless, which neither satisfies nor obstructs. A value, therefore, can be something so trivial as a cup of coffee to satisfy my thirst or so sublime as the truth of Plato's philosophy to satisfy my thirst for meaning in my cosmos. A behavioral test for a value is the human reaction to it, that is, whether the value is rejected or accepted. Human debate about whether something is desirable or undesirable, acceptable or unacceptable, is clear evidence that what is in question is the worth of the value.

In the twentieth century, a long and rather tedious debate has gone on among British and American ethicists about the relation between facts and values (Kerner, 1966; Hudson, 1970; Hanock, 1974). This controversy arose because scientists today make a great effort to formulate scientific statements in value-free language. However, if this model is followed in ethical and political discussions, it is self-defeating. Ethical and political talk deals not merely with the description of facts, but with how these facts are to be changed for the better.

This long controversy is still not over, but it has led to some points of agreement. First, it is clear that we cannot divorce ethical debate from all reference to facts (Toulmin, 1950), for example, every bioethical debate depends upon an accurate knowledge of the medical facts. Second, the debaters must give good reasons for their ethical positions in terms of these certified facts (Hare, 1952), that is, it is irrelevant in bioethical debate merely to talk about how one *feels* about abortion. There must also be reference to its consequences for those involved. Third, in all ethical discussions, people make reference to evident human needs, for example, it is good to be able to see and walk, bad to be blind and crippled, so that serious ethical issues arise when it is a question of blinding or mutilating a human being (Foote, 1959). Fourth, ultimately in ethical debates we get back to questions about value systems, that is, to our religious or philosophical view of the meaning and value of human life as a whole (Flew, 1964; Phillips and Mounce, 1965).

In chapters 7 and 8, we will take a definite stand on this facts-values issue. Here, suffice it to say that for us ethical values are rooted in the value of human persons and in concern to meet their basic needs in the human community in balanced and consistent ways.

Other psychologists have devised even more elaborate lists of natural needs (R. Fletcher, 1966). But some, such as Gordon Allport (1937), have objected to all such classifications as based too much on the notion of instincts. For Allport the innate tendencies of man are so broad, require so elaborate a set of cultural conditions to develop, and develop so much in the context of an individual personality with a personal biography that Allport wishes to avoid the notion of instinct altogether.

He speaks only of the development, differentiation, and integration of a personality in interaction with its natural and social environments (Grastyán, 1974).   Yet Allport cannot avoid discussing different *tendencies* of the organism in its effort to adjust to or control its environment.

Thus we can distinguish at least the following dimensions of personality, or levels of need (Ashley, 1972; Y. Maslow, 1970):

1. The *biological dimension* (Maslow's physiological needs). Human persons share with all living organisms the need to maintain themselves homeostatically in a dynamic relation with their environment, to grow and mature to full biological development as individuals, and to continue the species through reproduction. This is the level usually dealt with by biologists and physicians.

2. The *psychological dimension* (Maslow's safety needs and also his belongingness and love needs in their more emotional aspects). We are psychic organisms which sense, imagine, and feel. This is the level of need generally dealt with by experimental psychologists and psychotherapists.

3. The *ethical dimension* (Maslow's esteem needs, as well as the belongingness and love needs in their more developed aspects). This is the level of human free choice within the limits of an existing culture. It comprises the need of the individual both for self-control and for social relations beyond those determined by the family.   This is the level dealt with by lawyers, political leaders, and clergy acting as moral counselors.

4. The *spiritual dimension* (Maslow's need for self-actualization including needs to know and understand, to contemplate, and to create). This is the level of commitment, creativity, and transcendence at which we not only live within a culture, but criticize it, transcend it, and contribute to it. It includes all activity with a creative element in art or science or political innovation and, furthermore, religious activity as it extends to ultimate, cosmic meaning. This is the level dealt with by the inspiring teacher and spiritual guide.

Within each of these levels there is a complex of natural and cultural needs. Even at the biological level, where physiological laws predominate, there are still cultural determinations (e.g., kinds of food, forms of marriage, etc.), and at the spiritual level, where culture predominates, we still remain rooted in our biological, bodily nature (cf. 2.3).

The ethical problem we face is precisely to plan our lives and to engage in political decision in such a way that *all* these needs are to a degree satisfied in an integrated and consistent manner. This obviously requires adjustment of the priorities in regard to both aims and objectives and of the practical steps to be taken and demands the subordination, and even sacrifice, of less important needs to greater needs. The exact mix or proportion will depend upon both the culture and the individual.

Thus health as a value cannot be understood ethically in isolation from the whole hierarchy of values of which it is a part.

1.5 PRINCIPLE OF HUMAN DIGNITY IN COMMUNITY

In this chapter, we have tried to understand the *humanity* of the health seeker, which makes his or her health human and not merely animal or vegetative and not the mere functioning of a well-adjusted, well-oiled machine. This humanity can be summed up in three conclusions:

1. Health care must deal with human health humanely. Human health is that of a living organism of the human species, distinguished from other animals by its personhood, that is, its capacity for intellectual freedom which can be actualized only in a truly human community. Such a community must be based primarily on the sharing of human values — the communication of truth and love — and only instrumentally on material values.

2. Since human health can be achieved only in a human community, an ethics of health care is also a politics. In modern pluralistic society, a politics of ethics demands an effort to increase moral consensus by an ecumenical dialogue on a worldwide scale among all those who hold diverse values systems, religious or secular. The existing basis of such a consensus is the United Nation's *Universal Declaration of Human Rights* (1948), based on the principle of human dignity.

3. This *Principle of Human Dignity in Community* can be formulated as follows:

    All ethical decisions (including those involved in health care) must aim at human dignity, that is, the maximum, integrated satisfaction of the innate and cultural needs of every human person including his or her biological, psychological, ethical, and spiritual needs as a member of the world community and national communities which exist for this purpose only.

CHAPTER 2   THE RIGHT TO HEALTH

2.1   CONCEPTS OF HEALTH AND DISEASE

Overview

In the previous chapter we presented the dignity of the human person as the fundamental principle on which Christian ethics can seek agreement with other ethical systems.   Health is the aspect of this human dignity with which we are concerned in this book.   Hence in this chapter we will attempt to develop a concept of human health and disease that will take into account the multidimensional character of the human person in relation to community.   Since health is the ultimate goal of all health care, this concept of health and the human right to achieve it will serve as the specific principle in light of which we will develop an ethics of health care.

First, we will deal with the concept of the person as multidimensional (2.1) and then with the various kinds of health: biological (2.2), psychological, ethical and social, and spiritual (2.3) and how they are interrelated in total or integral health.   Finally, in 2.4 we will sum this up in the Principle of Totality and Integrity with has many applications in concrete medicoethical decisions such as donor transplant of organs.

Concepts of Health

The word *health* is etymologically related to the Anglo-Saxon word from which are derived not only *healing* but also *holiness* and *wholeness* (Goldbrunner, 1955; Lepp, 1966; *California Medicine*, 1970).   The root sense is that of "completeness," a whole which has all its parts. Such a whole can be considered statically as a *structure* with all its parts, with each part properly proportioned, and with all parts in their places. Thus a crippled person lacks wholeness or health because some part of his anatomy is missing or deformed.   But it can also be considered dynamically as a *functional* whole, in which all necessary functions are present and acting cooperatively and harmoniously.   Thus some sicknesses do not involve any lack of a part or organ or its deformity, but rather a dysfunction, where some needed function is suppressed or lack of harmonious balance between functions, as in diabetes or hyperthyroidism is present.

Since medicine has as its goal the fostering and restoration of health, it would seem the medical profession would be very clear on the definition of this goal (Riese, 1953; Tillich, 1961; Naegle, 1977). But one has only to ask the average medical student or student nurse the question, What is health? to discover that medical education devotes little time to developing such a definition. Medical schools and nursing schools somehow assume that students will pick up an adequate notion of health simply from their experience of dealing with sick and healthy patients. No doubt this sometimes happens, but such unexamined presuppositions can be dangerous. For a medical professional to be devotedly working toward a goal which is vague and ill-defined is as absurd as for a cancer research team to be looking for a cure without first trying to understand the nature of the disease (Wylie, 1970).

Henrik L. Blum (1974) in an effort to formulate a definition useful to guide health planning has proposed no less than eight definitions, each with experience-tested advantages and disadvantages, and then added a ninth definition of his own. In summary they are the following:

1. According to the *medical model*, "health is freedom from superimposed or unnatural influences." This concept has encouraged medicine to seek the causes of disease, but it has prolonged the dying process and has discouraged preventive medicine.

2. According to the *preventive or public health model*, health is still thought of as freedom from superimposed disease, but disease is seen as something against which barriers can be raised or whose invasion can be detected early and minimized and in which functional restoration can be pursued. This concept still fails to take sufficiently into account the social factors of disease.

3. The *humanitarian or well-being model* (such as that of the World Health Organization) places "man at the center of its concerns" and works for the survival of infants and mothers, the alleviation of malnutrition and cruel treatment, the ready availability of health care, and the provision of a safe and pleasant environment. This concept , too, has tended to prolong hopeless suffering and to substitute charity to the needy for justice in defense of the human right to adequate health care.

4. The *economic model* has thought of disease in terms of factors that might prevent entry into the work force, cause the loss of effective workers and homemakers, prevent the education of productive workers, cause losses from low productive performance, and affect cost-benefit ratios and thus lower the gross national product of a country. Such a concept has spurred on

practical efforts to raise the standard of health in many countries, but it also opens the way to extermination (calculated neglect) of poor risks and poor producers.

5. The *super biologic systems* model sees "disease as a natural phenomenon, and health as adaptation to the environmental demands to the degree to which the individual is capable." This view stresses normal growth, development, and functioning at physiological, psychological, and sociological levels. It has promoted scientific research, but has tended to result in great emphasis on the cure of degenerative disease in adults rather than in better health for those who still have a life to lead.

6. The philosophical model and the similar *mental health* model think of health as "the pursuit of the maximal capacity for self-realization or self-fulfillment." The concept has led to a deeper, more humane notion of healthful living, but it is open to interpretation in a selfish, individualistic sense and to neglect of less gifted and educated groups in the society.

7. The *ecological* or species-survival model displaces man from the center of things and sees human health as dependent upon our capacity to maintain the ecological balance of nature or to shift it cautiously to our own advantage as a species without destroying it. This view has not yet been time-tested, but it promises greater respect for limited resources, yet also may lead us to defense of the social status quo in favor of the developed nations.

8. The *Third World* model which stresses the survival of the victims of modern technology sees disease as the result of social oppression by the advanced countries and health as the result of a social liberation in which underdeveloped people will achieve greater productivity, learn to control population growth without genocide, and maintain their own religious values as against secularism. This concept emphasizes the need for universal social justice, but it tends to a kind of irrationalism.

9. Blum (1974) synthesizes the preceding concepts in his own working definition for a *health planning* model as follows:

> Health consists of the capacity of an organism (1) to maintain a balance appropriate to its age and social needs, in which it is reasonably free of gross dissatisfaction, discomfort, disease or disability; and (2) to behave in ways which promote the survival of the species as well as the self-fulfillment or enjoyment of the individual. (p. 93)

Briefly, "health is the state of being in which an individual does the best with the capacities he has, and acts in ways that maximize his capacities" (p. 93). He contends that this can be measured in terms of eight parameters: prematurity of death, departure from physiological norms, discomfort, disability to function, internal satisfaction, external satisfaction, positive health, and capacity to participate in social activities.

Blum's discussion is very suggestive and appropriate to his immediate practical purpose, but it leaves us uncertain as to a fundamental concept of health which might give unity to all these diverse aspects. For this we must seek further.

In the actual practice of medicine today *health* is most commonly defined (Spector, 1975) in terms of standard physiological parameters: the vital signs, various chemicals in the blood, electroneurological readings, and so forth, as well as by gross anatomy and histology. Moreover, the possibility of a complete physical examination and diagnosis of health by means of physiological tests and computerized calculations is anticipated and is partly practical already. Health, therefore, will soon be defined by a model of what is normal.

Such a model will raise some problems, however. First of all, it is obvious that an exact, universal definition of human health in these terms is impossible and that only a *range* of normal values can be achieved (Collen et al, 1969). In the case of some values, temperature, for example, the range from one individual to another is small; in others, weight, for example, it is large; but in all cases what is identifiably healthy for one individual is not necessarily indicative of a state of health for another person. Second is the question of how the model of normality is to be determined. The *normal* is not identical with the *average*, since it is quite conceivable that the majority of people today are not very healthy. The normal therefore is an *ideal* (Krutch, 1959). How do we determine such an ideal in a way that is not arbitrary, but which has a sound empirical basis?

This question brings us to the notion of health as *optimal functioning* (Means, 1955; Dalrymple, 1959; Dubos and Pines, 1965; Hayman, 1966; Dubos, 1968). Even health in the structural sense of absence of anatomical lession or deformity reduces to optimal functioning, since the axiom holds that structure is for function. The absence of a functionless part (e.g., perhaps the appendix) is not a defect of health, but even an advantage. Moreover, the deformity of an organ must ultimately be judged in terms of whether it is capable of optimal function. Even appearance can be considered one aspect of function since physical beauty has a social function. Thus, we say that a human being is healthy if he or she can function optimally. This implies that each organ and organ system of which the body is composed is functioning well and that all are functioning together to form a single life process, of which the diverse functions are harmoniously interrelated, although differentiated, phases.

This conception of health is a consequence of the basic conception of a human being as an *organism* (etymologically "a complex of instruments" or organs), that is, a *living whole composed of functionally differentiated parts*. A human being is thus a dynamic or *open system*.

A system is a "complex of interacting elements" (Bertalanffy, 1968), and a living system is dynamic or *open*, that is, is able to maintain *homeostasis* (dynamic stability, Cannon, 1939) in relation to its environment by regulating the input and output of matter and energy.

In such a system, as Bertalanffy shows, we cannot reduce the characteristics and behavior of the whole complex simply to those of the parts, because the parts in the context of the whole do not exist or act separately but in mutual interrelation and interaction. Moreover, in more complex systems there are several *levels* of organization which are in *hierarchical order*, so that the higher levels of function include the lower levels but cannot be reduced to them. The fallacy of reductionism is to attempt to explain these higher levels of functioning simply in terms of lower levels, or to explain the system merely in terms of its parts. To avoid reductionism we must always take full account of the interrelation and interaction of the parts and the levels of organization in the whole. The whole of the organism is not some mystical or extraneous entity added to the parts of the system, but is precisely the structural and functional interrelation and interaction of the parts.

Obviously, a definition of health in terms of optimal functioning of an open system cannot be complete unless we speak of the output of the system. A living thing cannot maintain itself in static existence; it must interact with the environment. This is especially obvious in the fact that living individuals must also reproduce in order to maintain the species, but it is also clear that living things modify the environment in their own interests. Thus animals build shelters and nests, fertilize plants on which they feed, and rid their environment of enemies. In fact, the earth environment as it now exists highly favorable to life has been largely the product of living things themselves who have modified both the soil and the atmosphere in ways favorable to life (Reid, 1970).

In the case of human beings, we must go a step further. Because man is a cultural as well as a natural being, his interaction with his environment is highly creative. He modifies the environment with conscious purpose, so that civilization is the production of a city, that is, an increasingly man-made environment (Roszak, 1972). Today, we are beginning to think of human beings living in an environment which is almost entirely artificial. For example, we are dreaming of men living on the moon or even on constructed satellites where nothing will be natural except the basic raw materials from which the total environment will be humanly constructed.

What is still more interesting is the fact that human creativity is not to be found merely through interaction with an external environment. Man creates not only external things, but also symbols which exist in his mind and feelings and which fulfill certain needs that cannot be fulfilled by what is merely objective, that is, outside his conscience (Cassirer, 1953). Ultimately, human beings have a need to assimilate, or draw into themselves in the form of information (i.e., symbols of order), the whole order of the external environment. Thus, scientists are constantly striving to re-create, as it were, the entire external cosmos within their own minds in the form of a symbolic system. The great importance, from a personalistic point of view, of this human life process is that such symbol systems carry communication between persons in the form of language. Human society is ultimately the sharing among persons of this communication by which we all come to live in the same symbol universe.

This internalization of the environment does not, however, render vain our interaction with the external environment. We can increase our scientific knowledge only by experimentation, by interaction with external things, and we can communicate only by languages which require an external medium. Moreover, scientific advance is also technological advance. To learn more about the world we often have to change it. By developing human culture we break down the barrier between mind and matter, between the internal and the external. Thus, the human organism as an open system is one which is progressively opening up to include other human persons and the entire cosmos, as scientific visionaries like Teilhard de Chardin (1964) and Alfred North Whitehead (1957 [1929]) have so vividly shown us.

In view of this conception of human functioning, we see that human health as optimal functioning means not only an internal harmony and self-consistency of function within the organism, but also the capacity of the organism to maintain itself in its environment — especially in the human case to extend itself creatively to the production of an ever-expanding culture. This is why the World Health Organization, in the definition given in 2.1 insists, "Health is a state of complete physical, mental and social well-being and not merely the absence of disease or infirmity."

Blum (1974) also ends his discussion (summarized earlier in this chapter) by the brief formula, "Health is the state of being in which an individual does the best with the capacities he has, and acts in ways that maximize his capacities." Similarly, Coe (1970) defines disease as "the subjective evaluation by the individual that something is wrong with him *as an individual* and usually first noted in terms of a reduced ability to perform social roles" (p. 144). Freymann (1974) in view of the reduction of acute disease in our times urges a redefinition of health as follows: "the presence of social function, that is, the ability to cope with and control one's environment to the maximum extent possible within the constraints of nature and circumstance" (p.383). We would stress that optimal human functioning is something more than the ability to cope with one's environment. Furthermore, we believe that the capacities of an individual are themselves open to improvement in view of our fundamental human capacity for intelligent freedom and creativity. Thus, it is clear that a definition of health in order to be precise must also itself be open, that is, be constantly revised in view of a deepening and enriching vision of human capacities for culture.

In 1.4 we saw that the levels of human needs can be placed in a hierarchical order from primary physical needs to higher or cultural needs according to Maslow's scheme of five needs, or more conveniently for our purposes, the four levels of *biological, psychological, ethical*, and *spiritual* needs. Health in the broad sense of the World Health Organization definition is thus "optimal functioning of the human organism to meet biological, psychological, ethical, and spiritual needs." The concern of the health care professions, however, is with health in the narrower sense of optimal functioning at the biological and psychological levels, yet in the context of the integration of all four levels. That this definition is closely related to actual professional practice is clear from the fact that most physicians concern themselves principally with biological functioning, but that some, the psychiatrists, deal with the psychological level, and that the ethical and spiritual levels are commonly the concern of other professions, especially of lawyers and clergy.

Concepts of Disease

Given this concept of health as structural and functional wholeness of the human organism in relation to itself and to its environment, a wholeness that extends even to the ethical and spiritual, to holiness, we can also approximate a more precise idea of the notion of disease (cf. Engelhardt, 1975a; Kopelman, 1975). The World Health Organization definition makes clear that disease and infirmity are not the exact contrary of health. Health, as we have defined it, is optimal functioning. For an organism to fall short of optimal functioning without actually being diseased or infirm is possible, because an organism can be healthy in a narrow sense without actually being used to its full capacity. However, without optimal functioning, the failure to function soon leads to dysfunction. A man can be healthy in this narrow sense and yet be lazy, half-alive through lack of full use of his capacity for living, but he will not stay healthy even in this minimal way for long because his faculties will atrophy.

In the history of medicine, as Owsei Temkin has shown (1963, 1973), there has been a constant pendulum swing between two concepts of disease: the ontological and the physiological. The ontological conception thinks of diseases as separate entities (devils, contagions, morbific matters, bacteria, genetic defects, neuroses, psychoses) which can be classified and named just as we name plants and animals. The organism is constantly fighting to throw off such diseases as alien invaders which disturb its own homeostasis. Those who think in these terms tend to diagnose diseases in terms of clearly classified and labeled entities and to treat them by seeking specific remedies (e.g., specific drugs, specific surgical procedures).

The opposite of the ontological conception, the physiological conception of disease, is that disease is a breakdown of internal functional harmony of the organic system due to hyperfunctioning or hypofunctioning of an organ. Thus, in this conception dysfunction makes the organism liable to invasion by external agents such as bacteria, but the bacteria are not the primary cause of the disease. Even trauma produced by external injuries in accidents may be the result of the victim's being "accident prone," since a truly healthy organism avoids such accidents. Hence classifying or labeling diseases is dangerous, because disease is essentially the condition of an *individual* who is internally maladjusted. The advocates of this position, therefore, tend to emphasize regimen or life-style and to use drugs and surgery secondarily to assist in the adjustment of the individual organism.

As Temkin shows, the central tradition of medicine, usually identified with that of Hippocrates the Greek "Father of Medicine," has always tried to reconcile these two extreme positions. In view of the account we have given of the organism as a dynamic system, it is evident that such a reconciliation should not be too difficult (Wylie, 1970). The physiologists are correct in thinking of health first of all as an internal homeostasis or harmony within the organism and disease as an imbalance. The organism as a system is constantly adjusting by means of feedback to changes in the environment, and these minor fluctuations are not diseases; rather they are health itself.

However, if the system exceeds a certain range of fluctuation, it cannot recover homeostasis without a major readjustment. This readjustment may be possible through the internal vital powers, but only at the cost of a period of sickness in which many normal functions must be minimized while the organism uses all of its energies to readjust. Such a disease is a time of acute illness. Or the organism may readjust but at the cost of permanent diminishing of function or suppression of some functions. Then the disease becomes chronic, or there is permanent crippling or handicap.

Finally, the adjustment may be greater than the organism can achieve, and death results. Death may be the result of acute disease or trauma, or it may result from aging. Aging is the gradual disorganization of the system as the result of repeated disease and trauma which become chronically debilitating because the organism is less and less capable of reaction and recovery as the result of imperfect recovery from many previous injuries.

From this point of view, death is always the result of disease, so that death cannot be said to be natural if by *natural* we mean, as the Greeks meant, the optimal function or health of the organism (Ferrater Mora, 1965). Physiologically speaking, the organism seems to be made to live forever, always recovering from any malfunction. Hence death is due to injuries done to the organism from the environment, not from any intrinsic tendency. A homeostatic system, by definition, is one which maintains itself perpetually when not interfered with.

Now we are brought to the other side of the picture. The organism is an open system which constantly interacts with the environment. Here is where the ontological theory of disease has relevance. The organism is homeostatic, but there are limits to its power of self-maintenace. Consequently, when the environment is altered beyond a certain normal range, the organism is unable to survive. Thus when the oxygen content of the air, the temperature, or the number of bacteria in the environment markedly changes, the human organism undergoes stress, then disorganization, and finally death. We can, therefore, think of diseases and classify them according to various external agents which overstrain the capacity of the organism to maintain itself. We can speak of diseases as entities such as plague or pollution or radiation sickness which affect all the individual organisms in a given area. From this point of view, disease and death are natural in the sense that the terrestrial environment is a part of the evolutionary process in which no individual, but only the species, is protected in perduring existence, and the species itself ultimately yields to the rise of new species. Without disease and death, natural evolution cannot go on (Nogar, 1963).

This organismic theory of health and disease has been central to Western medicine, but it has had a strong competitor in the mechanistic theory which goes back to the Greek Democritus. Even today, the mechanistic theory is very influential in the thinking of many biologists and in medical education. The mechanistic theory of health does not deny that an organism is an open system, but it tends to put emphasis on a reductionist understanding of such a system (Schubert-Soldern, 1962). For a mechanist, the parts seem to be more significant and more practically controllable than the whole. The whole is too complex either to understand or to manage, and its relational character seems tenuous and abstract. One can see and touch the parts, but the relations to mechanists seem largely mental constructs. Mechanists are more comfortable with anatomy or structure than with function or process. When they deal with process, they prefer to think of it as reduced to quantitative measurements of results. Their diagnosis tends toward ontologistic views in which disease is thought of as the result of alien bacteria, of organic lesions, and so forth. In treatment they incline toward a mechanical adjustment of parts by surgery or to use of specific drugs. This attitude is encouraged today by three factors: (1) the specialization in medicine which emphasizes the treatment of particular organs or organ systems, rather than the whole patient, (2) the increasing use of a multiplicity of drugs, of complex surgery, and of various measuring devices in diagnosis, and (3) the theoretical success of molecular biology which promises to give an account of the whole human organism in terms of its ultimate atomic parts.

Maintaining an organismic view in no way denies the mechanistic view, but includes it. The notion of dynamic system necessarily includes a detailed analysis of the parts, the interacting elements. To talk about vitalistic or holistic forces apart from the interrelation of the parts is unscientific (Koestler, 1969a). But an organismic view insists that the relations among the parts are just as real, just as scientifically observable and intelligible, as are the parts which are interrelated. Moreover, the parts themselves cannot be observed or understood in isolation, but only in the context of the system in which they exist. The eye or the kidney, the cell, and even the macromolecular gene cannot be understood except in the context of the whole organism of which they are parts. Medical specialization, therefore, can never be separated from a medical understanding of the whole person, nor can health or disease be defined except in terms of the whole *and* its parts.

One of the factors that has contributed to mechanistic prejudices in medicine has been the fear of teleology (see 1.4). If we speak of a homeostatic system, we necessarily introduce the notion of ends and means, since such a system tends to constantly achieve a normal state which is the end or *telos* Greek, namely, optimal functioning. The various vital processes thus are means tending to an end or goal. They have direction or inherent tendency. This is precisely what the Greeks meant by *nature*. The nature of a thing is its goal-direction tendency. For a living thing, such goal direction means its tendency to develop embryo-logically into a mature, fully differentiated organism — to carry on the various vital functions in an optimal manner, to reproduce itself, to maintain itself in the environment, and to modify the environment and itself in a life-enhancing, or creative, way.

The mechanist is uncomfortable with these concepts because they seem to him to introduce purpose into the natural world and to imply some kind of psychic dimension even to plants and minerals. Moreover, the mechanist argues that such thinking has been fruitless in scientific research, since scientific explanation is not in terms of purposes, but of agents that deterministically produce results according to fixed laws. In particular, the theory of evolution which has been so successful in modern biology seems to explain all living things purely in terms of agent-causes, the natural selection of those things most able to reproduce in a given environment, without any innate purpose.

The fallacy of this mechanistic rejection of teleology is twofold: (1) the supposition that purpose necessarily implies consciousness in that which tends to a goal and (2) the supposition that the identification of an agent-cause is a sufficient explanation of a process. Teleology simply implies that inherent in agent-causes are tendencies to produce directive or goal-oriented actions and processes. Bertalanffy (1968) and others have shown that homeostatic systems necessarily involve directed and controlled tendencies which involve feedback mechanisms. As he, Bertalanffy, states:

> . . . teleological behaviour directed towards a characteristic final state or goal is not something off limits for natural science and an

anthropomorphic misconception of process which, in themselves, are undirected and accidental. Rather it is a form of behaviour which can well be defined in scientific terms and for which the necessary conditions and possible mechanisms can be indicated. (p. 46)

In medicine in particular, some have actually wanted to eliminate the term *health* altogether on the grounds that is was normative — a value term, rather than a scientific value-free term. However, once teleology is admitted, then the *goal* becomes the norm or value from which the means to the goal are also evaluated. Once we have defined human health as optimal functioning and understood this as the satisfaction of innate and cultural needs, or the realization of potentialities, we have defined a norm by which the means to health can also be discriminated from what tends toward disease and death, that is, the suppressing or disuse of functions.

Social Construction of Illness

Recently, however, a very powerful criticism has been raised against all such definitions of *health* and *disease* by the sociologist Eliot Freidson in his book *Profession of Medicine: A Study of the Sociology of Applied Knowledge* (1971). Beginning with Talcot Parsons (1951), sociologists have been studying the medical profession as the typical profession and have been trying to specify not so much its technical as its *social* function. Freidson, basing himself on the sociology of knowledge of Peter L. Berger and Thomas Luckmann (1966), develops a theory of what he calls "the social construction of illness." He grants that there are some physical disorders (and perhaps some mental ones) which are unambiguously, and objectively, "illnesses," for example, a broken leg or smallpox. But he emphasizes that these disorders are only a small part of what our society considers to be illness and with which the medical profession deals. The actual definition of *health* and *disease* in any society is a "social construction" produced by many variable factors and essentially dependent upon how society, the medical profession, and the patient behave toward certain phenomena.

Furthermore, Freidson and other authors emphasize that today in United States society the tendency is to extend the area of illness to more and more phenomena which were previously given other labels:

> The medical mode of response to deviance is thus being applied to more and more behaviour in our society, much of which has been responded to in quite different ways in the past. In our day, what has been called crime, lunacy, degeneracy, sin, and even poverty in the past is now being called illness, and social policy has been moving toward adopting a perspective appropriate to the imputation of illness. Chains have been struck off and everywhere health professionalism has been raised to legitimate the claim that the proper management of deviance is "treatment" in the hands of responsible and skilled professionals. The labels of sin and

crime being removed, what is done to the deviant is likely to be said to be done for his own good, done to help him rather than punish him, even though the treatment itself may constitute a deprivation under ordinary circumstances. His own opinions about his treatment are discounted because he is said to be a layman who lacks the special knowledge and detachment that would qualify him to have his voice heard. (pp. 249-250)

If Freidson is correct, then it seems extremely unjust for a society thus arbitrarily to label people sick because they do not conform to average behavior in that society since, although thus relieved from responsibility for their deviance, they still retain (as Freidson makes clear) the stigma of that deviance. Consequently, some people today are demanding that society cease to label any behavior sick or abnormal unless it is obviously dangerous to others. Thus the psychoanalyst Thomas Szasz (1961), whom Freidson quotes with approval, argues that addiction to drugs and alcoholism should be treated not as diseases but as personal preferences which, if they do any harm, harm only the addict. Similarly the American Psychiatric Association (*New York Times*, December 16, 1973) has removed homosexuality from its list of mental illnesses in order to avoid stigmatizing the homosexual, whose behavioral tendencies should simply be considered personal preferences (Barnhouse, 1977).

This approach of Freidson and Szasz, while undoubtedly very useful in helping us uncover the social processes by which definitions of health and normality are constructed in different cultures, leaves us wondering whether all definitions of health are simply cultural artifacts. Obviously, the question raises a broad epistemological issue about *cultural relativism* which we cannot debate in this book. However, even Freidson admits that some conditions (e.g., broken bones) can be determined as abnormal by objective criteria which are transcultural. His real point is that we are too quick to extend such definitions to cover other conditions which are only *analogously* diseases.

Analogy is a necessary mode of thought and dangerous only when it is not recognized as such. In this book, we deliberately extend the term *health* from its strict medical application at the biological level to the other dimensions of human personality. This seems to us necessary if we are to do justice to the wholeness of the human person who can be sick in many different but closely interrelated ways. At the same time, we have tried to avoid the pitfalls pointed out by Freidson and Szasz by clearly distinguishing the different angalogical uses of health and disease in the four dimensions of human personality and to indicate the different criteria of normality appropriate to each.

Undoubtedly the application of such varied criteria is not always easy or unambiguous or free from arbitrary social construction (E. Cooper, 1972; Siegler and Osmond, 1974). Yet we may hope that with due respect for the cautions of the sociologists of knowledge we can constantly improve our transcultural statements of these criteria.

The theologian Paul Tillich (1967a) has also reminded us that, illusion prone as we human beings are, we can easily mistake for genuine health what he calls "unhealthy health." Of this unhealthy health Tillich says:

> . . . [it] comes about if healing under one dimension is successful but does not take into consideration the other dimensions in which health is lacking or even imperiled by the particular healing. Successful surgery may produce a psychological trauma; effective drugs may calm down an uneasy conscience and perserve a moral deficiency; the well-trained, athletic body may contain a neurotic personality; the healed patient of the analyst may be sick through lack of an ultimate meaning of his life; the conformist's average life may be sick through inhibited self-alteration; the converted Christian may suffer under repressions which produce fanaticism and may explode in lawless forms; the same society may produce psychological and biological disruptions by the desire for creative insanity. (p. 11)

Authentic health, therefore, must be multidimensional.

2.2 BIOLOGICAL HEALTH AND BIOLOGISM

This book cannot present even a sketch of the biological level of human functioning well-known, of course, to health care professionals. Biological and medical science are constantly adding details and precision to our knowledge of the tissues, organs, and secretions which constitute the human body: their chemical composition, structure, functional interrelations, and control and their differentiation, development, and modification by environment and through individual biography.

The important question for health care ethics is how this biological level of functioning can be considered as truly human and personal, as having profound moral and spiritual significance. In all cultures throughout human history, there have been tendencies toward dualistic theories of the human being, according to which body and soul (i.e., the biological and psychological levels of human functioning versus the ethical and spiritual levels) have been thought of as in essential conflict with each other. Generally, the body is thought of as the negative factor and the soul as the positive factor.

Underestimating the plausibility of this dualistic anthropology would be a mistake. We frequently experience the body as a burden, as something negative. This experience is true for two main reasons.

First, a great part of our biological functioning is involuntary and deterministic. We cannot voluntarily control much of what goes on inside of us. Even with medical advances, our biological life is veiled in mystery. Not being able to control this life, we find that it often becomes deranged and fails our human purposes. We find ourselves weary and exhausted, unable to do what we would like to do. We find ourselves suffering from pain and disease, and we are painfully conscious that eventually the body becomes subject to age and ultimate failure in death. Thus the body appears as a burden, a liability.

Second, the basic biological drives are urgent and inescapable. The need for sleep, the fear of insecurity, the demands of hunger and thirst, and the tension of sexual desire constantly urge themselves upon us. They are so insistent that we feel them as compulsions, limiting our freedom and sometimes overwhelming us against our will.

Since the dignity of human personhood consists essentially in our self-understanding and freedom, it is profoundly humiliating to us to be the helpless victims of our own bodies with their limited energies, their liability to pain, and their urgent and deterministic demands which arise from unconscious depths and disorganize our self-possession and freedom of action. Therefore, we experience the body as dragging us down to the animal level of unfree, instinctive, and blind action. In all religious mythologies this pull is often typified in the fear of sexuality as a regression to the primitive chaos (Neumann, 1964). The sex drive has always seemed especially mysterious. It subordinates the freedom of the individual to the imperious needs of the species. We feel ourselves severely disturbed at times by sexual passion, reduced to the level of the animal in heat, deluded by a promise of pleasure which is very brief, and which may be followed by the burdens of pregnancy, childbirth, and family responsibility. Thus, the woman whose biological functioning is more profoundly determined than the man's by the processes of menstruation, pregnancy, childbirth, and nursing and who in the human species is the more attractive or stimulating partner for sexual activity is in most cultures mistakenly regarded as somehow negative in contrast to the positive male, who is freer of such biological limitations for other activities (H. Richardson, 1971).

Thus it is understandable why dualism is so widespread. It is essential to certain religious systems (Buddhism, Gnosticism, Manichaeism) and has affected all of them (the Neo-Platonic influences in Jewish, Christian, and Muslim theologies). In the extreme form (Manichaeism), the body is thought of as intrinsically evil. In more moderate forms, the body is simply thought of as negative. It might be thought that such dualistic views are no longer common, since modern society emphasizes the value of sensual pleasure, the dependence of psychic functions on the body, and the qualities of male and female.

However, today dualism is reappearing under new forms. Thus, some (Lorentz, 1966; Ardrey, 1966; D. Morris, 1967; Koestler, 1968) have interpreted the theory of evolution to imply that in relation to our present environment the human body is archaic and outmoded. We were formed by evolution for a primitive environment where human beings had to be highly aggressive and very fertile in order to survive. Hence, we are now very badly adapted to modern artificial culture in which aggressive drives lead to war and antisocial violence, while excessive sexual drives and fertility lead to overpopulation and neurosis. This view has also been supported by the Freudian view that there is a basic antipathy between the demands of civilization and the human being's basic drives which results in modern man's liability to severe neuroses. To this Freud also added the notion of the death wish, an innate tendency of man to regress to the primitive and to ultimate extinction of the individual in the universal rhythm of nature (Menninger, 1938).

These ideas, especially when overpopulation is an increasing threat, have oriented many moderns to the view that the biological level of human life is a threat to human freedom (Hardin, 1974) and must be brought under radical control. Many think of the poor and the people of the Third World as primitives, living an instinctive, almost animal life, reproducing "recklessly" like rabbits. They also think of the traditional feminine role of the mother and housewife as having this limited, unfree, and subhuman character and therefore propose that the truly human life for men and women should be similar to that which upper-class men have always enjoyed, in which biological activities, and especially sexuality, are reduced to simple entertainment to be used or not used at will (Roszak, 1969).

From such discussions it is easy to conclude that the facts of human biology as such have no moral significance, but receive their moral meaning from the context of culture as a product of human invention and choice. Consequently many ethicists today (Curran, 1969; J. Gaffney, 1974; McNeill, 1976; Kosnik, 1977) emphasize that traditional moral theologians went too far when they attempted to establish moral norms on the basis of a distinction between behavior which is natural or unnatural for human beings considered as biological organisms. Such faulty arguments, they say, can be rejected as vitiated by the "fallacy of biologism" or "physicalism." On the other hand, defenders of such traditional positions (e.g., Grisez, 1964; W. May, 1977a) emphasize the opposite danger of a new dualism in which the animal and the rational aspects of the human beings are seen as unrelated or even inimical.

Certainly it is fallacious to argue that the moral character of human behavior can be settled simply by asking biologists what is natural or unnatural to animals or to human beings. In 8.1-3 we will discuss the important distinction between the moral and the physical specifications of an act. The morality of any act must be considered in the context of the activity of the human person as a whole since the biological level of function is only one level of the total system. Conversely, however, this consideration means that the spiritual or ethical meaning of a human act cannot be indifferent or neutral to its biological character. Every human act is an act of the whole person, involving spiritual, ethical, psychological, and biological dimensions. Every human biological function has human (and therefore spiritual and ethical) significance, and conversely even our most spiritual activities involve the body and must respect the structure and functioning of the body.

A sounder approach to this whole issue is provided by the Aristotelian tradition among the Greeks which, in opposition to Platonic dualism, insisted upon the unity of the human person of which body and soul are only complementary aspects (Allan, 1952). This approach is supported theologically by the insistence of the great monotheistic religions (Judaism, Christianity, Islam) on the creation of the body and of man and woman by God as essentially good and on the resurrection of the body as concomitant to the eternal life of the human person. Christianity goes even further by insisting on the Incarnation, through which God becomes truly a human being in bodily existence, and on the indwelling of the Holy Spirit in the human body as its temple, through which we become members of the Body of Christ (Owen, 1956; Pius XII, 1945). This same principle leads to the sacramental conception of the human body by which the basic biological functions become signs of spiritual events: birth is reenacted in baptism, eating and drinking in the Eucharist, and sexual union in the sacrament of matrimony.

This does not mean that Christianity rejects the truth found in dualism. On the one hand, it accepts a moderate asceticism (including celibacy for some) not as a rejection of the biological, but as an integration of the biological into the human whole (Goergen, 1975). On the other hand, it also acknowledges a certain moderate freedom of sensual enjoyment, provided that this remains within the limits of the teleology of these functions (Boulogne, 1953; Williams, 1974).

According to this Christian understanding of personhood, the biological level of man is only a part of human life, but it is truly human, and it has a genuine human value of its own (Goldstein, 1959; Longo, 1973). Hence, it cannot be suppressed or ruthlessly sacrificed to higher values or even trivialized as of no moral significance. Instead Catholic theology has always been concerned to find a middle way between the dualistic extremes of asceticism and antinomianism and to respect the intrinsic teleology of bodily structures and basic biological functions (Noonan, 1965).

2.3   THE HIGHER LEVELS OF HEALTH

The development of modern psychotherapy and of psychosomatic medicine leaves no doubt that while mental health is intimately connected with physical health it is not identical with physical health. In chapter 12 we will try to state more precisely what this differentiation and interdependence are. It suffices at this point to grant that there is such a difference, because mental disease is not describable in terms of physiological malfunction, but of impairment in the characteristic human ability to deal with the environment by *symbolic* activity and communication (Ruesch and Bateson, 1951).

Human beings far surpass animals in the capacity to use symbols (images, feelings, words) which stand for realities but which can be combined and ordered in many ways different from the relatively fixed order of real things (Pugh, 1977). We are aware that the images and concepts by which we represent the world do so only imperfectly, but that they can be verified and refined by our use of them as tools to change the world. Physical disease, especially dysfunctions of the central nervous system, can impair this symbolic activity, but it also can be disturbed by social and educational factors within the symbolic realm itself. For example, a physiologically healthy child can acquire prejudiced ways of perceiving reality and neurotic ways of reacting to it emotionally through his social environment. This environment cannot be adequately described in terms just of bodies in time and space, but also in terms of a symbolic communication system.

At this level of symbolic or psychic activity, however, are also differentiated levels of health and disease which are too often lumped together. To reduce human psychic health to emotional adjustment and maturity is a common fallacy today which can be termed *psychologism*. Psychologism assumes that a physically healthy person who also is free of those mental illnesses which are today considered the proper comptency of psychotherapy is totally healthy.

As we will show in chapter 12, psychotherapy has the modest goal of helping patients acquire that degree of self-understanding and emotional integration which will free them from unconscious psychological determinisms which hamper their daily practical life. Psychologically healthy persons are "in touch with their feelings." They perceive the world of ordinary activity as most people do — without manifestly absurd illusions or projections. They are free to choose between practical alternatives and do not have unrealistic expectations. They are responsible for the consequences of their actions.

At this point of freedom from psychological determination a whole new level of human activity opens up, the level of free, responsible, *moral* activity. Psychotics are incapable of moral action (at least within the area of the psychosis), while neurotics are severely limited in their freedom and responsibility. Only the free man or woman is a person fully capable of either moral good or evil. Recently Don Browning (1976) pointed out that problems of ethical counseling are often confused with those of psychological counseling. A good many of the clergy today seem to have abandoned their traditional role of helping people make ethical decisions in order to become amateur psychotherapists. In chapters 7 and 8 we will attempt to define more precisely the ways in which moral or ethical health differs from psychological health because of the centrality of freedom and responsibility at the ethical level of human functioning.

However, it is also possible to fall into still another fallacy, that of moralism (Tillich, 1955). We commit this error when we reduce all human failure to questions of right and wrong, attribute either mental or physical disease to the victims' sins, and attempt to heal them by moral exhortations. A more subtle form of this same fallacy is the assumption that the highest wholeness in the human personality is achieved at the level of practical ethical life. Some people identify the good person with the responsible, prudent, decent man or woman.

This is to ignore what is the deepest and most central in human personality, namely, that which is spiritual, intuitive, creative within us. While some psychotherapists of the Jungian and existentialist schools do concern themselves with this level, they do so only in order to free its activity of the impediments arising from neuroses and psychoses. To deal with this spiritual level of human existence in its own terms is the task of neither the psychologist, nor the moralist, but of the philosopher, theologian, and spiritual guide, as we will show in chapter 14. Spiritual health and disease, therefore, cannot be reduced simply to moral or psychological terms.

Even at this spiritual level we can fall into the fallacy of what the philosopher Jacques Maritain (1953) called "angelicism," treating human persons as if were were bodiless angels, or pure souls, as Plato and Descartes conceived the true human self. Human problems cannot be treated in purely spiritual terms, in which the lower levels of functioning, of human physiology, human symbolic activity, and human practical responsibility are ignored. It would seem today that this fallacy is again influential among those mystical and religious enthusiasts who attempt to heal all bodily, psychological, and moral ills by purely spiritual means.

Thus in trying to understand the fullness of human health we need to be on guard against those reductionist fallacies that ignore its many dimensions. For example, to determine whether alcoholism is a sickness without reductionism, or arbitrary social construction, we first have to define alcoholism in behavioral terms and then ask four questions. First, is it a biological disease in terms of biological criteria, for example, a change in physiology which puts a strain on biological homeostasis? Second, is it a psychological disease in terms of psychological criteria, for example, a persistent emotional conflict which restricts the victim's capacity for intelligent free choice? Third, is it a moral disease in terms of ethical criteria, for example, free choice of behavior that is contradictory to the full actualization of the person in community? Fourth, is it a spiritual disease by spiritual criteria, for example, closure to intuition, creativity, commitment? Moreover, we have to ask how these different levels of functioning are interrelated. The terms *disease* and *health* used at each of these levels in very different but analogous ways.

2.4   PRINCIPLE OF TOTALITY AND INTEGRITY

Integrity of the Person

Thus in summary we can say that human nature is an open system with several hierarchical orders of functioning. The term *integrity* indicates that in a perfect whole each part must be fully differentiated and developed. Furthermore, each part must be fitted into the whole and harmonized with it by correct interrelations and interactions with the other parts in the context of the whole. Integrity is lacking when a part is suppressed or unduly inhibited in function or when, on the other hand, one part is hypertrophied to the injury of others.

In a hierarchical order note that some parts are said to be higher because they are necessary to the unification and integration of the whole in the performance of its most complex and specific functions (e.g., the central nervous system) and that other parts are said to be lower because their functions are more integrated than integrating. Yet the lower parts may at the least be essential for the higher parts to function at all (e.g., the liver and the kidneys). In discussing Maslow's theory (1970; cf. 1.4) of the hierarchy of human needs, we noted the paradox that lower needs must be met before higher needs can be attended to. The reason is that lower functions are means related to higher functions as to their ends. We cannot achieve an end without the means, yet the end *measures* and integrates the means into a whole system. Since however the means are relative to the end, we cannot skip the means, but we can limit or restrict them so that they truly serve the end rather than overpower it.

This concept is expressed in the saying He lives to eat, but should eat to live, which means that we cannot engage in higher activities ("living") without eating. Consequently, eating is integral to human life. But eating is a lower activity, a means, not an end. When eating becomes an end, an absolute not measured by something higher, it destroys the integrity of human functioning.

We must not fall into the error, however, of thinking that only the higher values in this hierarchy are human personal values. We share biological and psychological needs with other animals, while ethical and spiritual needs we share only with other human persons. Nevertheless, all these needs and their correlative values, whether generically animal or specifically human, are *equally* needs and values of the human person, none of which can be destroyed without destroying personhood. I am a human person not only because I need love, but also because I need food.

Equally to be avoided is another error widespread today which concludes that since human sexuality and other bodily needs are truly human they differ *totally* in their meaning from animal needs. We do not assert our human identity by denying that we are truly animals with animal needs. A correct appreciation of the human person demands that we fully appreciate the *mutual* interdependence of all the various dimensions of human personality, all of which are essential to human personhood.

This hierarchical yet interdependent ordering of the four levels of human functioning holds also for any subsystem within each level. At the biological level, we find that the human body is divided into organ systems and these into organs, each having specific functions. The organ systems are commonly enumerated as follows: (1) nervous, (2) endocrine, (3) skeletal and muscular, (4) integumentary (skin), (5) alimentary, (6) respiratory, (7) circulatory, (8) excretory, and (9) reproductive. These systems are interrelated in very complex ways and not in any simple, linear hierarchy. Yet the nervous system (with the intimately related endocrine system) is obviously the one which coordinates the others and is the most directly involved in the psychological and higher functions. Obviously the reproductive system has a special importance (1) because it is directly involved in the evolutionary process by which the human species came to be and is continued and (2) because it is the source of the family and hence of the communal character of the human person.

At the psychic level of personality, there is a greater unification of function since we feel with our whole person in a unified awareness. Yet psychic life is also composite. Clearly the external senses are differentiated by their organs. Our other psychological functions have some kind of localization in various parts of the brain, although they also involve other centers and the endocrine system as well. Furthermore, as depth psychology has shown us, there is a differentiation in the field of awareness itself into an unconscious, a subconscious, a superego, an ego, and so forth. While some Catholic moral theologians (Curran, 1977a) suppose that the so-called faculty of psychology traditional in Christian anthropology is obsolete, it still remains valid in the light of modern empirical psychology when properly understood in terms of differentiated functions (Arnold, 1960; Royce, 1961), and is very helpful in understanding psychic integration.

At the rational and ethical levels still greater integration and unification of functions into the self-aware, conscious, free, self-controlling subject or person takes place. Even at this level there remains a differentiation into what have been traditionally called the reason and the will as distinct but ultimately correlative functions. Only at the spiritual level do the intellect and will come together in the "still point" (Johnston, 1971) or top of the mind or heart (in the Biblical, metaphorical sense) of the human person, in which peak experiences (Maslow, 1964) and basic decisions, commitments, and fundamental options take place to complete the total integration of the person.

Totality of the Person

The chief ethical question arising from this conception of the human person as an open hierarchical system is whether it is permissible in some circumstances to sacrifice one part or function in the interests of another or of the whole. Obviously, in medical ethics this is a recurrent problem as for example, in sterilization and organ transplantation. Traditionally, such cases were covered by the principle of totality, simply stated by St. Thomas Aquinas (1976 ed.) as follows:

> Since any member is part of the whole human body, it exists for the sake of the whole as the imperfect for the sake of the perfect. Hence, a member of the human body is to be disposed of according as it may profit the whole. *Per se*, the member of the human body is useful for the welfare of the whole body; *per accidens* however it can happen that it is harmful, for example, when a diseased member is injurious to the whole body. If, therefore, a member is healthy and continuing in its natural state, it cannot be cut off to the detriment of the whole. (II-II, q. 65, a.l,c.)

Aquinas applied this principle not only to the individual person considered as a substantial whole, but also by analogy to the community considered as a whole made up of many distinct but interrelated substances (persons). Thus, he defended capital punishment when undertaken by public authority for the sake of the common good, that is, the sacrifice of one member of the community for the good of the whole community (Mangan, 1949). However, in our day the experience of the totalitarianism of the Nazi and Stalinist regimes led Pius XII (1952) to stress the fact that this wider interpretation of the principle is only analogical, since the human body and the body politic are very different kinds of totalities:

> The community is the great medium ordained by nature and by God to regulate the exchanges by which mutual needs are met, to help each one to develop his personality according to his individual social capacity. The community, considered as a whole, is not a physical unity which subsists in itself. Its individual members are not integrating parts of it. The physical organism of living beings, of plants, animals, or men, possesses as a whole a unity which subsists in itself. Each of the members, for example, the hand, the foot, the heart, the eye, is an integrant part, destined by its whole being to be a part of one complete organism. Outside the organism it has not of its own nature, any meaning, any purpose: its being is wholly absorbed in the complete organism with which it is linked.
>
> A quite different state of affairs obtains in the moral community and in each organism of a purely moral character. The whole has not here a unity which subsists in itself, but a simple unity of purpose and of action. In the community the individuals are only collaborators and instruments for the realization of the ends of the community.
>
> What follows with regard to the physical organism? The master, the person who uses this organism, which possesses a subsisting unity, can dispose directly and immediately of the integrant parts, the members and the organs, within the framework of their natural finality. Likewise

he can intervene, when and as far as the well-being of the whole demands, to paralyze, destroy, mutilate, separate its members. In contrast, however, when the whole does not possess a unity except of finality and of action, its head, that is to say, in the present case the public authority, retains without doubt a direct authority, and the right to impose its demands on the activity of the parts, but in no case can it dispose directly of its physicial being. Moreover, every direct injury attempted against its essential being by public authority is a departure from that sphere of activity which rightly belongs to it. (n. 371)

In this discussion Pius XII in one respect widened the principle of totality by making it clear that it applied not only to the sacrifice of a diseased organ, but also to that of a healthy organ for the good of the whole body, for example, the removal of healthy testes to suppress the production of hormones which might stimulate the growth of cancer elsewhere in the body (Kelly, 1958). Nevertheless, he clearly intended to restrict the principle to the individual, so that theologians abandoned this principle as a justification for transplantation of organs from one person to another and developed a new justification on the basis of charity (Kelly, 1958). McFadden (1976) had made clear that the principle is to be understood not in terms of a *part* as a physical part, but rather as a *function*. Hence, this principle is not required to justify the cutting of hair or toenails, the removal of (apparently) nonfunctional organs such as the appendix and tonsils (even when they are healthy), and blood transfusions and skin grafts.

Bernard Häring (1973), although he accepts Pius XII's restriction of the principle to the individual, wants to interpret the term *whole* not to mean the "whole body," but the "whole person." He writes (italics his):

The traditional use of the principle of totality justified intervention in view of physical health and functioning. Medical ethics for the future must rest on an all-embracing concept of "totality": *the dignity and well-being of a man as a person in all his essential relationships to God, to his fellowmen and to the world around him.* (p. 62)

He goes on to insist that this includes the call from God for man to perfect his own nature:

Each intervention or medical provision that helps or enhances the whole-ness of the human person is right — be it a plastic heart or any other fantastic feat. If, for instance, genetic engineering can eliminate the XYY chromosomal anomaly and thus protect humanity from the heavy burden of dangerous criminal tendencies in a number of people, why should we object to it? (p. 64)

In our opinion, Häring is correct in thinking that it is not possible simply to speak of the good of the body, since the body itself is only a part of the person, and since any substantial part is entirely relative to the substantial whole. In the words of Pius XII already quoted:

Outside the organism it has not of its own nature, any meaning, any purpose: its being is wholly absorbed in the complete organism with which it is linked. (n. 371)

If such is true of an organ of the body, it is also true of the body itself as a substantial part of the person, the ensouled organism.

We also agree with Häring in this instance that God wills not only that man care for his body, but also that he perfect it, even by new medical technologies, as we will further explain in chapter 3. On this point it seems necessary to advance beyond the perspective of Pius XII (1950) who was very cautious about the implications of the evolutionary theory of human origins. The Second Vatican Council has opened the way to a more historical anthropology in which we need to take full account of two points: (1) human nature is not in every respect a finished product, and (2) we have a right and duty to perfect our own nature as well as the environment by every reasonable use of modern science. Hence we should not press Pius XII's language about the "essence of ideas and things" and "absolute value" too far, just as he warned us against pushing Aquinas's formulation of the principle too far.

Nevertheless, Häring's formulation risks being so vague as to have little value as a practical norm. If we take the person "in all his essential relationships to God, to his fellowmen and the world around him" as Häring puts it, we seem to have moved back into an analogical sense of whole, since this will include the social whole and even the cosmic whole.

Consequently, it seems necessary to reformulate the principle in such a way as not only to apply to the good of the whole person, but also to make clear what this good is. Häring is correct in saying that this human good is relational. We have shown in 1.2 that person is correlative to community. However, what is it that opens the human being to this common good?

We might be tempted to say that it is our highest, most personal powers at the spiritual level and perhaps also at the ethical and psychological levels. Consequently, we might argue that any part of the body at the biological level might be sacrificed to contribute to our higher functioning. Thus (to enter the world of science fiction) we might argue that in the future it may be desirable to use medical technology to reduce the human person to a brain floating in a nutritive and protective bath and communicating with other brains electronically. Such a brain would still be a person, capable of "all his essential relationships to God, to his fellowmen and to the world around him," if we define these relations in terms of knowledge, love, free choice, communication, and action on matter. Furthermore, such brain-human beings could reproduce artificially by some asexual, test-tube process or to go a step further might be maintained in deathless perpetuity.

Would this transformation of the human person into a brain-person be for the *good* of the person, a perfecting of human nature or an impoverishment? Intuitively, most people would probably call it an impoverishment. The sound reason for this insight is provided by our foregoing analysis of the complex, hierarchical, mutually dependent structure of human nature as a dynamic system. Human nature cannot be reduced merely to its highest functions, as the Platonists reduced the self to a simple, spiritual soul for which the body was a mere container or instrument.

The validity of this intuition is even clearer if we consider the historical, evolutionary character of human nature. Precisely because human nature is an organic bodily system with many levels of functioning, it could have been produced only by an evolutionary process. Its wholeness consists in the interdependence of higher and lower functions, of the spiritual and the bodily. Consequently, we cannot without qualification sacrifice the lower to the higher functions. This sacrifice might be to the advantage of the higher function, but not to the good of the whole person, since that good is essentially *complex*, irreducible to the good of one part, even if that part is the highest.

To be a perfect human being, therefore, is not merely to have the higher level functions but to have *all* the basic human functions in a harmonious order. This order requires the subordination of the lower functions to the higher functions but also forbids their total sacrifice, since in fact the higher functions depend also on the lower. Nor can this dependence be simply supplied by some means external to the person. For example, if we learn to produce babies in test tubes, the discovery would not of itself justify the elimination of the reproductive power of human persons as no longer necessary. Nor would the possibility of intravenous feeding simply justify the elimination of the human alimentary system. Human perfection requires that the human person reproduce and eat in a human manner. Such substitutions of external means of life may be justified temporarily out of necessity, but they are not perfections of human nature.

Reflecting on the fact that human bodily functions contribute to our higher functions not merely by supplying what is needed for physiological brain function, it becomes even clearer that they also supply part of our human experience which is essential to human intelligence and freedom. From our bodily feelings — our experiences of bodily movement, of eating, of sexuality, of bodily manipulation of the environment — our self-awareness and our relation to the community are developed. Thus, if a child were conceived in a test tube and gestated in an artificial womb and then raised in a laboratory, it is doubtful that he or she would have essential human experiences.

Some find it very inconsistent that the Roman Catholic Church disapproves sterilization as a suppression of a basic human function, yet lauds the practice of celibacy. We will deal with this question more fully in chapters 8 and 10, but here we note the important distinction between the ethical obligation to perserve all our basic human capacities (unless forced to sacrifice one to perserve the life of the whole) and the obligation to use one of these capacities in a particular way. Celibates do not castrate themselves, but freely choose not to use their sexual powers genitally. Nor does this choice mean that they fail to return interest on the gift committed to them by their Creator who made them men and women. Rather, they choose to use their human sexuality in such a way as to learn to love and serve a community wider than the family. This entails sacrifice, it is true, but sacrifice of secondary values rather than of essential values necessary for the complete development of their personhood (Goergen, 1974; Hinnebusch, 1974; Kiesling, 1977).

Totality and Integrity

The foregoing discussion of totality and integrity can be summarized as follows:

1. Primarily human wholeness is not a matter of organs but of capacities to function humanly.

2. Generally speaking, any particular human functional capacity can be sacrificed when necessary for the good of the whole person, that is, so that the person may better exercise all other human functions.

3. Secondary functions can always be sacrificed for more basic ones. For example, a finger can be removed to save the use of the hand, because the capacity of action given by one finger is secondary in relation to the capacity given by the hand as a whole.

4. However, primary or basic functional capacities cannot be sacrificed even to more important capacities except when it is the only way to preserve the life of the whole person. For example, the capacity for emotional feeling cannot be sacrificed to the power of scientific thinking. In order to think more effectively, we cannot sacrifice our capacity to think *humanly*. In the popular myth of the "mad scientist" we have a symbol of human intelligence become self-destructive.

Why then is it sometimes permissible to sacrifice one of these basic human capacities to preserve life? Because in this case it is not a question of sacrificing one basic capacity for another, nor for the better functioning of all other human capacities, but of sacrificing one function in order that the whole person should continue to function at all. Only in such extreme necessity does integrity yield to the good of the totality.

Of course, it is not always very easy to decide which human functions are secondary and which are basic or which are higher and which are lower. Nevertheless, ethics must seek to make such discriminations in view of our understanding the human system in its many dimensions and levels of organization. If we do not make this effort, either we will end by reducing human values to a single supreme value to which all others can be ruthlessly sacrificed as did the Greek dualists of old, or we will treat human values simply as equal items to be added and subtracted in the quantitative manner of utilitarianism. In either case the multidimensional concept of the human person developed in chapter 1 will be destroyed.

Thus the good of the whole person requires that all the basic aspects of human personality be simultaneously respected, even when it is necessary to subordinate or even sacrifice in some measure a lower to a higher function. Consequently, we would propose the following revised version of the principle of totality and name it the *Principle of Totality and Integrity*:

> The good of the whole human person, correlative to the common good of the community, should be the measure of the use, care, and preservation of its particular function such that lower functions may be sacrificed to higher functions only for the better functioning of the whole, compensating as far as possible for the proper value of each sacrificed function and never destroying the basic capacities that are definitive of human personhood except when necessary to preserve life itself.

Thus when we speak of the right to health possessed by each human person, or as some do of the right of quality of life, we mean that each person because of his or her inherent dignity as a person has the right to the help and care of the community in achieving this multidimensional health, which includes the biological and psychological health which are the proper concern of the health care profession. This right to human wholeness and integrity does not imply, however, that life is not worth living for those who cannot achieve this goal in its fullness. No one fully achieves this goal and many human beings fall far short of it, especially because the community does not provide them with the help they need or support the scientific research necessary to find ways to supply that help effectively.

CHAPTER 3 PERSONAL RESPONSIBILITY FOR HEALTH

3.1   PERSONAL RESPONSIBILITY

Will to Live Versus Death Wish

Chapter 1 pointed out that the human community is responsible for all that affects the full personal development of every one of its members. Chapter 2 explained further that this responsibility includes biological health, as well as the higher levels of human functioning which depend upon it. However, the primary responsibility for a particular individual's health rests in that individual, not in the community.

This fact is clear from the intensely personal character of health in all its dimensions. Biological health concerns that which is most individual and private to me, namely, my own body. My body, by its very materiality, is space-time limitations, is mine and mine alone. It identifies me as *not* anybody else. Someone can share a room with me, a table, a bed, even my clothes, but he cannot truly share my body. Sexual partners exchange the right to use each other's body sexually (in Biblical language, they become "one flesh," Mark 10:8), but even this intimate union has its limits. Ultimately, it is by reason of our bodies that each of us is alone in himself or herself, yet it is also by reason of them that we are in the world of things and persons (Merleau-Ponty 1962 [1945]).

My body is profoundly subjective not only because I possess it as my own and know it as myself, but because it is incommunicable. Much of what goes on in my body is hidden even from me, and even what I know of it I know for the most part in a thoroughly subjective way such that I cannot express it to you. All who consult a physician experience the difficulty of telling him how they feel. Bodily feelings are vivid, yet so vague and so hard to put into words! I am left frustrated and stammering because no one else can really know how I feel. I am the only final judge of whether I really feel well. When no medical test reveals anything wrong with me, but I do not feel well, then I *am* not well.

Even if my sickness is not physiological but imaginary, that imaginary sickness is real at the psychological level and is a psychological illness. At that level the criterion of health for the psychotherapist is how the client really feels about himself — it is the depth feelings underlying the surface feelings. At the higher ethical and spiritual levels, health also depends upon an individual's own conscience, or spiritual discernment. Thus, no one but the person ultimately can judge her own interior well-being.

Furthermore, this subjectivity is true not only of diagnosis, but also of treatment. The psychotherapist has constantly to remind the client: "No one, ultimately, can help you if you refuse to help yourself." Even the ethical and spiritual counselor must say, "God will help you by his grace, but you must open yourself to that grace." Does not Jesus say in Revelations 3:20: "Here I stand, knocking at the door. If anyone hears me calling and opens the door, I will enter his house and have supper with him, and he with me"?

Healing is a living process that must occur within the organism. It is true that at the extremity of life patients may be unconscious and purely passive to the surgery, medication, and injections thrust upon them, but these treatments seldom result in healing. Convalescence is an active process on the part of patients, and staying well is clearly something that they alone must do. No physician or nurse can make patients take pills, stick to a diet, or take necessary rest and exercise.

In a profound way the will to life and health is the fundamental element in all healing, and this will must be intelligent, that is, a realistic search for the means to health. A noted surgeon once said that he dreaded operating on patients who doubted their chances of recovery because in his experience such patients did *not* recover. Most doctors and nurses seem to believe that the patient's fighting spirit is a critical factor in favor of health.

Therefore, whether in working to prevent sickness, to maintain optimal health, to assist recovery from disease, or to rehabilitate oneself after a crippling trauma, a person must make a commitment to life and health. It might seem that no special commitment needs to be made, since every one of us has an instinct to live. No doubt the need to live, to grow, and to function well is innate, it is the very teleology of any organism. But in the human person whose inmost depth of being is not instinctive but free, this commitment is not a given; rather, it must be freely made by the person. Are not there persons who make the opposite commitment to suicide in open or hidden form?

Karl Menninger in his book *Man Against Himself* (1938) has shown that suicide is only the last step of an intensifying process of self-destruction, of hatred turned away from external objects and toward the self. Clinically, patients who attempt suicide often have a long previous record of psychosomatic illnesses such as hypertension or ulcers and of "accidents." Unconsciously they have been self-committed to death rather than to life. Menninger also believes that religious asceticism, whether Oriental or Christian, is sometimes only a mask for self-hatred.

Menninger and other neo-Freudians cite such clinical evidence in trying to interpret Sigmund Freud's paradoxical theory of the death wish as the instinctive opposite of the libido or pleasure principle. Freud

(1958 [1920]) believed that the death wish causes the human organism to regress into more primitive, compulsively repetitive, and ultimately passive types of behavior and that it is a "return to the bliss of the womb," the tomb of eternal night. Menninger is on less paradoxical ground when he interprets this instinct simply as the *aggressive* component of human behavior. He postulates that the pleasure principle leads us to seek satisfactions, and therefore the aggressive principle drives us to seek the destruction of every painful limitation on these strivings for pleasure. When these two principles are not working harmoniously for the organism, aggression may be turned on the self and thus become a death wish.

In sadomasochistic behavior, aggressive action and suffering of pain are invested with erotic overtones such that suffering and causing to suffer become intensely pleasurable. In self-hatred, satisfaction is sought through self-pity and the craving for attention and care from others. Some patients seem to enjoy being sick or at least to enjoy constant complaining, obscure ailments, medication, and even painful operations. A life otherwise empty is at least filled with the drama of disease and therapy (Brown, 1964).

This commitment to death means that everything associated with the medical profession becomes attractive to some persons and symbolizes their own unconscious drives. They often seduce medical professionals into satisfying their morbid needs. Physicians and nurses may be tempted to pander to these seductions, both because of financial gain and because it is flattering to be needed. In the home, such a neurotic person may induce the whole family to build its life around "tender loving care." We can only wonder whether the tremendous preoccupation of modern American society with the drama of medicine is not evidence that this neurosis has become social as well as individual.

The same sadomasochistic seductions appear in the ethical and spiritual arena of politics and religion. Jesus attacked the legalism of some of the Pharisees of his time, because these people, who were both political and religious guides, had imposed a moralistic scrupulosity that expressed self-destructive guilt. Puritan and Victorian morality exhibited similar tendencies. In the spiritual sphere such seductions are reflected in extreme dualistic asceticism with its hatred of the body, the self, and the world. Psychotherapists often are antireligious because they have been so shocked by the way in which moralistic religion seems to have maimed some of their patients.

Neurosis, however, is a counterfeit normality, and it is absurd to blame either medicine or religion as such for these aberrations, however widespread. Surgeons are not necessarily sadists, although sadism is unconsciously present in a few surgeons and leads to needless surgery. Nor are the clergy often moral sadists, although unconscious sadism may be found in moralistic sermons, unsound ascetical practice, and aberrant rituals.

Christian Affirmation of Life

The commitment to life, which overcomes such commitments to death, is an affirmation of the value not only of pleasure, but also of freedom, intelligence, creativity, and love. As Yahweh says through Moses in Deuteronomy:

> I call heaven and earth today to witness against you: I have set before you life and death, the blessing and the curse. Choose life, then, that you and your descendants may live, by loving the Lord, your God, heeding his voice, and holding fast to him. For that will mean life for you, a long life for you to live on the land which the Lord swore he would give to your fathers Abraham, Isaac and Jacob. (30:19-20)

Such a commitment to life has to proceed from the spiritual level, although it is ordinarily manifest at lower levels as well. This deep commitment can be so blocked that persons profoundly dedicated to life in their spiritual center can yet suffer from an unconscious will to death at the psychological level (Lepp, 1966).

The Old Testament presents the Jewish view as profoundly life affirming. It constantly emphasizes the idea that God gives his friends health, security, children, and long life and that God has created men and women for life and wishes to prolong it for them. Faced by the fact that the just often suffer persecution and martyrdom, the last books of the Old Testament affirm that God will raise his friends from the dead to everlasting life (cf. II Mach. 7:27-29). Jesus approved by saying, "God is God of the living, not of the dead" (Mark 12:27). St. Paul also teaches (Rom. 5:12 ff.) that death (and by implication disease and aging) is somehow a consequence of sin (cf. Wisd. 1:13-15). Thus disease, aging, and death are not willed by God, but only permitted by him as a punishment, the inevitable consequence of the sin of the human race which has committed itself to death rather than to life. St. Paul joyfully affirms that in Christ all may be born again to everlasting life.

Nor should this promise of life be understood in merely otherworldly terms. In preaching the Kingdom of God, Jesus taught us to pray it should "come on earth . . . as it is in heaven" (Matt. 6:10) and he revealed God's will for us by his miracles of physical healing and restoration to life even of the dying and dead. Health care professionals in the face of human suffering often experience a great longing to be able to extinguish pain, restore vigorous life, and close the door to death. They can be sure this compassionate yearning to fight for life and against death is a revelation in their own hearts of the fatherly heart of God. "If you, with all your sins, know how to give your children what is good, how much more will your heavenly Father give good things to anyone who asks him!" (Matt. 7:11).

When Jesus prayed in the Garden, "O Father, you have the power to do all things. Take this cup away from me. But let it be as you would have it, not as I" (Mark 14:36), he was affirming his own commitment to life, but expressing his willingness to endure death if the Father in his transcendent wisdom knew that only through death could we doubting men and women be convinced that God and his Son truly love us for our own sake and not for the sake of their honor or power.

Thus, a sound theology teaches that the Father and Christ desire only life, a desire which is fulfilled in the Resurrection. Following Jesus, who as St. Paul says was "never anything but 'Yes' " (II Cor. 1:20), Christians must always affirm life while being willing to endure the evil of death: (1) as witnesses to others that faith, hope, and love cannot be overcome by the fear and despair of death and (2) as sharers in Jesus' experience of death, by which we learn to be as unselfish, trustful, and hopeful as he was. However, the Christian endures death serenely not because death is good, but because resurrection and eternal life are good and destroy death forever.

We can also add that when Christians feel as did St. Paul in prison when he longed "to be dissolved and to be with Christ" (Phil. 1:23) they are not rejecting life, but longing to be freed of the barriers that constrict the fullness of life. A Christian can long for death as an inevitable crisis that has to be lived through in order to achieve full health and life, not as a Freudian regression to the peace of the womb which is only a tomb.

Thus it is essential to realize that Christian health care should never be directed to the passive acceptance of disease or death, as if they in themselves were somehow spiritual goods. Even a distinguished medical historian like Sigerist (1960b) falls into the error of thinking that Christianity thought of sickness as sacred. The evidence he cites only proves that Christian thinking is often distorted by the false sado-masochistic notions surviving from pre-Christian times or imposed by neurotic abuses of religious symbols. In authentic Christian belief, every individual has a responsibility to choose life and to fight for it. Christians must fight for life, for a full and abundant life, and must accept disease and death only as inevitable incidents in the battle, but not as its final outcome. Christian acceptance or resignation is not acquiescence, but rather a strategy by which good can be brought out of evil. Sometimes we can defeat our enemy only by patience, turning these evils into opportunities for growth and learning, but we should always see sickness and death as enemies. We should stand with St. Paul in condemning death as the ultimate evil: "and the last enemy to be destroyed is death" (I Cor. 15:26), especially if by *death* we understand the destruction of the human whole, that is, physical, psychological, moral, and above all spiritual death.

Spiritual death is nothing more than the commitment to this total death. By deliberately turning from the love of God and neighbor toward a false self-sufficiency, we commit spiritual suicide (Hillman, 1964). This self-sufficiency is so contradictory to the very nature of all persons, to their expansion into community, that it can only end in prideful despair and refusal to ask for any help beyond ourselves. Ordinary physical suicide probably seldom has this character of total death, because usually it seems to be an attempt to escape to some better life or at least to peace and sleep. But soul suicide is possible only as the hopeless shutting up of self upon itself.

The person who has made a spiritual commitment to life will strive to achieve wholeness in every dimension of personality. Some of course are so deceived by dualism that they do not realize that spiritual wholeness requires the care of our lower human functions. Thus we have had mystics who neglected ethical development, moral people who neglected psychological and physical health, and people concerned about psychological health who did not perceive its intimate connection with both ethical and biological health. But a true understanding of the commitment to life leads to a balanced concern for the whole personality, a respect for the Principle of Totality and Integrity (2.4).

3.2 PREVENTIVE MEDICINE AND LIFE-STYLE

When we speak of personal responsibility for health, many of us think simply of going to a doctor, but of course this is only a part of it. The famous ancient dictum attributed to Hippocrates was that the doctor should prescribe "regimen, medicine, and surgery" in that order, meaning by *regimen* the person's life-style of diet, rest, and exercise. Today, we are still living largely in a world in which medical technology remains at the curative stage rather than at the preventive stage. In the future perhaps the emphasis will shift from the hospital to the center for teaching people how to improve their life-styles.

If we look at current life-styles in terms of physiological and psychological norms, we are appalled by the extremely unhealthy kinds of lives many of us lead. Our advances in preventive medicine have been largely in the form of ridding the environment of infectious diseases and disease carriers. We have made little advance in removing other environmental pollutants (Dubos, 1959, 1976). Civilized man and especially twentieth-century man seems to be subjecting himself to more and more unknowns while relying on medicine and surgery to remedy the harm done.

First of all, modern life often leaves insufficient time for *rest*, not merely in the sense of lack of sleep, but also in the sense of too much stress (Dubos and Pines, 1965). It might seem that we have more leisure because machines have relieved us of much hard, servile labor. But this relief is more than offset by the strange routine of urban life that forces us, for example, to spend hours a day driving to and from work in the hazards of traffic. Clearly, as individuals, we are powerless to escape this sytem, but within it we do have some freedom to make choices that will gradually give our lives greater simplicity and more natural rhythm, free of excessive competition and the drive for success.

Reduced stress also will contribute to moral and spiritual health by making room for a contemplative atmosphere in our lives, for service rather than for ambition for power, for solitude and silence, as well as for more time to give to persons and less to things. Certainly, in past ages, men and women suffered from the burden of manual work, from fear of enemies, from disease and hunger. Yet there remained something of the natural rhythm of effort and of rest. Today, these natural rhythms are often broken up by artificial pressures and hectic overstimulation. As Rordorf (1968) and Kiesling (1970) remind us, we seem to have forgotten that the Jewish and Christian cultural traditions were profoundly shaped by the divine command to keep holy the day of rest and reflection (Exod. 20:8-12; Mark 2:27).

This stressful life can lead to addiction, the enslavement of human beings to the pursuit of intense pleasure or anesthesia as an escape from the pain of life (cf. 12.5). Not only is this addiction to be found in hard drugs, but also in smoking, alcohol, and tranquilizers (McAuliffe and Bosen, 1972). It is found in milder form in the common addiction to overeating and in a particularly corrosive way in the anxious twentieth-century pursuit of sexual pleasure. In moderation, none of these things is unhealthy, but in addictive form they become obsessive and destructive (Van Kamm, 1966). The United States population suffers from many physical and psychological illnesses as a result of these addictions. Venereal disease is not a negligible problem, but sexual addiction may have more serious consequences at the psychological and ethical levels, because it promotes a selfish hedonism that stands in the way of true interpersonal love or loyalty and subverts the human social order traditionally based on the family.

Finally, moderns lack proper physical exercise. Although sports are highly cultivated, they are more and more something to be watched, not to be played by the average man and woman. The average person does little manual work and seldom walks or dances. Illich (1976b) points out, "People who are solely dependent on their feet move at about three or four miles an hour. The United States now puts 45 percent of its total energy into the production, care, and use of vehicles. The typical American, in the course of a year, devotes 1,600 hours to his car — working to pay for gas and insurance, driving, etc. — and he travels 7,500 miles. So he travels about five miles per hour invested" (p. 66). To gain this one mile an hour of speed, he loses a lot of healthy exercise.

To assume personal responsibility for our health, therefore, each of us must have a scientifically based knowledge of the requirements of hygiene, good diet, rest, exercise, and moderation. These cannot be imposed from without. All of us need to design our life to meet personal requirements, which differ greatly. To be healthy, one's life-style must express one's own personality, and it must be one's true personality, not a false one, a resignation to being half alive.

The problems of mental health are similar. Today, we tend to live a life which is overstimulated as regards sensation and passive imagination, but impoverished in active imagination, in reflection and meditation. We have much input, much information, but often little integration of symbols and feelings. We live at the top of our heads, out of touch with our feelings.

As regards spiritual life, it is typical of many moderns that they try to live without clear commitments or goals, suffering from the emptiness, meaninglessness, and absurdity of life, in a loneliness that never seeks deep-level communication with others (R. May, 1958). Nor should we be deceived by a kind of pseudohealth which is sometimes observed in the comfortable modern personality whose life is filled with satisfactions and whose anxieties have been alleviated by psycho-therapy (Rieff, 1968). As in the past religion was sometimes the opiate of the people concealing the symptoms of acute misery with illusory consolations, so also modern life often conceals spiritual emptiness under cover of an illusory secular "happiness" as it is lived by the "beautiful people."

If we are to be healthy, therefore, we need the courage to break with the accepted norms of modern life and subject it to serious criticism. This brings us face to face with the ethical dilemmas produced by modern technology. Perhaps it is ridiculous even to talk about a natural way of life, as our counterculturists do. Have we in fact come to the point in human history when we have to replace nature with a world we have made, even with human beings who have fabricated themselves?

3.3 PRINCIPLE OF STEWARDSHIP AND CREATIVITY

"Be fruitful and multiply; fill the earth and subdue it. Have dominion over the fish of the sea, the birds of the air, and all living things on earth" (Gen. 1:28). On this one verse some ecological enthusiasts have placed the blame for our technological ravagement of the natural environment, but we must also note that in the next chapter of Genesis another tradition reports, "The Lord God took the man and settled him into the Garden of Eden to cultivate and care for it" (2:15). Thus although man is lord of lesser creatures, nevertheless his dominion over them, and over himself, is only a *stewardship* for which he remains responsible to the One Lord (Richardson, 1972; Anderson, 1975).

Classical theology based Christian ethics on the conviction that God endowed all human beings with one common nature which remains essentially the same throughout all history from Adam and Eve to the Last Judgement. We are stewards of this nature as of the world in which God has placed us. By studying the God-given structure and dynamics of this nature it is possible, so theologians in the past thought, to formulate unchanging moral norms binding for every time and culture. Stewardship demanded that we abide by these norms lest we destroy the garden of the world and the temple of our own body which were given us to "cultivate and care for."

Today this traditional conception of stewardship is open to several serious criticisms. First, since theologians generally accept the view that the Creator produced the human race by an evolutionary process, they have to take account of the fact that we are not finished master-pieces but rather a work in progress. Hence it is no insult to God's creative wisdom for us to suppose that we can further perfect the world and even our own bodies. Indeed, it is to God's praise that He has generously called us to be co-workers with Him in his creative task.

Second, we have come to realize that human behavior is less a product of natural instinct than of culture and social determinism. Human nature exists not in the abstract but in the flux of human history and of indi-vidual biographies where it seems subject to endless variations. How then can we formulate universal definition of human nature that is more than an empty commonplace?

Third, with the rise of modern technology, for the first time in history human beings have achieved a real dominion over nature. In principle, at least, the discovery of the deoxyribonucleic acid (DNA) molecule opens the way for us to produce life and to control evolution. Moreover, we are acquiring mastery of the building blocks out of which all material things are made and may soon tap the sources of energy which will make it possible for us to reconstruct our world.

The ethical implication of these discoveries seems to be that we can no longer base ethical norms on human nature, because that nature itself becomes a matter of our own choosing (Callahan, 1973b). We may be able to select from among various models of human nature the ones we prefer to construct, just as we do between various models of houses. The prophecy of Karl Marx (1964 [1844]; Dognin, 1970) that in our age man will become his own creator seems to be coming true. Perhaps we can even learn to reverse the aging process and make overselves immortal! Thus we are no longer stewards but creators.

Of course the Biblical story of the Tower of Babel (Gen. 11:1-9) and the Greek myth of Prometheus stealing fire from the gods remind us that this dream is not new. Before we totally succumb to it, we should take into account certain doubts expressed by scientists them-selves. First, it must be noted that these predictions of unlimited human dominion over nature are less convincing now than they were a few years ago at the time of the discovery of atomic fission and the genetic code. The ecological crisis has revealed that modern technology in its present form has its limits (Callahan, 1973c; Muller, 1974). Every tech-nological advance exacts its price in environmental pollution and depletion of energy resources. Moreover, since evolution has adapted human nature very nicely to its primitive environment, we cannot alter either that nature nor that environment without serious risks. We always have to proceed strategically, trying to gain a little more than we lose.

Again, the proposals for genetic engineering which we will discuss from an ethical point of view in chapter 11 are still largely theoretical (Davis, 1970; Karp, 1976). Even the improvement of the body by transplants or artificial organs is still in a very crude state. We have grasped certain basic principles of life, but these principles operate in life systems that are bafflingly complex. We will be able to unravel the details only painfully and by long and often frustrating research, as our slow progress in understanding cancer exemplifies.

Furthermore, there is one ultimate limiting factor which is still very little understood. Since our human creative intelligence depends upon the human brain, any alterations of body structure which might injure the brain will be disastrously self-defeating (Smythies, 1965). Can the human brain be significantly improved? So far as we know, the human brain is the most complex system in the universe. To build it would require far more information than to construct any other system, even the most complex computers so far invented. Yet the brain is relatively very small, and unlike a computer it is capable of self-development and some self-repair. In fact, as we think we constantly restructure our brain circuitry at the synaptic level (Rose, 1973).

Perhaps, then, our human brain is already near the limit of evolution. Hence any kind of improvement we can make in the rest of our body must be limited by the requirements of the brain. No doubt we could turn ourselves into brain-persons by replacing most of the other body systems with artificial organs to support the life of the brain. We could feed the brain with information and let it transmit its orders electronically. Yet this would eliminate much of the imaginative and affective life which plays so important a part in our motivation and interpersonal relations. Would we want, for example, to eliminate sexual reproduction and reduce sex to orgasms produced by direct stimulation of pleasure centers in the brain? This would indeed make us one-dimensional men (Marcuse, 1964). Thus the Principle of Totality and Integrity which we discussed in 2.4 warns us of the ethical limits to human self-creation.

While such warnings are in order, we believe it would be wrong to conclude as do such modern critics of technology as Jacques Ellul (1965) that modern technology is the temptation of the Serpent, a sin of pride and rebellion against the Creator. God would not have endowed us with creative intelligence and freedom if He did not want us to share in his creative action. We are divinely called not merely to preserve the old, but to produce the new. In *The Church in the Modern World* (1965c) the Second Vatican Council teaches us that technology is a gift of God for which we have stewardship like any other of his gifts.

Classical theology in its account of God's dominion was too much influenced by the Old Testament image of the monarch God jealous of his supreme dignity and power. In New Testament perspective we understand God as best revealed in Christ, who "though he was in the form of God, did not deem equality with God something to be grasped at, but rather he emptied himself and took the form of a servant" (Phil. 2:6-7). Such a God is not jealous of his power but calls us to share in his work of making all things new (Rev. 21:5). Our cooperation is not merely filling in details in a finished "plan of God." Rather He has called us to use our own initiative and originality in completing his work.

In our creative activity, however, we have to respect our own limits and the limits of the materials with which we must work. These limits are not set by God out of any concern for his own authority. God himself is "limited" by his own wisdom and love which forbid Him to do what is contradictory to his own nature. We are far more limited by the fact that our share in God's knowledge and love is finite. No matter how we may progress in science, freedom, and power, we dare not contradict our own human nature without destroying ourselves.

At any given moment in our history our limits are set by our knowledge. Once we understand some aspect of nature well, we can freely choose to improve nature and surpass it. But when we lack that understanding, our efforts to improve on nature may prove disastrous. The evils of modern technology are not the result of creative use of our knowledge, but of rash exploitation of a nature little understood. Above all we have failed to understand ourselves, our authentic needs and potentialities. To acquire the knowledge we need, research and experimentation, with all the risks they involve, are necessary, but even here we must proceed with reverence for the persons and the environment which are at risk.

As a result of these considerations, we can formulate the *Principle of Stewardship and Creativity* as follows:

1. We are ethically obliged to use our natural environment and our multidimensional human nature as precious gifts, with profound respect for their intrinsic teleology.

2. We are also obliged to use our creativity as an equally precious gift to improve our environment and our nature, with a caution set by the limits of our actual knowledge and by the risk of destroying that same creativity.

3.4   PRINCIPLE OF PRUDENT CONSCIENCE AND INFORMED CONSENT

Need for Truth

Clearly, modern medicine constantly involves both technological and ethical judgments. In modern medical practice we must ask not only, "Can it be done?" but also, "Ought we to do what we can do?"

The sociologist Eliot Freidson in his book *Profession of Medicine* (1971) has shown from a different point of view that the claim of health care professionals to make autonomous professional decisions about medical matters is invalid because the fact that their professional knowledge makes them experts about the techniques of medicine does not imply that they are experts in the *use* of these techniques, since this use involves social, political, and moral issues concerning which they are not experts.

Thus, Freidson's argument implies that individuals who seek the services of a medical professional cannot simply delegate to that professional those concrete decisions about their health on the grounds that the doctor knows best. For a woman to consent to a tubal ligation because the doctor advises it is to take the advice of someone who has special competence in medicine but not in ethics. On the other hand neither is the individual competent to decide such a question on her own unless she has adequate information about the medical aspects of the decision. There is thus a certain dilemma in medical decisions: Who has the knowledge both of the ethical norms and of the medical facts to make a wise decision? And how are these norms and facts to be related to each other? This dilemma requires us to discuss at some length the problem of *prudent conscience*.

Christian theology has always insisted that when it comes to concrete decisions to act or not to act in a given situation and to choose this or that possible alternative course of action each normal individual has the capacity and the responsibility to judge and to act on his own judgment which cannot be delegated to anyone else or to any institution — not to custom, to the law, or to advisers and not even to civil or religious leaders. The capacity to make practical judgment in matters involving ethical issues is what we call *conscience* (cf. Curran, 1977a). The Second Vatican Council (1965c) said of it:

> For the human being has in his or her heart a law inscribed by God. A person's dignity lies in observing this law, and by it he or she will be judged. Conscience is the person's most secret core and sanctuary. There the person is alone with God whose voice echoes in the person's depths. By conscience, in a wonderful way, that law is made known which is fulfilled in the love of God and one's neighbor. Through loyalty to conscience Christians are joined to other men in the search for truth and for the right solution to so many moral problems which arise both in the life of individuals and from social relationships. Hence, the more a correct conscience prevails, the more do persons and groups turn aside from blind choice and try to be guided by the objective standards of moral conduct. (m. 16)

Thus our responsibility is to follow our *informed* conscience; that is, (1) we must get as much relevant information about the facts and values involved as we are able to obtain in the situation of time and place in which we find ourselves, and (2) we must then make and carry out our decision in accordance with this information. Sin is the failure either to inform our conscience or to follow our conscience after informing it.

Thus in any bioethical question we have the responsibility (1) to learn the facts about the medical condition and other circumstances of the persons involved, as well as to reflect in the light of our own system of values on the human values and rights involved while also keeping our mind open to what we may learn from dialogue with those who believe in other systems and (2) to come to a concrete, personal decision that we will live by in spite of disagreement or pressures from others.

Persons who lack the information necessary to make a wise decision in bioethical matters will only make a good decision by chance; yet if such persons decide wrongly, they will have to suffer the consequences of the mistake no matter how sincerely it may have been made. Such persons are said to be invincibly ignorant.

On the other hand, persons who have deliberately failed to seek the information which they know is necessary for a realistic decision are said to be vincibly ignorant and are morally responsible for the consequences of decisions hampered by this ignorance. This can happen either through neglect (crass ignorance), through self-deception (affected ignorance), or through willful resolve to ignore the facts (malicious ignorance). Such avoidable ignorance does not excuse us morally for our bad decisions. This principle is clearly recognized by the law governing malpractice suits whereby a physician is held responsible only for mistakes in judgment he could have avoided. All health care professionals have the obligation to obtain the information they need through initial and continuing education, personal study, careful examination of the patient, and consultation with other professionals and perhaps even with the patient's family. This obligation applies not only to medical knowledge, but also to relevant legal and ethical knowledge.

Not only ignorance causes mistaken judgments. Ethicists point out that we are prevented from *using* the knowledge we may actually possess by various emotional factors. Thus fear, force, unthinking routine, neurotic compulsions, and prejudices cloud our judgment and limit our freedom to select among all available alternatives. Modern psychology and social psychology emphasize these limitations on human freedom and realistic choice. They have taught us how our social background, family training, professional education, and social position can limit our perception of reality. Theology also recognizes this limitation of freedom under the name of *original sin*, which according to current understanding is not merely one remote sin of Adam and Eve, but is also the whole burden of human sin from the beginning of human history built into our culture and its institutions, even our religious institutions (not to mention our health care institutions!) (McDermott, 1977). We suffer from the effects of this burden and have our freedom restricted by it (Curran, 1977a), but we do not become personally guilty of this sin until we begin to realize this blindness and enslavement and accept our chains, rather than struggle to be free of them.

Thus, all medical professionals need to take a tip from the psychoanalysts and realize that if they are to be psychologically free to make truly ethical and helpful decisions they must have insight into their own prejudices, biases, and unconscious motives. All physicians need to be alert to their own tendencies to dominate the helpless, to take sadistic pleasure in their power over the human body, and to avoid facing their own feelings of tenderness or fear of death. All these emotions are perfectly human, and when disciplined they actually contribute to ethical sensitivity and good judgment, but when they are unconscious, neurotic, and self-serving, they can lead to very unwise judgments. Thus an informed conscience must be supported by a good will and healthy, disciplined emotion. To think that cold-blood, scientific objectivity will lead to ethically wise decisions is an illusion, just as it is an illusion to think that sentimentality is helpful. An emotive ethics is not adequate, but it contains an important measure of truth.

Does full information before a decision definitely determine what the decision is to be? If it did, then there would be no such thing as *freedom*. Human beings are free not simply because they are relieved from any external coercion, but for two other reasons. First, usually there are many alternative means to a goal, some of which are clearly inappropriate, but many are often appropriate, each with its advantages and disadvantages. Second, it is possible for us to reconsider our goals and to redefine or even alter them in view of some higher goal. Thus morality always involves a choice, and that choice is not always between a clear-cut good line and a clear-cut bad line of action. It may be between two good lines of action, and there may also be many wrong ways that involve different degrees of evil.

Since knowledge of the factors involved in any decision seldom results in a determinant judgment that this or that action is best without qualification, it might seem that a rational decision is impossible. But knowledge is not the only factor involved in decision; there is also will, along with affection. Our decision will be ethically good only if we have a good will (supported, if possible, by healthy emotions) which inclines us to follow our best information and ethical insight, even if they are not conclusive. Hence, we speak not only of an informed conscience as if all we need is knowledge of the facts and of the law (legalism), but also of a prudent conscience, that is, of a virtuous way of using our information.

Certitude in Ethical Decisions

An informed conscience can still be mistaken about the *objective* goodness of an action because of invincible ignorance. The history of medicine is filled with disturbing episodes in which medical professionals followed a line of treatment and care in accordance with the best knowledge available at that time, but which turned out to be disastrously mistaken. Does this mean that they acted unethically? By no means, but they and the patients nevertheless had to bear the tragic consequences. The same is true also of ethical norms, and we should not be unduly disturbed when we find that a rule of conduct which once seemed sound later turns out to be inadequate for the protection of human rights. Thus in recent years the norms for ethical experimentation on human subjects (see 9.4) have become much stricter (HEW, 1975). Some people have the mistaken impression that progress in civilization means an easier, more liberal morality. In fact, the more knowledgeable we become of human needs, the more careful we are likely to be about the protection of human rights and, therefore, to propose more precise ethical norms.

As a result, as many health care professionals today know only too well, ethical decision may involve a real agony of conscience. We may be faced with the realization (1) that although we have tried to get adequate information, we still do not have all the facts or the clear understanding of values that we really need to make a decision that will be objectively correct, and (2) that even when we have acquired the best knowledge available, the best alternative may remain very unclear, because every alternative has advantages and disadvantages. Given such uncertainty, many people try to pass the buck to someone else. But by doing so, they do not escape responsibility; instead, they assume responsibility for the decision made by the other person, whose judgment may be even less trustworthy than their own. Such uncertainty also causes many to think that in practical matters an ethical decision is finally nothing but a leap in the dark.

This is not the case. We are always obliged to act with *moral* certitude. There may and usually does remain a theoretical or objective doubt as to whether what we decide will actually work out for the best, but there must be no practical doubt. My conscience must be certain that for me here and now the best thing to do is A, rather than B. Otherwise, I would be acting blindly rather than on the basis of the good will to follow the best information available.

How can we come to such a practical or moral certitude that here and now this is what we ought to do? After we have informed our conscience as well as possible in the time and place in which we are situated, it will probably become clear that at least some alternatives are excluded as clearly inappropriate means to ethical goals. Among those possibilities that remain, some may be attractive, but we may still not be sure whether they are right or wrong.

The great medieval theologians taught that in such doubts we are obliged to act *prudently*, that is, to choose that course of action which as far as we can discover will more probably be the most effective means to achieve our legitimate goals. To act otherwise would be unreasonable and therefore unethical. However, in the seventeenth and eighteenth centuries a more legalistic approach to morality came into vogue. Moralists tended to adopt the methods employed by lawyers who solved doubtful cases by recourse to general legal rules or what moralists called "reflex principles" (Connell, 1968) such as "A doubtful law does not bind" and "The accused is to be held innocent until proved guilty." Eventually this legal mode of reasoning was developed into the system called probabilism.

According to probabilism persons who are in doubt about whether a law forbidding a course of action they would like to take exists, or about whether a law applies in their case are free to act as they prefer provided that (1) their doubts rest on solidly probably reasons and (2) there is no risk of serious damage to others or to themselves. Proponents of the sytem argued that all reflex principles can be reduced to a single principle: In doubt the presumption is in favor of the existing situation: that is, we are free to continue our ordinary way of conduct unless new information or a clearer duty demands a change.

Although probabilism was bitterly opposed by Catholic Jansenists and some Protestant theologians on the grounds that only a rigorist application of moral law can protect us from slipping into the moral laxity to which the corruption of our human nature by original sin makes us liable, probabilism was finally accepted by all Catholic theologians, although we may still question the legalism on which both probabilism and rigorism rest.

Whether we follow the prudential method of the medievals or the legal method of the probabilists, it is clear that in regard to controversial ethical questions we need to maintain a balance between a rigid and a laxist approach to morals. When in doubt about whether a course of action is ethical, we should give the benefit of the doubt to existing custom, to established and well-known laws, to our usual way of acting, and we should do what has already been done as if it were well done. For example, procedures and policies well accepted in the medical profession should be used as norms of ethical behavior unless the contrary can be reasonably established. This *conservative* presumption is based on the fact that in human life what is customary and established at least has the merit of long experience, reflection, and survival We cannot change the world every day. On the other hand, we may also make use of the *liberal* presumption that we are free to do what seems most attractive and best for us subjectively provided that there is no clear law or reason against it or the rights of others to consider. Probabilism (Connell, 1968) leaves the individual conscience free in doubtful matters to follow more liberal views as long as they are not mere fads, but are supported by reliable authorities in ethics. For Catholics, this freedom supposes loyalty to the living Tradition of the Christian community in its authoritative expression by the popes and councils.

In the recent past, most Catholic health care professionals used a very simple method of arriving at this required moral certitude in bioethical questions. They had only to ask what was the Catholic position on abortion, sterilization, and so forth. The answer was easily supplied by the Catholic chaplain who referred to a standard manual in Catholic medical ethics. These manuals gave detailed and assured answers to almost every imaginable question based on the common opinion of standard authors in moral theology. The official directives of the various offices of the Vatican and especially of the popes were the ultimate and decisive word of such authorities. Among these directives the encyclicals and addresses of Pius XII (1962), written with great clarity and precision because of Pius' deep interest in the problems of Christian professional people and their dilemmas in our technological society, were quoted as the final authority in the field.

This strict dependence on official teaching had the disadvantage that it often led to a kind of unthinking obedience on the part of health care professionals. They became almost schizophrenic in the way they compartmentalized their Catholic principles and their scientific professional knowledge, without attempting to make any intellectual reconciliation of the two. On the other hand it had the advantage that a uniform policy in Catholic health care facilities could be developed, while the individual doctor or nurse had the security of a quiet conscience. This advantage did not mean that the duty of following one's informed conscience was abrogated, but only that the task of informing one's conscience was very much simplified. Probably a good many Catholic health care professionals wish that this simple way of achieving peace of conscience were still available, since they believe they have neither the time nor training to do any thinking about bioethical issues on their own.

However, since Vatican II, and especially since the controversy over Paul VI's encyclical *Humanae Vitae* (1968c), this peace of conscience has been greatly disturbed. For some health care professionals the change has meant a crisis of conscience; for others it has meant rebellion, confusion, or bitter feelings of betrayal. Occasionally, we hear recriminations of conservative Catholics against liberal colleagues saying, "If he doesn't accept the pope's teaching, why doesn't he get out of the Church? Some have, in fact, left the Church, either because they felt they could not dissent and remain sincere Catholics or to the contrary because they were disgusted with a Church too weak to expel dissenters. Understanding more clearly the function in Christian life of the official teaching of the pope and bishops and why dissent is possible even for a good Catholic and what the limits of both teaching and dissent are, are necessary elements in the ethical knowledge of any sincere Catholic. The following explanation of these topics, of necessity, is highly simplified and can be supplemented from current authors (Rahner, 1968c, a; Curran, 1969; McSorley, 1969; Costanzo, 1969; Halligan, 1969; Kippley, 1971).

Guidance by the Spirit

The Christian community or Church is founded on faith in Jesus Christ. Jesus is known to us only because the good news about him is preached and witnessed to us. Such witness, however, requires the continuance of the teaching authority (*magisterium*) of Christ and his apostles in a lasting way in the Church, and by the power of the Holy Spirit we are guaranteed that this witness of and in the Christian community will not fail (i.e., it is *infallible* until Christ comes again (Matt. 28:18-20; John 16:4-16; 17:9-26).

In nineteenth-century theology this *magisterium* (teaching role) was usually considered the exclusive work of the pope and bishops. They alone seemed to have had the right to teach actively, while the other members of the Church were merely passive hearers and learners. However, the Second Vatican Council (1964b) reminded us that Christ's threefold mission as priest, shepherd, and teacher is shared in appropriate ways by *all* members of the Church. Thus, while not all Christians have a special gift of teaching (I Cor. 12:29; I Tim. 1:7), by their baptism and confirmation all Christians participate somehow *actively* in teaching and witnessing the faith (Congar, 1976). For example, Christian parents have an important share in the active *magisterium* when they pass on their faith to their children.

This common witness to the faith (*sensus fidelium*) that flows from living a Christian life is not mere public opinion. When pollsters report that a majority of United States Catholics do or do not favor abortion or racial discrimination, we cannot conclude that this is the *sensus fidelium*. To discover that faith witness we would have to inquire what truths relevant to abortion or racism Catholics believed God has or has not *revealed* to his people. The *sensus fidelium*, therefore, is not human opinion, but the witness of the Christian community to the apostolic faith they have received and by which they live.

A special form of this discernment process is the witness given by those in the community who are especially dedicated to contemplation and intense prayer, which the Bible often refers to as the gift of prophecy (I Cor. 14:1-5; Acts 21:9) and which helps the community grow in depth and purity of faith and in the liveliness of hope. Thus Paul VI recently honored St. Teresa of Avila and St. Catherine of Siena as "Doctors (teachers) of the Church." Nor should we forget that a Christian artist like Michelangelo, a scientist like Teilhard de Chardin, or a philosopher like Gabriel Marcel help us by their human disciplines to express the faith in its full splendor.

In the Middle Ages theologians were recognized as playing a special role in the *magisterium*. Today, some suppose a good Catholic theologian should be content to explain and defend the pronouncements of the bishops and pope. Some recent popes have even urged theologians to keep silent about deficiencies in Church documents lest authority be weakened.   However, it is now generally admitted that the teaching mission of the Church will be weakened if theologians do not have the freedom to express their honest opinions.

Sometimes this freedom is called "the right to dissent," but more properly it might be called "the right of expert criticism." The charisma of the theologian is to witness to the faith by responsible, scholarly criticism which involves not only defense of official formulations of the faith, but also pointing out defects and proposing hypotheses for the improvement of such formulations — hypotheses which sometimes may seem very daring and novel. Of course, theologians as responsible members of the Christian community have the duty to use their gifts to build up the faith of the community (Eph. 4:11-13) by communicating to the public not only their criticisms and difficulties, but also the positive, constructive results of their researches.

The pastoral ministry makes a very special contribution to the Church's teaching effort. This ministry is not limited to the ordained, but is carried on by many men and women whose experience in applying the faith to actual life is essential if the Gospel is to be effectively preached to the poor and the little ones (Matt. 11:5; 18:5-14). For example, religious sisters and brothers have probably contributed more to the active *magisterium* in the United States than have the ordained clergy.

Finally a special leadership responsibility falls on the bishops with their priests and deacons in a local church and on the pope for the whole Church to unify all these different witnessing voices, to express their consensus in clear terms suited to our times, and to link this to the tradition of the Christian community throughout the world in its historical development.   Without such unifying leadership the spiritual riches of faith and insight contributed by the members of the Church would be dissipated and the community would be divided in its faith and life. Thus, while the role of theologians is primarily critical and analytic, the role of bishops is primarily pastoral and synthetic.

In particular, bishops have the hard task of reconciling partial and extreme views within the Church which might lead to heresy or schism. This they can best do not by condemnation, but by wise emphasis on those principal truths and values which keep a straggling flock moving toward its goal. In moral matters prudent bishops do not burden the freedom of individual consciences by insistence on secondary issues (I Cor. 10:23-33) since they recognize that the members of the Church are at many different levels of moral development, but rather constantly emphasize the primary goals of Christian life.

Sometimes, however, bishops and popes are confronted with dangerous crises in the life of the community in which as leaders and pastors they have the painful duty of using their authority "to bind and to loose" (Matt. 16:19; 18:18) to protect the community from disruption and to strengthen its public witness. This is why in extreme cases a bishop may have to resort, as did St. Paul (I Cor. 5:1-13), to excommunication or exclusion from Christian life of those who "will not hear the Church" (Matt. 18:17), observing, however, all the care for justice which today we call "due process."

As we have so far described it, this work of the *magisterium* is said to be "ordinary." This ordinary teaching, even as it is authoritatively formulated in the pronouncements of the bishops and pope, is obviously a combination of many different elements of unequal value. How, then, does it share in the infallibility guaranteed to the Christian community by the Holy Spirit's guidance? Immersed in the culture of their own times, most Christians seldom stop to reflect or discriminate the Gospel substance from traditions and opinions which are merely accidental aspects of their faith. Yet mature Christians do sense that some matters of religious thought and practice are essential and definitive of Christian commitment, while others are more or less peripheral and transitory.

Unfortunately, since the Reformation, polemics between the churches have led to a type of religious instruction for Catholics which tends to make them feel that loyalty demands of them equal adherence to every item of traditional Catholicism. Such faulty instruction is largely responsible for the present polarization within the Church between liberals and conservatives. This polarization is forcing us to discriminate between the unfailing Gospel in its inspired tradition and various human traditions which are passing away with the changes of time and the worldwide extension of the Church to include non-European cultures.

Clearly the ordinary teaching of the Church, along with such merely human traditions, must also include the whole revealed truth of Scripture and Tradition, otherwise the Word of God would not be unfailingly transmitted from one generation to another. Thus doctrinal minimalists who call into doubt everything in this ordinary teaching on the grounds that it is not "defined *de fide*" run the risk of eliminating all the certitude of the Christian community's faith witness. On the other hand, doctrinal integrists who identify every traditional belief or practice with the Word of God, who treat anyone who criticizes any pronouncement of a local bishop, a Roman congregation, or a pope as disobedient and disloyal to authority, run the risk of a great shock when they discover the Church has changed or contradicted itself.

It is necessary, therefore, to discriminate between those elements of the ordinary teaching of the Church which are the infallible Word of God and those which are simply human, perhaps even erroneous, opinion. To make this discrimination requires each of us, according to our gifts and situation, to engage in prayer, study, and reflection so as to note the signs by which God makes Himself known to the Christian community. Taken one by one these signs may not be completely convincing, but their convergence can bring us to a secure conviction that *this* is the Word of God. These convergent signs are simply the different kinds of witness to the faith already ennumerated. When the Scriptures, the faithful, the prophetic contemplatives, the theologians, and the legitimate pastors of the Church each in their own proper role give a concurrent witness, a Christian knows that to reject that witness would be to resist the Holy Spirit.

For example, the witness provided by the Second Vatican Council to the great truths of the Gospel by the pope and bishops in dialogue with theologians and representatives of religious orders and its reception by the vast majority of Catholics and, in the main, its general approval by the other Christian churches provides a secure sign of the Word of God and the presence of the Holy Spirit for all except a few integrists alarmed by changes in unessential matters. Nevertheless, the council did not go beyond the level of the ordinary *magisterium* by defining new dogmas.

Such ordinary teaching authority is all that Protestants generally recognize in the Church. The Orthodox and Roman Catholic Churches, however, also believe that when necessary an ecumenical council of the bishops has the authority to issue a definitive judgment *extraordinary magisterium*) on a disputed question of faith. Generally, the Orthodox believe that ecumenicity of such councils must be confirmed by the acceptance of the whole Church. Roman Catholics, on the other hand, believe that the Lord, by establishing St. Peter as the chief of his apostles (Matt. 16:13-20; John 21:15-17), indicated the solution to this need of the Church for definitive "binding and loosing" in questions of faith. Confirming the definitive teaching of the First Vatican Council on this matter, the Second Vatican Council (1964a) says of the infallible authority of such extraordinary teaching:

> This infallibility, however, with which the divine redeemer wished to endow his Church in defining doctrine pertaining to faith and morals, is co-extensive with the deposit of revelation, which must be religiously guarded and loyally and courageously expounded. The Roman Pontiff, head of the college of bishops, enjoys this infallibility in virtue of his office, when, as supreme pastor and teacher of all the faithful — who confirms his brethren in the faith (cf. Luke 22:32) — he proclaims in absolute decision a doctrine pertaining to faith or morals. The infallibility promised to the Church is also present in the body of bishops when, together with Peter's successor, they exercise the supreme teaching office. Now, the assent of the Church can never be lacking to such definitions on account of the same Holy Spirit's influence, through which Christ's whole body is maintained in the unity of faith and makes progress in it. (n. 24)

Although the power to make such definitive judgments extends to moral teaching with which the present book is concerned, it is not easy to point out any such definitive statements of the extraordinary *magisterium* on concrete ethical questions, although perhaps there are some general moral principles which have been so defined, for example, that Christians have other moral obligations in addition to the obligation to believe religious truths (Denzinger and Schönmetzer, 1963; Neuner and Dupuis, 1975). We should not conclude, therefore, that the Gospel teaches us nothing certain about Christian conduct. The correct inference is that to know God's will about what we are to do or not to do in order to follow Christ it is necessary to take into account all forms of Christian witness, among which the pastoral documents of the Church provide us with firm guidance. This ordinary teaching as expressed in such pastoral documents may be infallibly certain when confirmed by the convergence of other witnesses, but is not of itself equivalent to a definitive judgment by the extraordinary teaching authority (Thils, 1968), and hence it may in some respects be subject to correction.

Even very traditional Catholics need not feel insecure in this situation, since they will find that the main lines of Christian moral life are clear (National Conference of Catholic Bishops, 1976a), and that even in particular issues there is usually a course of action which enjoys such great probability of correctness that individuals may be quite safe in following it. However, in some matters in every one's life and in every age of the Church are moral dilemmas in which we must pray earnestly for the Holy Spirit's guidance to make courageous personal and communal decisions. Those who demand greater certainty than this and cry out for the pope to settle every moral question with an infallible definition are exhibiting scrupulous consciences weakened either by neurosis or by lack of real faith in Christ's promise to guide us by the constant presence of his Holy Spirit.

A Prudent Conscience

Nor do Catholic health care professionals need feel in medicomoral matters that they are sinking into a theological morass. They need only keep in mind that there are two different levels of moral certitude: (1) the level of principles and value priorities and (2) the level of concrete application of these principles to particular problems of moral decision. At the level of principles and values Jesus Christ has given to Christians ample light on what are "the weightier matters of the law, justice and mercy and good faith" (Matt. 23:23), and they are clearly expressed for us in the ordinary teaching of the Church. If professionals study the official pastoral documents of the popes and bishops in a spirit of faith, prayer, and reflection, they will discover there the chief ethical values at which to aim in making practical medical decisions. The clearer our understanding and appreciation of these values the surer will be our moral judgment. Without such understanding mere mechanical obedience to laws and rules will not yield prudent decisions.

At the second level of concrete application of ethical principles we enter into an area of complexity and difficulty where official Church teaching can be of great help, but where we should not expect perfect clarity or undebatable certitude. Health care professionals are well aware that the clarity and high probability of scientific laws are not to be expected in the application of these laws to particular medical decisions. It is painful to have to make a life-and-death medical decision without being sure how the principles in the medical textbook fit the particular case, yet such decisions have to be made every day. In the same way moral decisions cannot be made simply by referring to theological textbooks or to official Church documents.

In fact at the level of detailed application of basic moral principles conscientious Catholics may discover that the pastoral guidance provided by the pope, the bishops, and their priests seems inadequate to the problems with which the laity have to deal, either because these guidelines do not touch the precise problems with which the laity have to deal, or because in dealing with such issues this pastoral guidance seems to ignore experiences, objective facts, and special insights coming from other sources. Thus a medical professional may find that a pastoral document does not seem to be cognizant of medical and social facts which condition special medicoethical problems. Of course it would be unjust to assume that pastoral leaders do not make a serious attempt to be well informed on such matters, but nevertheless the gap between abstract principles and concrete cases may be painfully apparent.

In such situations loyal Catholics may find themselves faced with the question whether they should publicly criticize the adequacy of official Church teaching. We have already argued that theologians have the duty to carry on such criticism in a responsible and constructive way. So also do other Catholics whose special expertness or experience gives them the right to contribute to the development of magisterial positions (cf. National Conference of Catholic Bishops, 1968).

Granted this right to discuss authoritative pastoral teaching in the spirit of constructive criticism, is there also the right for a Catholic to *act* contrary to such official teaching? Since we are always morally obliged to follow a prudent, informed conscience, there is unquestionably not only such a right but a duty to act on our own best judgment even when in a particular instance this departs from official teaching (Curran, 1975). However, those who find themselves conscientiously obliged to dissent in this way have to take on themselves the responsibility for the consequences of their action. Nor is it fair for them to call on the pastors of the community to confirm and approve their dissenting judgment. When we do not take others' advice and counsel, we cannot justly blame them for refusing to agree with us.

The situation of a Catholic health care facility, however, is quite different from that of individual theologians carrying on scholarly debate and from that of individual Catholics forming their personal conscience. A facility supported and approved officially by the local bishop has the responsibility of bearing a public witness to Christian values as these are interpreted by the local bishop. Therefore, its policies need to be correlated with authoritative pastoral teaching. In the United States such teaching is proposed in the *Ethical and Religious Directives for Catholic Health Facilities* (1971) issued by the United States Catholic Conference (USSC) with the approval of the National Conference of Catholic Bishops as promulgated and interpreted by the local bishops. These *Directives* have been rather severely criticized by some theologians and have required some additional official interpretations with regard to abortion (CTSA, 1971; cf. O'Donnell, 1972; Keefe, 1973), sterilization, and cooperation (cf. chapters 9 and 10), but still remain in force. Of course, in accordance with the Principle of Subsidiarity (8.2-2) Catholic health care facilities have the responsibility (1) for interpreting the *Directives* in their application to local situations, preferably through a Christian identity committee (cf. 6.5) and (2) for working for changes in these *Directives* on the basis of their own experience and reflection through representatives to the pertinent committees of the Bishops Conference (*Directives*, 1971).

The fact that the pastoral guidance of the Church at the level of concrete application leaves considerable room for individual and institutional judgment makes it obvious that the effort of Christians to acquire and act on a prudent conscience involves no little risk and conflict. Hence a vital factor in such efforts is self-criticism of our own maturity of moral judgment. We have to be aware of our own biases, narrowness of experience and outlook, and half-conscious motivation. Consciences have their own psychological and spiritual pathologies, as do our emotions, and they have often been weakened or distorted by defective ethical education.

There are persons who have a rigid conscience, that is, they demand a clear set of laws which they can apply almost mechanically to concrete situations. Without such security, they feel heavily burdened. Some physicians, for example, who are disturbed by present ethical debate in the Catholic Church suffer from this pathology. More extreme is the scrupulous person who not only demands excessive certitude, but also can never achieve it, no matter how clear the rules. Such persons constantly beg for reassurance from some external authority as to what is right or wrong and are tortured by neurotic guilt which is not based on any real guilt. This neurotic guilt can be so compulsive that it interferes with rational ethical judgment. Both of these pathologies may require psychotherapy and spiritual reeducation. Persons who begin to realize that their conscience is seriously rigid or scrupulous have an obligation to seek help, since such pathologies tend to be progressive (O'Flaherty, 1966).

On the other hand, there are lax, insensitive, callous consciences. At the extreme are those psychopaths who seem incapable of keeping in mind the possible consequences of their actions for others or even for themselves. But callous conscience is also found in cynical persons who have been so scandalized by the hypocrisy of others and so weary of their guilt over their own frequent sins that they no longer bother to try to inform their conscience. More common among health care professionals are those whose moral sensitivity has been hardened by the routine of suffering. Most of us also have a tendency to avoid moral responsibility by shifting decisions to others or by blundering ahead into action without making a firm decision. We act *in doubt*, swayed by popular opinion, by the last person who talked to us, or by the mood of the moment. For these reasons, the study of medical ethics and regular, orderly discussions with others about ethical issues are necessary to help us be ethically balanced and decisive.

Moral Decision in an Immoral World

In spite of all our efforts to come to principled moral decisions with which we can live in peace of conscience, we may occasionally find ourselves with a *perplexed* conscience — a state not necessarily pathological but rather the result of the human condition in a sinful world wherein finding our way is not always easy. Some Protestant moralists who stress the total depravity of human nature argue that since no matter what we do our actions are distorted by our sinful condition we should "sin bravely" (to use a paradoxical but often misunderstood expression of Luther's), that is, with trust that God will forgive us no matter what our actions are as long as we have faith in his mercy. Of course, such theologians are not denying that we still have the Christian obligation to do the best we know how and by no means intend to excuse sin, but only to underline our total dependence on God's mercy (Thielicke, 1969).

Traditionally Catholic moralists deal with this obvious fact that we live in a world so distorted by sin that often human conscience is perplexed and obscured by having to distinguish between the objective evil of such acts as divorce and the subjective excusability of persons living in a culture where divorce is an accepted custom. Jesus himself seems to have made some such distinction when he argued that Old Law permitted divorce "because of the hardness of your hearts" (Matt. 19:8). Recently, however, Charles E. Curran (1968, 1972) has proposed a theory which he terms "moral compromise." While he does not accept the extreme pessimism about human nature as proposed by some Protestant theologians, he does wish to emphasize that we have to act in a world into which sin has introduced a disorder which makes it impossible even for the just man always to act in a way completely consistent with the just order of things intended by God. Thus Curran (1977a) recently writes:

> Sinfulness for the Christian always remains present in our human existence. I am not understanding sinfulness in this case as the individual single acts of a person or even the sinfulness of the person placing the act but

> rather the cosmic and interpersonal aspects of sinfulness which become incarnate in the world in which we live. Sometimes the presence of sin forces us to act in a way which would not occur if there were no sin incarnated in the structures of human existence. (pp. 185-186)

Curran goes on to argue that given this sinful condition some actions which would have been objectively wrong may become objectively right. At the same time he does not believe this situation excuses the Christian from working to overcome the sinful situations which make such compromise necessary:

> The theory of compromise recognizes that sin affects the objective order as well as the subjective order. However, compromise also recognizes that the Christian is called to attempt to overcome the reality of sin as well as acknowledging that sin will never be completely overcome this side of the eschaton. Meanwhile, the presence of sin occasionally forces us to do things which under ordinary circumstances we would not do. The word *compromise* tries to indicate the tension involved in recognizing even in the objective order the fact that sin is present, and the Christian tries to overcome it, but at times the Christian will not be able to overcome it completely. (p. 186)

We would agree with Curran that the sinful condition of our world affects moral decisions not only subjectively by reason of our moral blindness or lack of freedom, but also objectively. As Curran correctly points out, St. Thomas Aquinas (1976 ed.) also taught that after the Fall war, slavery, and private property became objectively part of the natural law, although they are contrary to that law in the original intention of God. However, we must be very clear that legitimate compromise consists in accepting a lesser good in order to avoid a greater evil. It cannot be a consent to use an evil means to obtain a good end. We need to remember that the Christian struggle against the evils of this world cannot be effectively carried out by becoming a party to the injustices by which this world achieves its goals (cf. 8.1-2).

Consequently, it is never permissible to choose the lesser evil as such. We must always choose an appropriate means to our goal, and an evil act, by definition, is an inappropriate means. Ordinarily, if there is no good means, we should not choose any.

But what if not to choose also seems to be an evil because we have an obligation to act? This might be the case with a physician who feels he has a responsibility to help the patient whom he cannot neglect, and yet finds something about the needed treatment ethically dubious. The famous case is the physician who must decide whether to let both mother and child die in delivery or to save the mother by directly killing the child. (We discuss this case in 9.2.) Traditionally, moralists advised the physician simply not to act, because it is unquestionably evil to kill the innocent child. But the physician has been so educated that he believes he always has a grave obligation to do what he can for the patient and cannot simply stand by and let nature take its course. Thus he has a perplexed conscience. He must come to moral certitude.

He cannot simply act in doubt, trusting in God to forgive him for his sin. Of course, God will be willing to forgive, but the physician is making his own repentance more difficult by adding imprudence and presumption to his other sin.

To resolve this perplexity, the physician should work it out prudently as follows: "Either course of action involves evil, but my obligation is to do the *better* (not necessarily the stricter) thing. I may later realize that my understanding of the ethics of this matter is mistaken, and I have made the wrong choice. If so, I will have to suffer the consequences, and I will regret the mistake, but I will not reasonably consider myself guilty, because I have moral certitude here and now that as far as I can see this is the better thing to do."

However, this reasoning avails only when persons are in an actual situation without the opportunity to inform their conscience better through study or consultation. When there is time for study and thought, we have the obligation to try to resolve the perplexity so as to find a mode of action which is simply good. It is possible that not only the individual but also the whole Church may at a particular time be unable to resolve some such perplexity, for example, the contraception controversy (Noonan, 1966). Nevertheless, we still have the duty to work toward a resolution.

Ordinarily, traditional moral theology in speaking of the lesser evil was not talking about the informed conscience, but rather about the problem of a counselor who sees that a client is determined to do something evil. In such a case, the counselor (according to most theologians) could tell the client that it would be better to do something less evil, if in so telling the counselor might dissuade the client from the greater evil (e.g., to be sterilized rather than to commit an abortion). This is quite different from the problem of conscientiously perplexed persons of good will who can always achieve moral certitude by doing what seems to them the better of two alternatives, both of which seem somehow wrong.

Closely related to the problem of a prudent conscience is the notion of *informed consent*. When we ask another person to cooperate with us or even to allow us to act upon his person, for example, when a physician asks a patient to take a prescription, to undergo surgery, or to act as the subject of an experiment, we have to respect the other's human dignity according to the Principle of Human Dignity in Community (1.5). However, by this principle the other person, because of her own personal responsibility for her health, may not consent without an informed conscience. Obviously this implies that a health care professional has the duty to supply the patient with the medical information necessary for the patient to make a prudent decision. The health care professional has no right to ask the patient to cooperate or submit to any medical procedure without first obtaining informed consent from the patient or if the patient is not competent to give this consent the informed consent of the patient's guardian. In chapter 9 we discuss in more detail some of the difficulties that may arise in making sure that this ethical condition is properly satisfied.

In view of the foregoing discussion, we can now formulate the *Principle of Prudent Conscience and Informed Consent*:

1. In every free decision involving an ethical question, we are morally obliged as follows:
   a. Prudently to inform ourselves as fully as possible in our practical situation as to both the facts and the ethical norms. The Catholic Christian must give special weight to a Gospel understanding of human values derived from prayer, the Scriptures, and Tradition. In this Tradition, the official guidance of the pope and bishops takes first place.
   b. To inform a morally certain judgment of conscience on the basis of this information.
   c. To act prudently according to this informed conscience.
   d. To accept responsibility for our actions whether conscientious or not.

2. Also, if we request the cooperation of others, or if our action affects their personal integrity, we must ask their permission after making sure that whatever relevant information we have is also communicated to them in a manner they can understand and which permits them to make a free decision. If they are not competent to accept this responsibility for themselves, then we must fulfill the same duty toward their guardian.

3.5   PATIENT'S RIGHTS

Choosing a Physician

Since each of us has the primary obligation of caring for our own health, each also has the obligation to seek and choose professional people to help advise us concerning health care. Yet this does not mean that we can surrender to others the responsibility of making decisions about our health. Professionals are our helpers, not our keepers. Frequently, health care professionals fail to realize how difficult for ordinary persons this selection of a physician may be, or how uncertain such persons are about their own rights in dealing with a health care institution. Health care professionals have an educational responsibility to help clients know how and where to seek health care and how to protect their own rights in doing so.

No one is a good judge in his own case, is a saying that expresses the fact that health, precisely because it is so personal a value, is something about which it is hard to be objective. We tend to delude ourselves both as to how well we are and as to how sick we are. Even if we were all physicians ourselves, we would still need the advice of others, since most physicians do not dare diagnose themselves or their families. Psychotherapists usually undergo therapy as part of their training and return to it from time to time. Moral guides know that if they are to be of help in making sound moral decisions they must engage in public discussion and be open to guidance themselves by responsible authority. Finally, good spiritual guides recognize their own spiritual blindness and their need for the spiritual guidance of others, above all by the Spirit. Thus to be whole and healthy, each of us must be humble enough to seek help from others more expert, or at least more objective about our problems, than we are.

Not only humility, but also courage and hope are required. Richard H. Blum (1964) in arguing that perhaps one out of three persons who need to see a doctor fail to do so lists as causes for this failure not only economic and educational obstacles, but also fear, apathy, shame, and self-punishment as important psychological and moral factors that prevent people from getting the health care they need. The most dangerous aspect of any diseased condition is that it may make the victim despair of health or afraid to seek help to obtain health. At the psychological level, neurotics and alcoholics notoriously deny their problems and resist therapy. Physically sick people also seem to have an almost instinctive dread of recognizing their illness and facing the pain of its cure. Even hypochondriacs who seem only too eager to claim sickness are probably best understood as persons who use the illusion of one disease to hide from themselves some other sickness, perhaps at the psychological, ethical, or spiritual level, which it would be even more painful to face.

Perhaps the reason for such resistance to the truth about ourselves is because we are organisms who tend, once an acute crisis has passed, to adapt to a chronic disease by integrating it into our way of life. Once such a distorted integration has become fixed, we sense real peril in returning to the acutely painful crisis that might be provoked by a new effort to become really well. Hence we dread physicians and avoid them as long as possible. Thus both psychological and physiological diseases are allowed to hit bottom before we can submit ourselves to treatment. The same principle holds at the ethical and spiritual levels, so that most profound moral and spiritual convictions are brought about only after a deep conviction of sin. Jesus noted that it was the publicans and whores who were most likely to enter the Kingdom of God (Matt. 21:31).

Even when we have the humility and courage to seek a physician, we are faced with two very serious ethical problems in choosing a good one. The first arises from the fact that our choice may be very much restricted by the complex organization of modern medical care and the maldistribution of its services. Should we submit to this restriction of our freedom or do we have a moral obligation to resist it? This socio-political issue is discussed in some detail in chapter 6.

The second ethical issue in choosing a physician or a health care facility arises from the fact that today there is widespread doubt about the competence and the character of health care professionals. Some like Ivan Illich (1976a, 1976b) have launched an attack on the whole system of health care in the United States. Others (R. Blum, 1964; Annas, 1975), without going as far as Illich, have criticized vigorously the way that American health care professionals live up to their pro-fessed standards. Of course, these criticisms have been heatedly refuted by others, for example, Harry Schwartz in the *Case for American Medicine* (1972). Yet with due allowance for polemics, we cannot deny that in the United States as in most countries the average citizen does not find it easy to obtain satisfactory health care.

Although Americans are convinced, and with reason, that the billions of dollars we spend each year on health care goes to support the most advanced medical technology and professional education in the world, we also realize that this by no means proves that the average citizen is receiving health care of high quality. The life expectancy of our citizens is lower than in a number of European countries and has not improved notably in the last twenty years. In some of our states the death rate is twenty-five percent higher than in other states.

Available studies (cf. R. Blum, 1964a; Freese, 1975; Levin, 1975) of the actual competency of physicians in practice commonly turn up alarming percentages (from 30 to 50 percent) of physicians whose com-petence is substandard, while a similar percentage of hospitals do not meet minimal accreditation standards. Again estimates show that a high percentage of surgery (50 percent in some hospitals) is unnecessary and explainable only by incompetence or greed. Finally, the same studies show that among professionals, physicians rate highest in drug addiction, alcoholism, and psychological disorders. When we add to this the grow-ing evidence that a considerable percentage of physicians have an income well in excess of members of other professions, we must regretfully admit that in choosing a reliable and competent physician and a high-quality hospital we are at risk.

Protection of Rights

The ethical issue raised by such risks are dramatized by the very titles of recent books like Freese, *Managing Your Doctor* (1975); Levin, *Talk Back to Your Doctor* (1975); Annas, *The Rights of Hospital Patients* (1975); and Sagov and Brodsky, *The Active Patient's Guide to Better*

Medical Care (1976). These books advocate a very critical, even suspicious and aggressive, attitude on the part of the patient toward the health care professional and the health care facility. This seems in strong contrast to the attitude of *trust* which has been traditionally regarded as the basis of every profession (a tradition we will defend in chapter 4). Yet these authors, with evidence to support their position, argue that persons who fail to take this distrustful stance toward the medical profession today are failing in their responsibility to their own health.

Certainly it is true that in every age many, perhaps most, people have been quite irresponsible in selecting medical guides, as well as political and religious leaders. The very fears that prevent people from seeking help also cause them often to prefer the quack (medical, psychological, ethical, or spiritual) to the competent guide who they suspect may make them face a painful reality. The quack knows how to exploit these fears, this flight from real diagnosis and cure, in order to gain control over the patient. Not all quacks are incompetents since very able guides can easily be tempted to use their own gifts to gain power for themselves, as the history of illicit medical experimentation evidences.

To escape enslavement to the incompetent or exploitative professional, we need to be conscious of the rights which are correlative to our responsibility to choose professional help prudently. George J. Annas (1973) has summed them up as follows:

1. The right to the whole truth
2. The right to privacy and personal dignity
3. The right to refuse any test, procedure, or treatment
4. The right to read and copy medical records

He further concretizes these rights in the form of *A Model Patient's Bill of Rights* (Annas, 1975) to which we refer the reader for details.

Annas correctly argues that the rights he proposes all rest on the fundamental concept of informed consent, which we have previously discussed in 3.4. If the patient is to give free consent, then the patient must also be able to refuse any test, procedure, or treatment. As Annas interprets the right to privacy and personal dignity, it also amounts to the right of patients to refuse to be involved in any professional procedures which make them objects to be examined or discussed for the benefit or convenience of professionals or students rather than for the patients' own therapy.

If this consent is to be not only free, but also informed, then the patient has the right to the whole truth including access to read and copy medical records. Many professionals deny these rights on the grounds that the patient is not able to understand the technical information known to the physician and may be harmed by it. Annas rightly says that such difficulties do not disprove patients' rights to know so that their consent may be fully informed, but only establishes the professional's duty to communicate this information in ways that are hepful, not harmful, to patients.

Among the things patients have the right to know is the competency and ethical integrity of the physician or health care facility to which they may entrust themselves. The authors already cited give a great deal of good advice on this subject. Generally, they agree that the first consideration is medical competency. In the present state of affairs, they believe such competency is most likely to be found among physicians holding assignments to a medical-school affiliated hospital, since they are most likely to be well educated and up-to-date in knowledge and skill. Similarly, these authors generally recommend us to choose a larger, accredited, medical-school affiliated hospital, whether it be a public or a nonprofit private institution, and to avoid small proprietary hospitals.

We are also recommended to begin with a primary service physician who is concerned for our total health and who should be a family practice specialist rather than a general practioner. If a family practioner is not available (and they are still scarce), then an internist for adults, a pediatrician for children, and perhaps a specialist in adolescent medicine and one for geriatrics need to be chosen for the various members of the family. Through these primary service physicians the need for further specialized care can be ascertained and suitable specialists sought. However, all these authors emphasize that no matter how excellent we may find our physican we should never hesitate to ask for consultation when doubts arise, especially when surgery is in question.

Thus the underlying ethical issue of trust again emerges. Is competency the primary consideration in choosing a physician as these authors insist? Certainly it is the *specific* qualification most people seek in any professional, including their physicians. However, if physicians are not also trustworthy in the sense that they are sincerely dedicated to helping the patient get well, then their medical competency is dangerous, as in the case of brilliantly competent surgeons eager for more bodies on which to demonstrate their skill.

Thus the notion of competency as used by these authors is somewhat ambiguous. They evidently presuppose their competent physician is a trustworthy user of his competency, not one who abuses it. Hence they insist on the great importance of a careful choice of the physician of primary service, since it is this physician who is most concerned for the patient as a whole person. Also they prefer physicians who work in institutions where not only their skill but also their professional dedication to patient welfare is most likely to be tested and evaluated by peers.

We should not, therefore, lightly accept the idea that our personal responsibility for our own health is satisfied merely by assuming a critical attitude toward our physicians and demanding our rights from them. Such a responsibility also includes willingness on our part to trust our physicians once we have chosen them prudently, to make good use of their advice, and to cooperate with their healing efforts on our behalf.

While we should never be afraid to protect our rights and to insist that physicians give us all the information we need to give informed consent to treatment, we should also give them a deserved respect, as long as they deserve it.   Trustworthy and competent health care professionals do us a very precious service, for which they deserve profound gratitude, good reputation, and fair and prompt payment.

While retaining our primary right and responsibility to give informed consent or refusal to any kind of professional health service, we should also remember the commendatory words of Scripture:

> Hold the physician in honor, for he is essential to you and God it was who established his profession,
> From God the doctor has his wisdom, and the king provides for his sustenance.
> His knowledge makes the doctor distinguished, and gives him access to those in authority.
> God makes the earth yield healing herbs, which the prudent man should not neglect;
> Was not the water sweetened by a twig (when Moses sweetened the bitter waters in the desert), that man might learn his power?
> He endows men with the knowledge to glory in his mighty works,
> Through which the doctor eases pain and the druggist prepares his medicines;
> Thus God's creative work continues without ceasing in its efficacy on the surface of the earth. (Sirach 38:1-8)

PART II

THE HEALING PROFESSION

CHAPTER 4

THE HEALTH CARE PROFESSION

4.1 WHAT IS A PROFESSION?

Overview

While individuals have primary responsibility to care for their own health as well as for the psychological, ethical, and spiritual aspects of their personal development, such development can be achieved only with the help of other members of the community. In advanced communities, such help is furnished by persons who have chosen and been educated for the special social roles we call the professions. In Part II we will consider the chief ethical issues involved in the choice of the health care profession as a vocation and in the educational preparation needed to fulfill the demands of so difficult a vocation.

Because the health care profession is only one among several professions basic to the culture of any advanced community, it is necessary first to consider the nature of the professions in general, then to define the specific role of the medical profession, and finally to identify its interrelations with other professions. Since our chief thesis in this chapter is that medical education must include the development of basic ethical attitudes, and since we also will argue that these attitudes have their root in the relation of trust between professional and client, in chapter 5 we will deal with the specific character of this relation in the health care situation. Finally, since today the profession of medicine, like that of teaching, is exercised largely in institutional settings, in chapter 6 we will consider the ethical issues raised by the social organization of health care.

In this chapter we will first deal with the concept of a profession in general and then with the health care profession in its specific task. However, traditionally this profession has been rather narrowly identified as "the medical profession" and with the role of the physician as a medical doctor (M.D.). Our overall emphasis is on the health team, but in this chapter we will deal with the older and narrower concept, considering the historical ideals of the medical profession in 4.2 and the education of physicians as it transmits these ideals today in 4.3. Our concern here is not with the scientific knowledge and technical skills so essential to this profession, but rather with its ethical ideals and standards.

We repeat here what we said in the Introduction: Our purpose is not to pass moral judgment on the shortcomings of the health care profession in meeting its own standards, but is rather to identify some of the ethical issues that are most acute for the progress of this profession today, and to suggest some directions in which Catholic health care professionals can give witness and leadership in the resolution of these issues by the profession and by the public.

Depersonalizing the Professions

W. J. Reader (1966) provides insight into the development of professions as we understand them today:

> The professions as we know them are very much a Victorian creation, brought into being to serve the need of an industrial society. But, like so much else in Victorian society, they took on some of the outward forms of older and very different institutions. (p. 2)

The older medieval professions were divinity (theology), physic (medicine), and law. They were "person professions" (Goode, 1969) centered on a counselor-client relation. They did not produce goods for sale or works of art for enjoyment, but worked to heal, guide, or protect some person in a life crisis. Industrial society has greatly fostered the professions (Taylor, 1968), but it has also depersonalized them. No longer are they centered on conviviality of persons (Illich, 1972b), but on the productivity of an impersonal system. They no longer deal with better interpersonal communication, but with more efficient exchange of energy.

This slow depersonalizing transformation of the professions is reaching its completion today just as industrial society itself seems about to yield to a new postindustrial society (Touraine, 1971; Bell, 1973). Neither progressive Capitalism nor revolutionary Marxism has been able to fulfill the promises of scientific technology to produce a society of abundance and freedom. Even this promise begins to seem illusory in view of the ecological doomsday predicted by some authorities (Meadows, 1972).

In postindustrial society, the source of power will no longer be economic ownership (whether capitalist or socialist), but rather *knowledge and its communication*. Such power means a still greater role for the professions (Bottomore, 1972; Brzezinski, 1967). This knowledge can be used to bring about greater social conformism and dependency on the professionals, or it can be used to open the system to wider and more genuine social participation by all. In either case, the professions must be radically reconstructed.

Will professionals become technocrats whose technological mastery must extend itself to behavior control? Or will they become the persons who helps others to transcend the depersonalization of technological systems in order to free them from what Touraine (1971) calls "dependent participation"? If we choose the latter alternative, then the professions must again be personalized. They must be reconstructed so as to eliminate the threefold depersonalization that they have suffered in the epoch of industrial society.

First, *clients* have been depersonalized by the proliferation of specialisms. They are no longer thought of as organisms, but as collections of organs (Freymann, 1974). There is healing for the parts but not for the person such that the very meaning of *healing*, that is, "to make *whole*," has been lost. Around each profession has grown a host of "para" or "semi" professions (Moore and Rosenblum, 1970; Purtilo, 1973). Yet the result is not so much integration as competition and confusion. Even the efforts at interdisciplinary healing teams never quite seem to succeed in getting it all together again.

Second, *professionals themselves* have been depersonalized by a loss of clear identity. This loss is notoriously true for the ministry (Gustafson, 1965) and is now evident in medicine, law, and teaching (Freund, 1965; Wittlin, 1965; Freidson, 1971). A recent study showed that psychiatrists, psychoanalysts, and psychiatric social workers all do much the same thing, yet are considered members of three different professions (Henry, 1971). What is even more confusing is that many ministers, lawyers, and physicians counsel clients in ways not easily distinguishable from those used by psychotherapists (Freeman, 1967).

Contributing to this confusion of identity today is the tension within the profession between the goals of research and the goals of practice. There is even the threat that many areas of professional practice may soon be handed over to computers (Comfort, 1972; Freymann, 1974). How then can a professional make that kind of personal commitment always regarded as a mark of a profession if it is not clear to what he is professed?

Third, the validity of the professional-client relation is being questioned. Professionalism seems to imply an elitism that is ultimately socially destructive. Thus Ivan Illich (1971), studying the problems of underdeveloped countries, has launched an all-out attack on schooling and the concept of the teaching profession and is extending the same criticism to medicine (1976a). He contends that the industrial model for organizing the professions has progressively restricted access to knowledge and skill, placing them in the hands of elites on whom the public is more and more dependent, but from whom the public receives less and less adequate service. The result is that our service institutions have become "production funnels" which proliferate subordinate professions and paraprofessions. Illich wants to free people from such production funnels by giving nonspecialists easier access to the information now the prerogative of professional elites. He argues that both Capitalist and Marxist politics are based on the same invalid professional ideal, and that the Third World is desperately striving to make the same mistake.

These three depersonalizations are most easily illustrated in the case of the medical profession, but they also occur in the most unlikely profession — the religious ministry which has always claimed to be concerned for the whole person. In recent years many priests, ministers, and rabbis have deserted their calling in discouragement and confusion. How painful to realize that, while claiming to serve, the clergy have accepted elitists status and are neither sure of their own role nor competent to give interdisciplinary guidance to other professionals in the service of persons (Underwood, 1972).

Personalistic Concept of a Profession

Today the term *profession* is used for almost any prestigious occupation (Goode, 1969; Wilensky, 1964) because it has the aura of an ideal. It is a symbol rather than a reality. The distinguished sociologist Howard S. Becker (1960) writes:

> The symbol systematically ignores such facts as the failure of the professions to monopolize their area of knowledge, the lack of homogeneity within professions, the frequent failure of clients to accept professional judgment, the chronic presence of unethical practitioners as an integrated segment of the professional structure, and the organizational constraints on professional autonomy. A symbol which ignores so many features of occupational life cannot provide an adequate guide for professional activity. (p. 46)

Nevertheless, the sociologists have devoted much time to developing a good empirical definition of a profession. Robert K. Merton (1960) very succinctly says that the social values that make up the concept of a profession are as follows:

> First, the value placed upon systematic knowledge and intellect: *knowing*. Second, the value placed upon technical skill and trained capacity: *doing*. And third, the value placed upon putting this conjoint knowledge and skill to work in the service of others: *helping*. (p. 9)

Bernard Barber (1965) proposes the following "relativistic" definition:

> Professional behavior may be defined in terms of four essential attributes: (1) a high degree of generalized and systematic knowledge; (2) primary orientation to the community interest rather than to individual self-interest; (3) a high degree of self-control of behavior through codes of ethics internalized in the process of work socialization and through voluntary associations organized and operated by the work specialists themselves; and (4) a system of rewards (monetary and honorary) that is primarily a set of symbols of work achievement and thus ends in themselves, not means to some end of individual self-interest. (p. 18)

Similarly Kenneth Underwood (1972) says:

> These four concerns — concern for persons, trained skills, values and basic theory, and public responsibility — are the central themes of professional ideology always mentioned in the sociological literature on the professions and the professions' statements of purpose. (p. 422)

A recent work (Moore and Rosenblum, 1970; see also Greenwood, 1966) offers a definition which admits of degrees of application in terms of a scale of professionalism. A professional must rate high on the following six operational attributes:

1. A professional practices a *full-time occupation*.
2. He is committed to a *calling*, that is, he treats his occupation "as an enduring set of normative and behavioral expectations."
3. He is distinguished from the laity by various signs and symbols and identified with his peers — often in formalized *organizations*.
4. He has esoteric but useful knowledge and skills through specialized *education* which is lengthy and difficult.
5. He is expected to have a *service orientation* so as to perceive the needs of his clients relevant to his competency.
6. He has *autonomy* of judgment and authority restrained by responsibility in using his knowledge and skill.

The problem with these definitions (which fundamentally come down to Merton's "knowing-doing-helping") is that they fail to clearly distinguish the original group of person professions from other highly developed occupations which do not deal *directly* with persons to which the term has been extended. Today, engineering, architecture and the other arts, and business are considered professions since they also involve knowing, doing, and helping (Lynn, 1965). Yet their immediate objective is not personal but productive. This obliteration of the distinction between the person professions and productive occupations is characteristic of industrial society and its depersonalization of the professions. If they are to be repersonalized, this distinction must be drawn once more.

This need for distinction has been seen by Harrop A. Freeman (1967) in his insistence on the importance of the counselor-client relation in the professions and by the sociologist William J. Goode (1969) who, in our opinion, gets to the heart of the matter when he writes:

> Specifically, I suggest that a category of occupations is set apart (as a profession) by a primary variable, upon which a considerable number of structural consequences hinge: whether the professional must symbolically or literally "get inside the client," become privy to his personal world, in order to solve the problem that is the mandate of the profession. (p. 307)

If we accept this view, then research scientists and scholars are not professionals because they are directly concerned with knowing, not with doing, with theory, not with practice. The work of laboratory experimentation may seem like a doing, but its purpose is to test a theory, not to apply it practically.

To call the technologies and the arts (engineering, business, fine arts) professions is confusing and dangerous because this designation disguises the fact that they are productive of things, not directly helpful to persons. Certainly we should promote the humanization of the technologies by educating their practitioners to be more sensitive to the human uses to which their product will be put, but this humanization of technology will be hindered if we continue to follow the old tendency of industrial society to lump the technologies and the person professions together under one name and to judge them all in terms of productivity.

A true profession, therefore, is rooted in theory but aimed at practice, and a practice that is not productive of things external to persons, but directly a service to persons themselves. Furthermore, this service is not applied to persons who receive it passively but is a facilitation of those persons' own activity. It aims at healing them, at making them whole, at freeing them to act on their own. Counselors should not act on clients, nor dominate them, but enable them to become fully, autonomously themselves. Thus a profession cannot properly be elitist. It communicates power rather than enforces dependency.

Finally, we cannot speak significantly of professional help in the full sense unless it is concerned precisely with those problems that are deeply personal, that are matters of life and death. Therefore such help engages both counselor and client in a profound responsibility both to each other and to the larger community. In terms of this conception of a profession, we need to think about the reconstruction of the professions and of professional education for the future.

Health Care Counseling

In this book, we are concerned with the way this personalistic concept of a profession applies to the health care professions since, although health care counseling has much in common with other types of professional counseling, it is also quite distinct from them.

Orginally, the term *counseling* pertained to the dimension of rational, moral, and ethical functioning (Freeman, 1967) and in particular to the legal profession, as the British use of the term *counselor* shows. Obviously, it also found a place in the religious ministry, since the rabbi was in fact a kind of religious lawyer, and this role was passed on to Christian priests. Yet, as we argued in chapter 1 and will develop more fully in chapters 14 and 15, the specific type of counseling proper to the ministerial profession is something deeper than the ethical level and pertains to the spiritual dimension of the human person. It can also be argued that the teaching profession in its work of arousing the creativity of the student also reaches to this same level of intuitive life.

The medical professional often performs one or the other of these types of counseling proper to the other professions. A physician may have to discuss with a patient certain ethical and legal issues, for example, those involved in an abortion decision. Sometimes a physician is involved in a patient's spiritual struggles about death and the meaning of life. Often physicians must play the role of teacher, helping patients to a better understanding of their body or psyche. Yet all these involvements are incidental and substitutional. A prudent physician is quick to refer the patient to experts in other professions when it becomes clear that the issues are ethical or spiritual, rather than medical.

The proper task of the medical professional is to deal with problems at the biological and psychological levels of human functioning. Obviously, at the psychological level counseling of a certain type plays a major therapeutic role, although some deny this (cf. chapters 5 and 12). At the biological level, however, it is not so obvious that the physician's role in still primarily that of a counselor. Yet if we acccpt the thesis argued in chapter 3 that all persons have primary responsibility for their own health, then it becomes clear that the physician's primary responsibility is to help patients make good health decisions, which requires a counseling process. We cannot make good decisions about how to care for our health unless we have the required information. In more complicated cases, this information can be obtained only by consulting a physician. To some extent the physician in giving this information is playing the role of a teacher, but more is involved than that, since the information required is not abstract biological truth but a concrete assessment of personal health and the possible ways of dealing with the problems it presents. This kind of guidance is what we require from a physician whom we can trust, and it engages the physician in a special type of counseling.

J. G. Freymann (1974), a doctor, calls this basic counseling relation on which the whole medical profession is built "trusteeship". He argues that technological progress in medicine has temporarily obscured the importance of trusteeship, making it appear that the physician is a scientist-technician rather than a counselor, but that this same technological progress will eventually expose what it covers up. Soon not only the process of treatment, but also diagnosis itself will become the work of technicians, while physicians will be freed once more to deal personally with patients. Moreover, physicians will be dealing not with patients so sick that they cannot think, but with responsible persons concerned to stay well. In such situations, the physician will play the role of health counselor:

> The degree of which a modern patient seeks these two attributes — knower-doer and trustee — in his doctor varies. The victim of an acute catastrophe may need and want only the knower-doer. But the less

clear-cut the clinical picture, the more the patient looks for both. He wants a knower-doer who can solve those problems for which there is an answer. But he wants a trustee who can comprehend *all* his problems and help him to face them, no matter what the outcome. The former calls for a scientist, but much of what the pure scientist can do now will be taken over by the technician-computer teams. The latter calls for a physician or a nurse, for no matter how man-like computers may become, I do not think trusteeship will ever be automated. (p. 313)

The nursing profession is truly a profession because it shares in this counseling task of the physician. Today (cf. 6.4), the role of the nurse has become very ambiguous, but Freymann (1974) is certainly right in saying that the medical profession has always had the double dimension of cure and care, and hence always requires a distinction between the curing task of the physician and the caring task of the nurse. What is common to both cure and care is that the patient must consent to both and cooperate actively with both, so that both physician and nurse must enter into the trustee relation with the patient.

Nor will this basic relationship be eliminated as patients in the future come more and more to relate to a health team rather than one-to-one with a personal physician (R. Wilson, 1963). We have shown in chapter 1 that personal relationships always have a social character. Group psychotherapy has proved that personalism need not be eliminated just because the one-to-one relationship with a therapist is expanded into a more complex social relationship.

However, we must face the fact that the account of the professions as rooted in the counselor-client relationship is very far from the reality of the professions in our society today. We have already cited (2.1) the contention of Eliot Freidson (1970, 1971) that the professions are no longer characterized by service to the client, nor by fidelity to a body of expert knowledge, but instead by a drive for autonomy. Hence the medical profession is often unresponsive to the health needs of the public, because the public has no way to make its needs effective in the face of this professional autonomy.

Freidson is not alone in this opinion. Thus Jeffrey L. Berlant (1975) denies that the medical profession in the United States and Great Britain arose to meet a social need, but rather that it developed as a "commercial class" dedicated to achieving monopoly control. He argues that historically the medical profession has gone through all the steps characteristic of any commercial class such as (1) creation of a commodity, (2) separation of the performance of its service from any necessary satisfaction of the client's interests, (3) creation of scarcity, (4) monopolization of supply, (5) restriction of membership, (6) elimination of external competition, (7) price fixation, (8) unification of suppliers, (9) elimination of internal competition, and (10) development of group solidarity and cooperation. Of course, similar disparaging accounts can be given of the other professions including that of teaching and of religious ministry which are supposed to deal with spiritual values. We will consider these socio-logical criticisms of the professions in more detail in the following section.

4.2   TRADITIONAL IDEALS OF THE MEDICAL PROFESSION

Priest or Scientist?

To make sure that the personalistic concept of the medical profession which we are defending is not a mere ideal, we need to look briefly at the crosscurrents of purpose which have been at work in the historical development of the profession.

The standard histories of medicine (Sigerist, 1951; Ackernecht, 1955; Garrison, 1960) commonly divide this history into the prescientific period and the scientific period which begins only in the seventeenth century with Vesalius and Harvey, Michael Foucault in his fascinating book *The Birth of the Clinic* (1973) shows that the crucial step was taken as a result of the efforts of the radical wing of the French Revolution to abolish all professions including the medical profession as a means to establishing a classless society. The resulting chaos in health care then led to the reestablishment of the medical profession and its hospitals on a new basis under the domination of the scientific ideals of the Enlight-ment.

Freymann (1974) has also shown that from 1700 to 1850 health care was fragmented and the profession at a low ebb until the Age of Pasteur with its emphasis on the scientific education of doctors to fight acute diseases. Only now, Freymann believes, is the profession entering the Age of Darwin and Freud with the emphasis on an ecological, positive health approach. Thus, medicine as an effective scientific technology is a very recent development in human history.

On closer examination, however, it becomes evident that this division into prescientific and scientific periods is somewhat misleading because it is only a manifestation of two aspects of the medical tradition which have always coexisted and still do. Even today, along with orthodox scientific medicine, there is a vast field of heretical medicine, ranging from naturopathy, faith healing, homeopathy and chiropractic to osteopathy and acupuncture, not to mention countless forms of pure quackery. These therapies evidently supply a complement to orthodox medicine because they seem to meet health needs which it does not. Nor is it any secret that even within orthodox medicine the field of psychotherapy is a borderline area which many medical doctors consider unscientific.

This duality, as we examine it more closely, turns out to reflect the mind-body or psychosomatic duality of the human being who is sick. In early times, the learned professions all took their origin from the one rather confused profession of priest (or perhaps priest-king). Priests were looked on as custodians of sacred wisdom and power over the forces of nature, a gift from the gods who alone possessed cosmic secrets.

In Greece (whence modern Western medicine is directly descended) the first father of medicine was Asclepius (Kerenyi, 1959), who was the "mild god" so kindly that he was to prove the greatest rival of Christ as Christianity spread throughout the pagan world (Edelstein, 1945). Asclepius's priests presided over shrines (the first clinics) where the sick came to worship, to sleep, and to have their dreams interpreted. The symbol of the medical profession today is still a staff with entwined serpents because the serpent, symbol of wisdom and the healing power of mother earth (i.e., nature), was the cult animal at these shrines. Today in the city of Rome, the Hospital of the Benefratelli of medieval origin is built on an island in the River Tiber over remains of a shrine of Asclepius transferred from Greece in classical times. A great snake is still to be seen carved on the ancient ruins.

This myth manifests a basic truth about the medical profession: the physician to this day retains something of a priestly ministry in the service of the healing forces of nature. We have shown that something similar is true of every profession, because all professions deal with the sacred dignity of the human person and rest on the sacred covenant of trust between client and professional. This priestly ministry is especially true of the medical profession because its direct relation to life and death gives it a fundamental, primitive character. Our trust in the physician is almost like our trust in our mother, a primordial confidence in our life support.

No wonder then that even today the physician (witness the myths of television doctor shows) is a charismatic figure, surrounded by a priestly atmosphere. While this trust can be abused and exploited, it is valuable when it is authentic. There is no healing without trust. Thus the most significant distinction in understanding the history of medicine is not between scientific and nonscientific medicine, but between authentic medicine and quackery. Authentic medicine has both priestly and scientific dimension.

Why did it take until the seventeenth and even the nineteenth century for the rapid development of this scientific side of medicine to begin? The empirical rational method was already well understood in the time of Hippocrates about 400 B.C. Hippocrates rejected the designation of epilepsy and other ailments as sacred diseases and attempted to explain them biologically. In the next century Aristotle, himself a son of an Asclepian doctor, the physician of Alexander the Great, in *De Somniis* demythologized the notion of dreams, often used to diagnose diseases, by giving such psychic phenomena a physiological explanation. This tradition of scientific medicine was further developed by Hellenistic doctors like Galen and by medieval Arabian, Jewish, and Christian physicians. Yet before Harvey the practical fruits of this scientific approach were sparse. Why?

One explanation is that the scientific aspect of medicine was held back by its priestly aspect. (A. White, 1960 [1896]). However, it is not inevitable that these two aspects should hinder rather than complement each other. Others have pointed out that scientific medicine could not get far until the development of chemistry and biology. But why were these sciences also so slow to develop? Perhaps the better explanation is that given by some Marxist sociologists and other authorities. Greek thinkers clearly recognized the method and value of empirical science, but they were discouraged from engaging in experimentation in science and clinical practice in medicine by a social system based on the sharp division between the liberally educated freemen who despised manual work and the slaves or serfs. This barrier between theory and practice, between the spiritual realm and the realm of matter, was the major obstacle to the development of science and scientific medicine.

Evaluation of the physician to the status of a learned professional more and more separated from the suffering patient was intensified by the university education of the Middle Ages. Nevertheless, the Christian concern for the poor began to break through this Greek contempt. Glaser (1970b) has shown that Christianity, particularly in its Roman Catholic form, has been the religion most concerned to provide organized health care because of its belief in personal charity and of the integral relation of the body to the human person. However, in spite of practical efforts to realize this Christian ideal, the state of scientific knowledge and the level of social organization were so low that until the end of the Middle Ages the chief efforts were directed more to caring for the sick and dying than to healing them.

Only with the Renaissance and the development of Christian humanism in Catholic Europe and Calvinist emphasis on work as a vocation in Protestant Europe was the concern for the practical and material clearly seen to have religious and ethical values. Thus was the groundwork for the rapid rise of empirical science and modern medical technology finally laid. Undoubtedly the secular Humanism of the Enlightenment built well on this basis, but it did not lay its foundation stones. The role of the French Revolution was essentially negative. It broke down the old, fixed patterns of the medical profession so that the new model might develop fully (Foucault, 1977).

Does the old tension between the liberal and the service aspects of medicine exist today? At first sight such a suspicion seems absurd. Certainly the modern physician is above all interested in practice, and no class of doctors has greater prestige than surgeons (King, 1972) who certainly get their hands dirty! However, if we look more closely, we see that the emphasis on the specialist as against the general practitioner, and the building up of a pyramid of paramedical professionals in the service of the physician meditating between him and the patient in his misery, is the modern version of this class distinction.

The Christian Physician

On the other hand the rise of psychiatry and psychosomatic medicine in the twentieth century has meant a strengthening and development of the other, priestly aspects of medicine in which the physician as counselor becomes less the scientific technologist and more the artist in direct contact with the patient. The current debates about the humanization of medicine reflect the resurgence of this other aspect of the medical tradition which has never died and which, we can be confident, will always be part of medicine. Many of the real needs of patients which nineteenth-century medicine tended to abandon to the medical heretics are now being recovered as legitimate concerns of the orthodox medical profession. These debates, however, are still going on, and the problem of the personalization of health care is far from solved.

Therefore, the charismatic character of the doctor, which arises from the priestly side of medicine, but is also enhanced by the miraculous power of scientific technology, should be respected. In all professions the charismatic atmosphere is an important element of the professional relation, and is essential to the healing process. This atmosphere makes it possible for the patient, often distrustful, to place the necessary trust in professional help. It also gives medical professionals a sense of personal dignity, dedication, and responsibility that immeasurably contributes to their satisfaction and persistence in a difficult vocation.

It is also a guard of other ethical values, since nothing is likely to keep medical professionals from abusing their position for financial or other gains as this sense of self-respect. It would be disastrous if the increasing mechanization of medicine or the reduction of the medical professional to an anonymous functionary in a government bureaucracy would destroy the priestly charisma of the profession.

On the negative side, however, as with the clergyman, overemphasis on the special status of the doctor is open to great abuses. The doctor can become an unquestioned, dogmatic authority in medicine and in all other matters as well. The medical profession often jealously defends its authority and its prerogatives, refuses to discipline members of the profession, and claims the right to settle ethical and social questions that affect the profession on the grounds that laymen have no right to opinion in such matters (Freidson, 1971).

Therefore, the doctor who wants to develop a sound ethical judgment must (1) have a profound respect for the medical profession as a vocation that has both scientific and priestly aspects and (2) have a clear understanding of the limits of this profession and of its interrelation to and dependence upon other professions which also deal with the human person.

Christian health care professionals are called by their faith to understand this vocation in a special way, as professionals of other religions or philosophies of life are called by theirs. Christians think of life as a gift of God and the body as a marvelous work of divine creation to be reverenced as a temple of God. They also think of the human person as not only a living body, but also as a body living with spiritual life open to a share in the eternal life of God. Consequently, the Christian health care professional thinks of sickness as an evil desecrater of the temple. Even when sickness cannot be overcome, the struggle against it can be lived through as an experience that can further moral and spiritual growth. Thus the Christian physician or nurse is truly a minister of God, cooperating with Him in helping suffering human beings overcome their suffering in order to live more fully.

The Christian medical professional finds a model in Jesus Christ, the Healer (McNutt, 1977). While physicians do not have supernatural or miraculous powers, they do have medical skill which is also a gift of God and can imitate Jesus' compassion for the patient and his reaching out to the most neglected, even the lepers. This Christian attitude cannot be a matter of mere pious words; rather it is a profound dependence on God who gives the physician and nurse the inspiration, insight, and courage to carry out their work as professionally and as skillfully as possible.

Moreover, one should not make the mistake of thinking that the ethical aspect of medicine pertains only to its personal, priestly side. It also penetrates its scientific aspect. A scientific approach to disease is built on the devotion to objective truth and the courageous, persevering effort to advance this truth through research and criticism. The history of medicine is unfortunately replete with examples not only of outright quackery, but also of superstition and self-delusion. Eminent physicians have sometimes become so enamored of their own theories and personal reputations that they have continued to defend their theories and even to counterfeit evidence concerning them long after their fallaciousness was evident. Others have stubbornly refused to face new facts and new theories. Yet, on the whole, the scientific approach with its insistence on objective evidence and critical review by peers has a splendid record. This scientific integrity has been very effective in limiting the excessive charismatic pretensions of some physicians.

Dedication to objective truth and scientific integrity is an ethical value of the highest order. Nothing is gained if the effort to humanize or personalize medicine interjects an unhealthy sentimentalism or occultism into the practice of medicine. Sound ethical judgment can only be based on critical, scientific knowledge.

On the negative side, however, the scientific method as now understood and practiced often tends to reductionism, that is, the assertion that the scientific method is the exclusive road to truth. Since the scientific method deals only with the limited aspect of reality that can be measured and experimented upon, such a reductionist attitude can compel physicians to ignore and deny facts and experiences outside these rather narrow limits. When reductionism is rigidly applied, the patient is treated as a soulless machine. In the history of medicine, this mechanistic approach has been profitable to the degree that it has used the scientific method intensively, but it has ultimately limited the advance of medicine. Again and again, biologists and physicians sensitive to the holistic character of living organisms and the human person have revolted against reductionism and opened new, broader, and more fruitful lines of research.

Thus sound ethical judgment must completely respect scientifically established medical facts, but it cannot rest on these facts alone. It must be open to all humanistic approaches to understanding and evaluating the human condition.

4.3   MEDICAL EDUCATION AND ITS BIASES

Progress in Medical Education

In view of the complex history of the medical tradition, it is obvious that medical education needs to do justice to these various aspects of the profession if it is to prepare medical professionals to make good ethical judgments. Most medical professionals tend to think all their lives in the categories learned in medical or nursing school. This outlook has become so much a part of them through the intensive experiences of their training that they never reexamine it or question it. For them it has become self-evident. This is a dangerous attitude because it stifles creativity and growth.

In the medical profession, as in other professions, it is widely recognized that educational institutions often have glaring biases and defects. The medical profession in the United States took the lead in self-criticism in this regard. The famous report by Abraham Flexner, published in 1910, led the way for reform in medical education. Flexner emphasized (1) the need for professional self-criticism; (2) the unity of scientific research and medical practice; (3) the advantages of the university-associated medical school; (4) the great importance of a sound, liberal education, rich in the basic sciences as a preparation for medical school; (5) a systematic or logical, but not overburdened, ordering of the curriculum, with some limited elective freedom for the student; (6) an emphasis on laboratory and clinical work; (7) the great importance of constant research in special institutes; and (8) the adequate financing and use of a full-time medical staff. On the whole, these recommendations still remain sound. However, many authorities today would reject Flexner's emphasis on logical ordering of the curriculum, with theoretical study of the normal body preceeding clinical contact with the sick body. They would argue that from the beginning of the program theory should be balanced by clinical experience.

Freymann (1974) has showed the great practical influence of Flexner's report, coupled with establishment of Johns Hopkins University and Medical School in 1873 under the leadership of John Shaw Billings and Daniel Coit Gilman. This medical school became the model for all American medical education and fixed on it the ideal of scientific research according to the German pattern and the concept of scientist-physicans working in teaching hospitals devoted primarily to the diagnosis and cure of acute diseases.

While Flexner placed strong emphasis on a sound general education as the basis of scientific medical education, he did not provide equally for the personalistic aspect of the profession. Thus his curriculum has little room (1) for discussion of the nature and limits of the profession itself, (2) for study of the counseling skills needed by a physician, (3) for study of medical ethics, and (4) for sociology and ecology. Clearly, Flexner assumed that such matters are best learned by imitation and experience and need not be formally taught. But what model is the student to imitate? Experience has shown that it is the specialist oriented to scientific diagnosis who is the attractive model admired and imitated, rather than the physician concerned for the whole patient and master of the *art* of health care (Becker et al., 1961; Becker and Greer, 1963; Balint, 1964; Evans, 1964; Lippard, 1975).

For fifty years this pattern has persisted and intensified. Few medical schools have yet provided for the essential personalistic elements of a physician's education, although their incorporation into the curriculum is frequently discussed, with little effective action (Merton et al., 1957; Bloom, 1963; Knight, 1973; Veatch, 1973b; Hiatt, 1976; Ingersoll, 1976; Pacoe et al., 1976).

The training of nurses has been forced into the same pattern, with the result that today the nursing profession is undergoing a severe identity crisis (Fagin et al., 1976; Levine et al., 1977; cf. also Corwin and Taves, 1963). In the United States the physician's role has been masculine; the nurses, feminine. The result is that the nursing profession has had to struggle to achieve that autonomy which, we have seen, characterizes a full profession (Christman, 1965; Stein, 1967; Ehrenreich and English, 1973a, 1973b, Pankratz, 1974; J. Ashley, 1976). This power struggle has forced many nurses out of an expressive or caring role into an instrumental administrative or technical role (McLemore and Hill, 1965; Leonard, 1966; L. Smith, 1966; Pankratz and Pankratz, 1967; Mussallem, 1969; AMA, 1972). Furthermore, the relation of the registered nurse to the practical nurse and other auxiliaries is far from clear.

The view that the nurse has a role complementary to that of the physician rather than subordinate to it (Freymann, 1974) has not yet been generally accepted. Obviously, it cannot be unless the education of nurses provides them with adequate preparation in the personalistic aspects of health care. Fortunately, in the last fifteen years the nursing education has become more and more insistent on (1) good general education, (2) emphasis on the sociological aspects of nursing, and (3) some emphasis on personal-relations techniques (Heidgerken, 1965; Levine et al., 1977).

Medical and nursing schools operated under Catholic auspices have done little more than other schools in regard to most of these points, although many (not all) have been seriously concerned enough to require a course in medical ethics. However, such courses have often been seriously inadequate for several reasons. (1) They have been treated simply as a requirement, often taught by a nonspecialist (a chaplain) and intruded into the curriculum without any real connection to it. (2) They have often been offered very late in the course of study, frequently in the senior year to extremely busy students, and as a result have had little influence on the actual thinking of students. (3) They have stressed a few prohibitions (birth control, sterilization, abortion) rather than the everyday work of the physician or nurse. (4) They have often been presented as a list of unchanging moral rules rather than as the formation of a critical Christian conscience.

The result has been that Catholic physicians and nurses often exhibit either a rigidity of moral outlook or a kind of ethical schizophrenia. Their concern is to conform minimally to official Catholic teaching so as not to be guilty of mortal sin, but in their everyday work as medical professionals they think in purely secular terms.

Biases

In view of this neglect in medical schools of explicit attention to the ethical aspects of medicine, what is the ethical outlook of the medical profession at present? The empirical data of a study by Amasa B. Ford and associates entitled *The Doctor's Perspective: Physicians View Their Patients and Their Practice* (1967) led the authors to the following well-grounded interpretations:

1. Most physicians have a "strong sense of vocation" rooted in the original priestly character of medicine and reinforced in American culture by the Protestant Calvinist stress on vocation. Yet this religious motivation has been covered over: "The vast growth of science and technology in the four hundred years since Luther has obscured the specifically religious conception of most vocations. The physician seldom speaks of God any more when discussing his concern for the

patient.   Yet he still finds satisfaction in measuring up to personal standards.   Vocation, thus, has come to have an ethical rather than a religious basis and to be rewarded by satisfaction rather than by salvation.   To be effective, the physicians of this study have said 'they must be motivated and competent and must show concern for the patient" (p. 140).

2. But another important component of this motivation is the physicians' sense of specific competence, that is, they have an important and well-defined service to offer.   Much of physicians' personal satisfaction in their work depends upon this sense of competence.   Competent physicians are happy physicians.

3. Doctors are very convinced of the necessity of a "modern individualism," or a professional one-to-one concern.   This conviction has been influenced by American economic attitudes, but it also penetrates even deeper.   Most physicians believe they must "care for the whole patient," and a minority of physicians are also highly socially conscious.

4. Physicians tend to think *pragmatically*, so their basic attitude can be characterized thus: "The physician sees himself as a profesionally competent person who is in a social position to apply scientific knowledge and to exercise impartial control over the situation in order to achieve the rational goal of curing or helping a sick patient.   The patient's part of the job is to trust the doctor and cooperate with him" (p. 144).

This element of control implies that the physician retains a detached concern or benevolent, affective neutrality and that the patient should be cooperative and trustful.   Physicians on the whole are not very sophisticated about the question of control from a psychological point of view.

Furthermore, the study showed that physicians on the whole do not regard themselves as scientists, but rather as applied scientists, and that they do not clearly experience a dichotomy between the scientific and the humanistic or affective aspects of medicine.   Their satisfactions are not theoretical but pragmatic.

5. Physicians take much satisfaction in their professional position as a mark of achievement.   This study tended to show that this sense of achievement is more important for physicians than monetary rewards, which they do not like to think of as a primary motivation.   However, they resent (a) failure of patients to pay, or failure to receive what they consider just acknowledgment and recompense for the burdens of responsibility, of long education, and of long hours which they have to bear and (b) limitations on their independence, because these restrictions remove important symbols of their professional position.

Moreover, while physicians gain some satisfaction from scientific interest in their work, they gain more from the therapeutic results. Physicians get more satisfaction from giving to the patient (in a parental, nurturing sense) than from a mutual relation. Perhaps some in this way alleviate a sense of guilt over their higher social status. An important element of satisfaction or dissatisfaction is found in the sense of consistency between personal and professional ethics. The modern physician is not inclined to moralize: this factor is associated more with older general practitioners than with younger specialists. And yet this study gives evidence that physicians do have a common sense of ethical purpose.

This well-done study indicates some possible ethical biases which medical professionals need to be aware of and which medical education should strive to balance if the medical profession is to make good ethical judgments.

First, on the whole, physicians fortunately continue to exhibit the dualistic balance between the scientific and the humanistic, but this balance is constantly imperiled by the fact that their scientific training is explicit, detailed, and specialized, while their humanistic and moral training is left largely to examples and symbols transmitted to them without explicit reflection or criticism. Physicians thus assume that, while science is exact, ethical discourse is vague, subjective, a matter of opinion. On the one hand, this assumption leads to a kind of moral skepticism and on the other to a dogmatic rigidity, since no method of dialogue or research for critical consensus is available.

Second, physicians tend to take a pragmatic view whereby what is most valued is an immediate, practical solution (cf. also Freidson, 1971). In ethical matters, this pragmatism often causes physicians to act so that (1) they will not be made to feel guilty if an action is taken against their professional or personal standards, and (2) they will not seem inhuman toward the patient, yet will not get too involved in the emotional or social problems of the patient, and (3) they will not go beyond the limits of the patient to wider social problems.

Third, because the motivation of physicians is so bound up with their sense of vocation, autonomy, and competence, they resent interference in their own decisions. They believe that only the physicians are in the position to make medicoethical judgments and that they can be relied upon to be decent and humane in these decisions (Freidsen, 1971). This belief tends to lead physicians (as, for example, in the problem of the dying patient) to follow as their primary rule: help the patient, but to interpret help as the duty to keep trying by every technique available to improve the patient's condition. They can then rest assured and without guilt that they have done all they can do. This attitude leads to deeply felt but simplistic attitudes toward ethical questions.

Fourth, physicians are often resentful that so much is laid on their shoulders. They cannot understand why a wider sociological, religious, psychological, or interrelational view should be their responsibility. Physicians believe that such concerns are someone else's business. Moreover, when medical students select a specialty with its even more well-defined area of competency their limits of responsibility become even narrower.

None of these attitudes is wrong. Undoubtedly they are the result of the medical professional's need to live by a clear motivation, with limited responsibilities, and to have sufficient freedom for action and personal judgment. However, if they result in a closed attitude which renders the physician incapable of learning from others or sharing in a team effort to improve ethical treatment of health problems on a social scale, they are harmful biases that can lead to gravely mistaken ethical judgments.

CHAPTER 5 PERSONALIZING THE HEALTH CARE PROFESSION

5.1 THE COUNSELING RELATIONSHIP

Overview

In chapter 4 we argued that at the heart of every profession there is a counseling relation between persons and that this relation takes on a special mode in the health care profession. We also pointed out that many health care professionals are untrained or not specifically skilled in how to develop and maintain such a relation. Yet ethical decisions about health matters depend first of all upon a cooperative effort of patients and professionals without which patients lack the information they need for an informed conscience. Ethical decisions also depend upon peer relations between members of the health team who must pool their information and expertise. Such cooperation between patients and professionals and between professionals and colleagues demands trust and effective communication which are rooted in sound personal relations. Therefore, unless we establish and maintain such relations in a health care facility, there is little hope of ethical, humanistic health care.

In this chapter, we will first try to define more precisely the exact nature of professional-patient relations and then in 5.2 we will deal with the ethical problems of professional communication and confidentiality. In 5.3, we will touch on one basic aspect of peer relations in the health team, that is, the problem of peer discipline, leaving other aspects of this important question to later chapters. We again remind the reader that what is said of the physician-patient relation must be understood also to apply to nurses and other members of the health team in ways appropriate to the specific role of each.

Models of Professional-Patient Relations

Szasz and Hollender (1956) identified three basic models of the doctor-patient relation: (1) the model of activity-passivity, for example, the surgeon operating on an anesthetized patient; (2) the model of guidance-cooperation, for example, the physician prescribing medication

106

and the patient taking his pills regularly, and (3) the model of mutual participation, for example, the patient engaging in a program of diet and exercise with supervision by the physician. They point out that in all three cases the physician as well as the patient achieves certain satisfactions. Thus the doctor derives a sense of power from the activity-passivity model, a sense of paternal superiority from the guidance-cooperation model, and a sense of friendliness and usefulness from the mutual participation model. In a course of treatment for a particular illness there may be progress from one model to another.

Siegler and Osmond in a fascinating book entitled *Models of Madness, Models of Medicine* (1974) have refined Szasz and Hollender's analysis by identifying eight common models of a therapeutic relation.

1. The *medical model* whereby the physician diagnoses and treats the disease of a patient who is relieved of blame, who is free to take time out to be treated, and whose role is to trust and cooperate with the physician.

2. The *impaired model* whereby the physician must get the patient to accept permanent and incurable defect and then rehabilitate her for a life as normal as possible.

3. The *psychoanalytical model* whereby the therapist assists the patient to come to a greater self-knowledge, even of unconscious motivation, and to develop a more effective way of living.

4. The *psychodelic model* whereby the patient undergoes a trip, an unusual experience, during which the patient needs guidance in order to achieve personal growth.

5. The *family-interaction model* whereby the patient is only a part of a family system which is disordered (the patient may be the member) and whereby the therapist tries to improve the quality of the system.

6. The *social model* whereby the real problem is reform of the social order which is causing the problem. The therapist is a social reformer and the patient perhaps a corevolutionary.

7. The *conspiratorial model* whereby the patient is a victim, not merely of social disorder but of an actual effort of suppression, and the therapist becomes an advocate to expose the conspiracy.

8. The *moral model* whereby the patient requires moral reeducation and conversion of behavior under the guidance of a moral director.

In view of our discussion of the differences in professional roles it seems that the social, conspiratorial, and moral models are not directly appropriate to the work of the health care profession but pertain rather to the work of ethical counselors who deal with the level of conscious, free, responsible behavior, whether it is personal (moral model) or social as well (social and conspiratorial models). The conspiratorial model, although concerned with political behavior, has also a psychoanalytical aspect, since it involves the unmasking of hidden political forces just as psychoanalysis unmasks unconscious personal motivation. On the other hand, the medical, psychodelic, and family-interaction models clearly deal with the psychological level and are the concern of psychotherapy. The psychodelic model also raises questions for the spiritual or pastoral counselor. Similarly, the family-interaction model is suggestive for ethical counselors because the family is the basic unit of social life. Finally, the medical and impaired models obviously deal chiefly with the biological level of human functioning.

Psychotherapeutic Models

From our bioethical perspective, issues are raised first by the medical and impaired models at the biological level and then by the psychoanalytical, psychodelic, and family-interaction models at the psychological level. Psychotherapists are well trained in the problems of the counselor-client relation and are generally well aware of the ethical issues that arise. Some of the more detailed issues are discussed in chapter 12.

However, here we need to ask what is the ethical basis of the remarkable dependence of mentally and emotionally disturbed persons in relation to their therapists? Following Siegler and Osmond, we can summarize the significance of this relationship by a more detailed account of the psychoanalytical model.

In the psychoanalytical model the client comes to the therapist because of painful anxieties that make normal life difficult or impossible, with the goal of trying to resolve emotional conflicts whose unconscious origin is unknown to the client. The therapist's responsibility is not to diagnose the illness by labeling it, but to help the client come to an understanding of the causes of his problems and to cope with them more effectively. To achieve this the therapist must gradually win the client's trust and help the client step by step to interpret the symbolism of the symptoms. The therapist must grant the client the right to have her behavior interpreted as symbolic rather than judged morally and to have the client's sufferings counted worthy of sympathy. The therapist must help the client not to act out symptoms, but to discover their underlying meaning and thus to come to a deep and realistic self-understanding. Finally, the therapists must reeducate the client and help him terminate dependence on the therapist. To do this the therapist must personally arrive at self-understanding through the same process.

The client must come to trust the therapist, speaking more and more freely, cooperating by undertaking the task of working through symptoms, rejecting escape from the process by suicide or even by a flight into health. The client's will to get well and become independent of the therapist must also be reinforced. This process depends upon an intense one-to-one relation in which the patient withdraws from the familial and social situation in which she has become ill.   It also demands toleration by family and society of the patient's temporary withdrawal from ordinary relationships and responsibilities.

The dependence of the client on the therapist is essentially a recapitulation of the parental relationship, but a healthy one rather than the unhealthy one from which the client has suffered.   The therapist is a good mother in taking on the attitude of what Carl Rogers (1951) called "unconditional benign acceptance" and also a good father in the increasing role of interpretation and confrontation with reality.   The libidinal, erotic elements of the transference of the client to the therapist are gradually turned toward the real love objects of the client's independent life.   By no means is it easy for clients to come to such total trust in their therapists, since they have learned to distrust any mother or father.   Yet if clients are to get well, they have a moral obligation to try to trust, cooperate, and negate in this working through.   Clients must accept the tasks (1) of trusting the therapist and (2) of trying to recover health and normal independence.

On their part, therapists undertake the moral burden of being faithful to this trust reposed in them by their clients.   Therapists must listen, not judge, and (to a degree) must sympathize.   Therapists must set limits on acting out by clients and must insist on working through.   They must approve and reinforce the clients' progressive achievement of insight and gradually confront them more and more with the demands of reality.   Finally, therapists must be willing to let even favorite patients go.   In order for therapists to be ethically true to this trust, they must be personally aware of any tendency toward countertransference (i.e., the development of a relation in which the therapist begins to use the patient to meet the therapist's own emotional needs) and must strive to keep this human tendency within limits.

Today these mutual duties, which clearly involve considerable virtue on the part of therapists and a desire for virtue and willingness to grow through suffering on the part of clients, are often formalized in a contract made at the beginning of therapy.   In this contract, therapists make sure clients understand and accept the goals and limits of therapy and are aware that they can hold a therapist liable for the therapist's half of the contract.   Thus therapists are unethical when they fail to make such a clear contract (which is an aspect of informed consent as discussed in 3.4) or fail to adhere strictly to it. Therapists should *not* assume moral obligations beyond the limits of this contract.   Thus analysts ought not to normally undertake any responsibility for patients' acting out of their symptoms outside the therapeutic setting.

Such limitations raise certain difficulties, however.   We might list the chief ones as follows: (1) What if the patient is contemplating suicide?   (2) What if the patient is contemplating some act injurious to another party, for example, physical attack, theft, adultery, or divorce?

(3) What if the patient proposes sexual relations with the therapist? (4) What if the patient refuses to work seriously at the therapy or needlessly delays its termination? We will discuss these problems at greater length in chapter 12. Here we need only to point out that these actions constitute a breach (perhaps not culpable) of the contract on the part of the client. They relieve the therapist from his contract, but they leave him obliged (not as a professional, but simply as a citizen) to prevent harm to a third party or to prevent an insane person from harming himself. Consequently, the therapist can discreetly inform the family or others to guard against suicide or crime. In cases 3 and 4 the therapist can also terminate therapy. If the patient gets worse or needs commitment, consultants should be called in or the family informed so that the commitment process can be undertaken.

Other forms of psychotherapy do not rest on such a close relation between therapist and client, but they present the same essential issues.

Medical Model

In strong contrast to the psychotherapeutic models is the medical model, although today the patient enters both models in much the same kind of setting — a private office, clinic, or hospital. In the medical model the professional goal is to treat a physical illness so as to restore normal physical functioning to the degree possible. The physician first seeks to diagnose the disease, then to prescribe a course of treatment (in which the physician is assisted by nurses and others) through medicine, surgery, nursing, or change of regimen. The physician must also make a prognosis and if possible offer the patient hope. The patient, on the other hand, is relieved from blame for his or her condition and from ordinary responsibilities to work and family, but is expected to be cooperative with the professional staff. Families and society are expected to support the patient psychologically and to contribute to the expenses.

In this model the patient is not expected to be as active as in the psychotherapeutic models except in rehabilitative stages of treatment which pertain more characteristically to the impaired model. This patient passivity raises the main ethical issue characteristic of this model. If we were correct in arguing in chapter 3 that the health care professional is only a servant to the patient because primary responsibility for the patient's health remains the patient's, then it follows that the professional has no rights over the patient, except those given by the patient's informed consent. Hence, ethically speaking, an implicit or explicit contract must regulate all that goes on in the medical model.

What are the essential features of this medical contract? First, the contract *limits* the obligations assumed. In the medical model a physician does not assume the role of a psychotherapist or of an ethical or spiritual counselor. In our efforts to repersonalize medicine we should not demand that the medical doctor assume all the roles proper to a complete health team. Of course physicians need to be aware of nonphysical factors that may be affecting the patient's health in order to refer them to other members of the health team.

Nevertheless, the physician who provides primary care stands in a special relation to the patient (Somers and Somers, 1961). Studies show that fifty percent or more of patients seen by primary care physicians are not suffering from any physical dysfunction. Some physicians regard such patients as hypochondriacs, are bored with their complaints, and get rid of them as fast as possible, or (sorry to say) keep them coming back for an easy fee. Other physicians patiently try to alleviate excessive anxiety by prescribing a placebo or tranquilizer or using a little amateur psychotherapy or a dose of fatherly advise.

However, the implied contract between a patient and the primary care physician obligates the physician to undertake a serious effort to help the patient discover the nature of the problem and the type of help which is appropriate to it, medical or otherwise. The patient who does not feel well comes to a physician as a first, obvious step in an effort to determine the source of the discomfort. If the possibility of a physical cause can be eliminated, the patient then has the information necessary to take the next step — seeing another type of counselor or other action. But if the physician fails to listen or to make an adequate examination or sends the patient away confused or with a placebo or tranquilizer, the patient still lacks the necessary information for rational decisions (Bok, 1974). Physicians who deal in an evasive manner with patients are only reinforcing hypochondriacal tendencies.

A well-known study of hospital care (Duff and Hollingshead, 1968) showed that a high percentage of patients were incorrectly diagnosed because of the failure of physicians to listen carefully to patients' complaints and to recognize nonmedical factors in their conditions. It is also well known that in clinics which provide free service physicians tend to prescribe tranquilizing drugs in a startling high number of cases (Schwartz, 1972).

Second, the medical model, like other professional relations, is based on trust. The physician, therefore, must establish trustworthiness within the limits of the contract. As it relates to this trust, the contract should have three elements.

1. *Concern.* Fundamental to the contract is the physician's concern for the patient's well-being. Trust will never exist if the patient believes that the physician is concerned only about the fee or is acting out of mere routine like a machine or a bureaucratic functionnary. The physican must communicate her interest in the patient as a person, not as a kidney or a heart, and a willingness to do for the patient whatever is professionally possible, not limited by mere self-interested motives.

For this reason Paul Ramsey (1970b) has rightly emphasized that the professional contract is something more than a contract; it is a "covenant" in the theological sense. In the Old Testament, God made a covenant with his chosen people based not on their worthiness but on his generous love for them in their need and confirmed by a promise not to desert them even if on their part they did not meet all their own obligations. The professional contract is analogous to such a covenant in the sense that the professional undertakes to help the client not because the client is ethically worthy of help, nor even because he is able to pay for the service, but primarily because of human need and the essential human rights based on need rather than on merit. The professional contract also implies the promise to continue the care of the patient even when the patient is no longer able to insist on its fulfillment.

However, this concept of covenant should not be exaggerated. God Himself insists on the responsibility of his people to respond to their own obligations under the covenant. Hence the physician also has the right to demand cooperation from the patient. Moreover, the physician's contract is not universal, but limited by his own competence, so that the physician is not obligated to do more than inform the patient when a problem exceeds his competence and refer him or her to another specialist or another type of nonmedical counselor.

2. *Knowledge and skill in medicine.* Health care professionals have the fundamental responsibility, within their specialities, to be expert in both the science and the art of health care, up-to-date in knowledge, experienced, of good judgment, and skilled in procedures. Personal warmth does not substitute for medical expertness. However, reciprocally, it may be said that this knowledge and skill cannot be put to their best use if the other humanistic elements are not also present. Professionals communicate such expertise to patients by evidence of their education and licensure, by reputation, and also by the care and thoroughness with which they deal with patients.

3. *Communication.* Since patients retain fundamental rights over their own bodies, and the fundamental knowledge of how they feel not only at this minute, but also throughout the day and in varied situations, physicians cannot hope to make a proper diagnosis, carry on successful treatment, or make an accurate prognosis without adequate communication with patients. Barnlund (1976) makes this observation about communication:

> When one turns to ask what is currently known about communication between medical personnel and patients, the answer is itself mystification — very little. Here is a profession founded on science, dedicated to truth, committed to inquiry, concerned with the relief of suffering, yet either oblivious or unwilling to examine its own communicative behavior. Is this simply a mote in an otherwise scientific eye? Or is it a defensive assertion of the medical mystique and the preference to do as one pleases? (p. 273)

Health Care Fees

To these basic ethical obligations of the medical doctor, we can add a fourth which applies also to the psychotherapeutic models: to set or refuse an appropriate fee (Glaser, 1970a). In our capitalist society it is assumed that a professional should be paid as any other worker is paid according to the laws of supply and demand. It is assumed that a service is just as much a commodity for exchange with a value measured in monetary terms as is any other product. Consequently, some persons argue that there is nothing ethically wrong with organizing the medical profession on the basis of profit just as we do any other industry. They believe that the stimulus of the profit motive has been the chief cause of the rapid technological development of American medicine. Harry Schwarz (1972) contends that if the free market were permitted to prevail in health care the economic efficiency of our American medical system would be greatly enhanced and inflation in medical costs reduced.

Furthermore, some argue that the fee is actually a part of therapy since it causes the average person to refrain from asking for unnecessary services which might overload the system and deprive others in real need from getting proper attention. Moreover, the fee promotes a cooperative attitude on the part of the patient and thus shortens the time of treatment. Psychiatrists in particular insist that in their experience the client who does not have to pay a fee is very likely to waste more time before getting down to the painful task of working through resistances.

However, the question can also be raised as to whether this capitalistic assumption is a realistic and practical fact. At no time in the history of medicine has the market system operated fully in the professions because there have always been people who desperately needed professional help but who could not pay for it. Either the professional had to provide free services or payment had to be made by a third party. In chapter 6 we will discuss the various ways of organizing medical systems to meet this inescapable difficulty.

If the account we have given of the nature of a profession is correct, it should be clear why profit cannot be the primary basis of any profession, but must be considered a secondary and highly variable feature. The medical profession, like any true profession, must rest not on bargaining but on trust, and it provides a service that is concerned with life and death, matters so precious as to be priceless. No monetary value can be set on the spiritual light given by a priest, the defense of human rights provided by a lawyer, the risk of his own life provided by a soldier, or the search for truth shared by a teacher. Nor is there any price for the service of a physician in the battle to live.

Just because the health care professional performs so precious a service it cannot be bargained for. Hence in the past the fundamental principle in all professions was that the professional must be ready to give services free to those who were in need but could not pay. Jesus said with regard to religious ministry, "The laborer is worthy of his hire" (Luke 10:7; cf. I Tim. 5:18), but he meant by this that his disciples should live from hand to mouth, "freely giving what you have freely received." St. Paul followed this same principle in his own way by supporting himself by manual labor, so that no one might accuse him of preaching for gain (I Cor. 4:12; Acts 18:3). Thus religious professionals deserve to be supported by the public so that they can provide services purely on the basis of the need of the client.

The same principle applies to all true professions because they provide services which are life-and-death necessities. Hence professional fees are not payments measured by the value of the service provided (which is truly priceless), but a *stipend* to be measured only by what professionals need to live in a manner which will free them to work without distraction. Therefore, medical professionals who set their fees so high as to accumulate wealth in other businesses which distract them from their profession are charging too much.

It is generally stated in official codes of medical ethics that medical fees should be adjusted to the ability of the patient to pay. The assumption is that richer patients will be charged enough to compensate physicians for what they lose in low fees or none at all which are charged poorer patients. The inadequacy of this as a principle becomes apparent when the fees are paid by a third party such as an insurance company or the government. Experience shows that in such a situation physicians are tempted to charge as much as they can get, with a resulting inflation in health costs. The ability-to-pay principle is not unjust as long as it remains within the bounds of the more fundamental principle that professionals are public servants who have no right to expect in return for services anything more than a standard of living which will make it possible for them to perform those services with liberty of mind, health of body, and adequate fulfillment of family and social obligations.

A Christian physician, lawyer, teacher, or religious minister can only conclude that a professional living is essentially a modest one in which simplicity of life-style and freedom to be available to serve others is the only honorable measure of remuneration. Nor can the argument be accepted which is so often put forward that since physicians spend long years of difficult study, work long hours, and assume great responsibility they deserve to make money. The rewards of any profession are to be found not in some extraneous gain, but in the satisfactions of knowledge and of interesting and absorbing work and in the joy in a baby delivered or a sick patient restored or a dying patient made comfortable and serene. Such an ideal is not easy to realize, nor is it often realized in its purest form, but even when imperfectly realized it is what has given the medical profession its own vitality and health.

5.2   PRINCIPLE OF PROFESSIONAL COMMUNICATION

Listening and Truth Telling

We have stressed that in health care, as in all professional relations, adequate communication between professional and client is a fundamental ethical requirement.   In the medical model opportunities for such communication may be rather sharply restricted, but they are still crucial.   Within these limits what are the duties of physicians and nurses?

The first obligation is to listen to the patient.   Yet in the medical model often while professionals concentrate on filtering out medically significant information patients are attempting to express their malaise in a rhapsody of symptoms, fears, fantasies, evasions, cries for attention, and so forth (Barnlund, 1976).   The work-pressured professional cannot afford to sit and hear a long and rambling discourse from a self-pitying patient.   Even the psychotherapist, who has a special interest in all sorts of behavioral clues, must insist that patients "get to work" without evading the therapeutic process.   Somehow professionals must cut through the noise and get at the real message, but they need to remember that "the medium *is* the message," that is, the way patients are (or are not) communicating may be the most significant symptom.

Therefore, no matter how busy they may be health care professionals may not ethically rush through interviews or simply rely on laboratory tests.   They have the responsibility to acquire the art of medical dialogue by which they can help patients say what needs to be said.   The first rule of this art is for the professional to repeat back to the patient what the professional has heard that seems significant and to ask whether it is what the patient meant.   This feedback not only reassures the patient, but can also gradually train the patient in giving relevant information.   A second rule is to obtain the patient's cooperation by explaining the purpose of questions, since unexpected and cryptic questions are threatening and confusing to many patients.   If physicians are unable or unwilling to learn this art of dialogue, then they must learn to work in a team which includes other professionals with such communication skills.

A professional must not only hear, but also *believe* patients who, like all of us have the basic right to be believed until they lose that right by clearly proved deception.   Hence the temptation of some busy physicians and exasperated nurses to jump to the conclusion that a patient is malingering has to be resisted.   While what a patient reports may not be objectively true, it is subjectively so because it expresses what the patient really *feels* and is therefore medically significant and important.

Of course, professionals also have the right to require honesty and frankness from clients.   When they suspect deliberate deceit, they should deal with the situation explicitly and directly as a breach of the patient's contract with the professional. However, also involved in most illnesses are psychological factors that may cause communication to be distorted by unconscious elements of self-deceit, denial, confusion, or panic. Psychotherapists in particular have to deal with this perplexing inability of some patients to communicate openly, but therapists also experience in themselves something of the same ambiguity. Appleton (1972) is of this opinion:

> Psychiatrists advocate honest and open communication by physicians with patients but too often do not practice what they preach. Their reasons for silence include uncertainty about the cause, treatment, and prognosis of psychiatric illnesses and unwillingness to depress, demoralize, anger, or alienate their patients. (p. 743)

This observation applies to all health care professionals, who cannot expect truth from their patients unless they are equally truthful with them. Lack of frankness by professionals is usually excused as concern to spare the patient, but is just as often the result of unconscious fear on the part of the professional. In chapter 13 we will discuss the problem of telling the truth to the incurable or dying patient. Here it suffices to say that the fundamental principle in all such situations is that the patient has the right to the truth, however difficult the professional may find it.

Confidentiality

Patients have the right to the truth about their health because they have the primary responsibility for their health. They also have the right to privacy about those aspects of life which do not directly affect others. Human community is based on free communication which is impossible if we cannot share confidences with some persons in whom we choose to confide. Hence health care professionals have a serious obligation to maintain such confidences that protect the patient's right of privacy.

How is a professional to act when questioned by others about a patient's condition? Can confidentiality be protected by lying? All Catholic moralists agree that it is always wrong to "lie," even to protect confidentiality, but not all agree on how to define *lying*. Some (Dorszynski, 1949; Curran, 1975) distinguished between a *falsehood*, that is, a false statement, and a *lie*, which is not only a false statement but also one made to someone who has the right to a true answer. Consequently, they hold that someone who has a duty to keep a secret can answer falsely to inquirers. It seems better to say with Knauer (1967) that the meaning of any human statement must always be determined from the context in which communication occurs. Consequently when persons ask questions which they have no right to ask, any answer to such questions, taken out of context would be literally a false statement and when *in* context would be not a false statement but a *meaningless* one, that is, so ambiguous that it does not even reveal whether the speaker is concealing something. Thus health care professionals who are questioned about confidential matters may without lying or even falsehood reply in any way that protects confidentiality. However, this cannot excuse the physician from frankly answering questions put by a patient or the patient's guardians, because these persons have the right to know.

It is not easy to draw the line between what individuals have the right to keep private and what they may have the duty to make public. Hence, the contract between professional and patient should determine this as exactly as possible. If professionals are convinced that in order to do the best for a patient they need to discuss the case with consultants or before other members of a team or of the professional staff, the professionals must obtain the informed consent of the patient. Generally, this consent is implicity contained in the contract. Thus in most mental hospitals it is assumed that voluntary (or even involuntary) commitment implies the right to discuss the patient's condition and progress with other members of the therapeutic staff.

However, such assumptions are easily open to abuse. Books have been published by physicians and psychiatrists about their famous or notorious patients, living or dead (Chayet, 1966). In our opinion, much greater care must be taken to obtain explicit consent from patients with regard to matters that may be embarrassing to them, especially as we move into an age of medical teamwork and computerized records. Most patients (when they are incompetent, their guardians) are ready enough to permit the therapeutic use of information, but they should have the opportunity to restrict the use of this information when entering into contractual relations with the professional. It should not be too difficult for a physician or for a health care institution to work out a regular procedure by which patients are informed of their rights to privacy and asked for explicit consent for any necessary use of confidential information.

Nevertheless, the right of privacy, sacred as it is, has limits set by the rights of other persons and by the individual's own limited rights of self-disposal. Patients may behave in ways which directly injure themselves and indirectly or directly injure others. For example, patients may commit suicide, seek ways to continue their chemical dependency, spread contagious diseases, or commit acts of theft or aggression against other patients or the staff. Some may become so seriously incompetent as to become a public danger on release from an insitution, for example, the epileptic bus driver who refuses to change his job (Davidson, 1968).

In all these cases, the family or society has an obligation to prevent harm both to the patient and to the public because all are members of a community which exists for the good of each of its members in relation to all others. Hence, generally speaking, professionals have not only the right but also the duty to communicate information necessary to prevent serious harm to the patient or to others, even when it is given to them in confidence, to those who may be able to prevent this injury (Cass and Curran, 1965; Davidson, 1968).

Thus, professional secrecy is not as absolute as the secrecy demanded of a Catholic priest who may not reveal what he has learned in confession as regards the sins or defects of a penitent even to prevent harm to a third party. Nor is it even as absolute as that given by law to the confidences between accused criminals and their lawyers. In the first case the penitent is revealing personal moral responsibility before God which is beyond human judgment. In the second case the accused is protected in his or her rights by the adversary process. In medical matters, however, the patient has no need to reveal to the professional anything which is essentially incriminating but usually only what may be a matter of embarrassment. However, moral fault may incidentally be revealed: for example, when the patient voluntarily admits an intention to commit a crime and when the medical condition has moral implications (addiction, venereal disease, illegitimate pregnancy).

When what is revealed is an intention to commit a crime (including suicide), the professional has the obligation to reveal to appropriate persons whatever information is necessary to prevent such a crime. When no crime is contemplated, but there is probable danger of harm which can be prevented, the professional should discreetly do what is likely to be helpful in preventing such harm. Ordinarily this should not be done without first warning the patient of exposure if the patient refuses to desist. For example, the professional should keep the fact of addiction confidential if the patient is willing to cooperate with treatment, but may be forced to make it known to the family if cooperation is refused. A professional should protect the confidence of someone illegitimately pregnant unless the intention to secure an abortion is evident, in which case the professional may be forced to inform the parents of a minor or the father of the child. In the case of venereal disease of a minor, confidentiality should be maintained unless the minor refuses treatment. In other situations professionals should first seek to obtain the cooperation of the patient and only proceed to inform the third party when this cooperation is refused and the damaged feared is both serious and probable since the benefit of the doubt is in favor of confidentiality upon which the whole influence of the professional over the patient depends.

Certain very serious problems about confidentiality have been raised recently by the requirement of private and government health insurance plans that physicians report the nature of a patient's illness as a condition of receiving payment and also by the computerization of health records. It is clear enough that a physician does not have the right to give information of this sort without the patient's permission (Annas, 1975).

However, this leaves the larger question of how patients are to obtain the benefits to which they are entitled without giving such permission. In our opinion, the insurance or public agency has the right to ask proof from patients that they have used funds for a legitimate medical purpose, but the agency also has the duty to design adequate controls which do not require detailed information which might be embarrassing or injurious to the patient. Computerization of health records should always require the patient's permission, and even when permission is given, care must be taken to limit the availability of these records to a few definitely authorized persons. Similar problems are raised in the case of peer review, a process which is becoming more and more widespread and which is discussed in 5.3.

Some professionals (Szasz, 1974a, 1977) argue for an extreme individualistic and libertarian position. For example, they contend that addicts should be permitted free access to alcohol and drugs and some even believe that suicidal persons should be permitted to take their own lives if they wish. The basis of their opinion is this view: "Freedom is doing what you want with your own life," and "Immorality is only doing harm to another, nonconsenting adult." We have shown in 1.2 that the very nature of personhood implies involvement in a community. Self-destructive behavior is not merely of concern to the person in question, but to all with whom his or her life is intertwined. In fact, psychology seems to show that such behavior is an unconscious cry for help (Schneidman et al., 1970). To let such persons destroy themselves because they claim that is what they want is actually to ignore this cry that comes from the true self. The real answer must be a social concern for persons in their real liberty, which consists in becoming more open to others, not more closed. To achieve openness, we must gain the trust of the alienated.

In view of this discussion, we can formulate the *Principle of Professional Communication* as follows:

Health care professionals have the responsibility:

1. To strive to establish and preserve trust at both the emotional and rational levels

2. To share the information they possess which is legitimately needed by others in order to have an informed conscience

3. To refrain from lying or giving misinformation

4. To keep secret information which is not legitimately needed by others, but which if revealed might either harm the patient or others or destroy trust.

5.3   PEER RELATIONS AND PROFESSIONAL DISCIPLINE

Health care professionals need good personal relations not . only with those they serve, but also with their colleagues on the health team. Problems of leadership and accountability, of common decision making and cooperation in carrying out decisions, of adequate communication and mutual support not only have psychological importance, but also are profoundly ethical in nature.

We will touch on some of these issues in chapter 6 and in the concluding Part V of this book. Here, we will deal only with the especially sensitive issue of peer discipline because in any group the problem of mutual responsibility is crucial. If health care professionals do not care enough about each other and their common enterprise to accept the painful task of maintaining group standards in a fraternal and humane way, they cannot hope to personalize health care.

The recent phenomenal rise in the number of malpractice suits seems proof that the health care profession is currently in need of stricter discipline. The Commission on Medical Malpractice of the Secretary of the Department of Health, Education, and Welfare (HEW, 1973) concluded (with some dissenting voices on the commission) that the main factor in this increase in litigation has been the increase in the number of medical injuries, real or apparent, perhaps in part due simply to the increasingly complex and risky procedures of modern therapy. But the commission also concluded that malpractice suits frequently result (1) from poor communication between physicians and patients and hence from inadequately informed consent on the patient's part, (2) from patients' frustration because physicians seem unresponsive to their complaints, (3) from patients' unrealistic expectations about the benefits of treatment, and (4) from growing public conviction that consumers need to defend themselves against arrogant, self-serving professionals. It is noteworthy that the first three of these factors (and perhaps in large part the fourth) reduce to a failure in communication in which, as we have seen, physicians are often not well trained. Furthermore, we are led to wonder why other members of the health team do not notice or correct such misunderstandings.

Two opposite remedies have been proposed for the malpractice problem. One answer is *peer review* (cf. Luft, 1976). It is argued, plausibly enough, that in a field so highly technical as medicine no one is competent to evaluate professional performance except peers in the profession or even in the same medical speciality. Professionals should judge their peers, set penalties and rewards, and if necessary expel serious and incorrigible offenders from the profession.

On the other hand, some authorities (Annas, 1975) argue that peer discipline has never been successful in protecting the patient or even in maintaining high standards of medical competence. A profession, they contend, is too concerned with its own autonomy to be very diligent in disciplining its members. A built-in bias works in favor of protecting members of the profession rather than in the interests of patients. Consequently, these critics believe that the disciplining of a profession must first of all be the concern of those who suffer from malpractice or neglect. Health care consumers must know and defend their own rights by all available economic, legal, and political means.

The former of these two positions was adopted long ago by the American Medical Association and the American Psychiatric Association for their membership, but has been implemented rather perfunctorily. As a result some twenty-five states have recently extended the authority of state licensing boards to include reevaluation of physicians' performance. Moreover, within various specialities and health care facilities, committees are being set up to monitor and improve professional performance (Symington, 1977; Sullivan, 1977).

The latter position is favored by two groups of very different opinions. Those like Harry Schwartz (1974) who defend the existing medical establishment on the grounds that the free market is the best regulator of medicine logically support the idea that consumers are the ultimate judges of whether the health care they pay for is satisfactory. On the other hand, radical critics of the establishment like Illich (1976a) favor the same conclusion for a very different reason, namely, that medical information should no longer be monopolized by an elite but should be made available to all.

Since we have taken the position that the primary responsibility for health must remain with each person to whom the professional is only a servant, we also believe that the ultimate right to call the medical profession to account must be in the hands of those the profession exists to serve. This is why the users of health services have the fundamental right to the final word in regulating the profession through public law.

In this matter it seems that the physician and the lawyer are in a somewhat different position than the minister, teacher, and scientist. These latter professions deal with objective truth as such, and the public has no right to silence the voice of truth. But the lawyer is an officer of the court, that is, he or she is subordinated to the legislative and judicial officers of the government who represent the people in determining the law. The medical professional also does not stand for truth as such, as a scientist must, but is providing a service to human physical or mental health, a service which must ultimately be judged in terms of its practical enhancement of human well-being. Consequently, the medical profession must accept a public, practical evaluation of its services. Of course, health care professionals in their secondary role as scientists have a right and an obligation to speak out for objective truth about biological and medical matters, but this does not give them complete autonomy in the realm of medical practice.

There are many views as to how the rise in malpractice suits and the great increase in insurance rates which it produces can be remedied.

Some blame the legal profession because the courts have too much extended vague legal rules such as those which relate to the time allowed plaintiffs to report injuries, the application of the *res ipsa loquitur* ("The injury is sufficient evidence of fault") doctrine to medical injuries, the doctrine of informed consent, and liability based on oral guarantees of good results (cf. Illich, 1976a; Harolds and Block, 1966), and because lawyers find malpractice suits very profitable since they receive a high percentage (usually thirty to forty percent) of the damages awarded according to what is called the contingent fee system.

Others blame the medical profession not only for the poor communication just mentioned, but also for the unwillingness of many physicians to testify against peers. It is admitted by all including the American Medical Association that physicians and other medical professionals have the duty to testify in such cases out of justice not only to the claimant, but also to the physician and the profession itself. Compassionate concern for a colleague does not excuse a professional from frank and honest testimony as to the colleague's competence or responsibility when this is in serious question as long as due process is being observed.

The medical profession and every learned profession must have a genuine but limited autonomy. As health care users become more knowledgeable about what is and what is not good medical care, they will become increasingly able to detect serious incompetence or negligence in the service they receive. But at best, this awareness will raise questions; it will not be sufficient in most cases to pass judgment. *Res ipsa loquitur* in some cases of medical malpractice, but not in most. I may have my doubts that an operation recommended by my surgeon is really necessary, but all I can do to find out is either to ask him for more convincing answers to my questions or to consult another professional.

It would seem, therefore, that a satisfactory system of discipline for the medical profession must be a combination of both peer discipline and consumer discipline. A medical review board must include both professional peers with requisite technical knowledge and experience and also health care users (along with legal advisers) who are concerned to see that the medical professionals are more concerned for the served than for their own self-interest as the servants. At the same time, it is essential that medical information be made more easily available to all users so that each can know and defend his or her own rights and interests.

Since it is medical professionals who now have this information, they have the responsibility to undertake the educational task of informing the public so that the public can defend itself against the professionals themselves. Since professionals are inevitably biased in favor of defending their own autonomy, and since any work of public education is difficult in the face of inevitable public apathy, the prospects of such an educational program are not bright. It looks like the public does not want to assume personal responsibility for its own health, but prefers to take pills or have surgery rather than to exercise or stop eating, drinking, and smoking too much.

In the face of this dreary reality, many otherwise compassionate and humanistic health care professionals are inclined to lapse into paternalism. They argue that the profession will have to do what it can for the public on the basis of its own expert judgment while defending itself against annoying or even dangerous lay intrusion into health affairs.

We believe that Christian professionals cannot accept this paternalistic and defensive position. The real remedy for malpractice and unjustified malpractice litigation is a more personalized practice of medicine which will reduce misunderstanding between professional and patient and will correct human failure by professionals through mutual cooperation and discipline within the health team itself. The notion of fraternal correction is part of the Christian ethos (Matt. 18:15-18). Applied to a profession, it means that the members do not simply ignore or hide the defects of colleagues out of indifference or self-interest, but are seriously concerned to help them overcome these defects and repair the consequences. It also implies that even those workers in subordinate positions have a right and an obligation to correct superiors and that the superiors have an obligation to listen to such corrections.

If such mutual support and discipline are to be possible in a health team, it must rest on a profound mutual trust and respect which can be built up only by persistent effort. One of the marks of a Catholic health care facility, therefore, should be this striving to establish the personal relationships within the staff and administration which will be the basis for such professional cooperation.

CHAPTER 6 SOCIAL ORGANIZATION OF HEALTH CARE

6.1   ORGANIZATIONAL MODELS AND PRINCIPLE OF SUBSIDIARITY

Overview

Today health care is no longer a matter of a person-to-person relation between physician and patient, nor simply of health teams located in separate health care facilities, but a great network of interrelated institutions.   In this chapter, we will deal with this social organization of health care, first explaining some of the organizational models which are under current discussion and then developing the Principle of Subsidiarity and Functionalism which is the ethical foundation of any social organization, and in 6.2 will also consider the question which some are raising as to whether the type of medical care now dominant in the United States requires not reorganization but radical revision.

Since in our actual situation the hospital is the chief feature of modern health care, we discuss the hospital as an institution in 6.3 and as a system of interpersonal relations in 6.4.   In 6.5 we delineate the special features of a hospital based on a Catholic value sytem.   Finally, in 6.7 we discuss some of the resources currently available by which health care facilities can achieve greater humanization and personalization.

Models

Up to this point we have been developing the model of a health care professional as a person competent in the art and science of medicine and motivated to serve other persons each of whom have primary responsibility for his or her own health.   The Christian health care professional finds this model in Jesus himself who came to heal and "not to be served, but to serve" (Matt. 20:28).

Since we have argued that individuals have responsibility for their own health and the health care profession a responsibility to be of service in this pursuit of health, we must now ask whether society as a whole has the responsibility for the health of each of its citizens and hence for the promotion and regulation of the health care profession in pursuit of universal health.

American culture is paradoxical in its prevailing attitude toward this question. We long ago accepted the principle that government should promote and regulate universal free education for all children at least through high school, but for some reason we have hesitated to accept wholeheartedly the principle that government should promote and regulate universal free basic health care. Only since World War II have local and federal governments become involved in the issue of comprehensive health care. The medical profession itself through what was long its principle representative, the American Medical Association, has shown itself extremely hesitant about supporting any such principle (Greenburg, 1965; Stevens, 1971).

We Americans generally tend to compare ourselves to our main competition, the Communist and Socialist countries. As we have already pointed out (1.3), this comparison is actually a juxtaposition of two religious value systems: Secularism in the First World and Marxism in the Second World. Consequently, since medical education is often woefully negligent of the social sciences, many physicians tend to identify all social issues in terms of two opposing models: Free Enterprise versus Socialism.

It is more helpful to follow the lead of Alford (1975) who points out that three models of the social organization of health care are being debated in the United States. The first of these is the *pluralist* system which actually exists, but which some people regard as no system at all. Its regulatory principle is the market in which persons with health needs compete for the services of health care professionals, principally on a fee-for-service basis and professionals compete to sell their services. However, today these professional health care providers no longer act merely as individuals, but are organized in a whole spectrum of health care institutions of which the hospital is the chief one.

Each of these health care facilities requires the cooperation of many medical specialists assisted not only by nurses but also by many different kinds of technicians and auxiliaries (Sloane and LeRoy, 1977). Furthermore, an increasing number of physicians are organized in *group practice* of various types in some of which they are prepaid by patients a fixed salary or a fee based on the number of patients served (capitation). Thus, in a pluralist system there is no single organizational structure but a plurality of health providers, some acting individually, but most acting through some institutional group.

The difficulties with this present system have become very apparent in recent years (Burns, 1973; Stevens and Stevens, 1974; Mechanic, 1974). It is an inefficient system because it does not provide for long-range planning and it wastes resources in overlapping services and duplication of expensive plant and equipment (Somers and Somers, 1961). More serious still, this model has not provided access to adequate medical care for many socially and geographically disadvantaged groups. Nor has it demonstrably raised the general level of health in recent years.

Finally, it seems subject to ever-mounting costs which promise eventually to absorb at least ten percent of our gross national product (McGinnis, 1976).

Some defenders of the system (Schwartz, 1972; Cronkhite, 1977) argue that the medical profession cannot be blamed for the unhealthy American way of life over which physicians have little control, nor for mounting costs which have been largely produced by government intervention in the form of Medicare and Medicaid, an intervention that prevents the market system from operating effectively. These defenders propose no remedy but the extension of private health insurance systems, with the government providing only for catastrophic illness. To such arguments others respond that without government intervention the poor will be even more neglected (Mechanic, 1974; Halberstam, Stevens, and Outka, 1974), and that the medical profession has itself destroyed free-market controls by monopolistic practices and by creating unnecessary demands for expensive modes of treatment.

Other defenders of pluralism avoid polemics and look for ways in which free-market mechanisms can be brought into play to afford better cost control and greater effectiveness in meeting real rather than artificial needs. While some (Sloan and Feldman, 1977) doubt professional monopoly is really the major factor in raising health costs, others (Havinghurst, 1977) assert this and call for restrictions on such monopolistic practices on the part of medical societies as the use of ethics codes to prevent advertising and limit access to information by which consumers might be able to make competitive choices (Benham, 1977). Other economists (Altman and Weiner, 1977) believe some degree of government regulation is inevitable, but advise that it should not emphasize planning so much as provide economic motivation for hospitals to control costs, for example, by budgetary measures, limits on new hospital construction, and encouragement to shift to more outpatient care.

Because of such difficulties with our present pluralist model, a second *centralized* (or regional) model has been widely proposed and defended (Ellwood, 1974). In this model, the country would be divided into regions in each of which all health care would be organized in a unified system. At the bottom of the pyramid would be a large number of primary care physicians with their auxiliaries who would care for the great majority of health problems requiring only a minimum of specialized knowledge and equipment. For cases exceeding such care there would be a second level of hospitals or other facilities with complete staffs of specialists and advanced equipment. Finally, for cases of still greater difficulty, there would be a third or even fourth level of institutions equipped to give the most advanced care in which medical education and research would be located. In such a system, long-range planning would be possible, and this system could move the focus of health care from its present emphasis on the cure of disease toward emphasis on prevention, so that each region would become a health maintenance organization (HMO).

The rationality and apparent efficiency of this model is appealing to many, but its critics point out defects. In such a system, bureaucratism seems inevitable. The experience of Czechoslovakia which has adopted this method in a very well-planned form (Freymann, 1974) or of Great Britain or Sweden (Anderson, 1972; Kohn and White, 1976) or Quebec (DeMarchai, 1975) shows that such systems continue to have many difficulties including the rise of health costs, complaints about delay in service, discontent of professionals, and considerable rigidity and conservatism (Mechanic, 1968). Moreover as Freymann (1974) has shown, such a pyramidal system tends to exaggerate the prestige attractions of specialized medicine at the top of the pyramid, rather than attract able physicians to the bottom of the pyramid in personal contact with the health needs of most people, which should be the objective of personalistic medicine.

Alford (1975) points out that it is a mistake to think of the pluralist model as free enterprise and the centralized model as socialism. Because of the monopolistic control by the medical profession, the pluralist model is in fact a free enterprise system only in a very limited degree (Freidson, 1970). In such a model, health consumers are seldom in a position to make intelligent choices between competitive alternatives either because they lack information or because these alternatives are very limited (Burns, 1973).

On the other hand, the centralized model is by no means incompatible with a free enterprise system as it now operates in the United States (Fein, 1973; Beckhard, 1974; Spivak, 1975). The American way of life has moved toward a high degree of rationalization and monopoly in industry as well as in government. Such centralization, as Alford points out, has not changed the class structure of American society in any radical way. It would be perfectly possible to set up a centralized model in such a way as to leave a considerable choice to both the consumer and the provider. It could even include voluntary health insurance and fee-for-service features. What is essential to such a system is that it be centralized on a regional basis and bureaucratically planned.

Alford, as well as Smith and Kaluzny (1975), and Freymann in his own way (1974) suggest a third kind of model which Alford frankly calls utopian and Smith and Kaluzny call *participatory* (see also Rosengren and Lefton, 1969; Hydebrand, 1973). Such a model is based on the view that there must be planning (as in the centralized model), but this is not the same as a planned society (Arnold, 1971). In a planned society, whether it be governed by a democratic bureaucratic elite or by a Marxist bureaucratic elite, individuals have their health cared for, but lose any real control over how it is to be done. In a market system, individuals have scarcely more control because they lack the information or alternatives to choose from. What we need, therefore, according to those who seek a third model is a system in which consumers play a real role in the planning process (Sheps, 1974).

The great problem in adopting the participatory model is the resistance of health care professionals. They have been educated to believe that the maintenance of high-quality health care demands professional autonomy and forbids interference by laypersons. Freymann argues that such barriers to a participatory model can be overcome by a change in medical education to move the ideal of the physician away from the exclusively scientific model toward a more humanistic model. Indeed, a humanistic model is superior even scientifically because it relates the individual ecologically to the environment. Other researchers (Annas, 1973, 1975; Blum, 1964) believe that a participatory model can come about only by educating consumers to know and aggressively defend their rights. Our line of argument would lead to the conclusion that the essential steps to developing a participatory model are (1) assumption of responsibility by each person for his or her own health, (2) restoration of a sound professional-client relationship, and (3) education of medical professionals to be able to work in this relationship.

Some of the proposals for a national health care plan currently under discussion by the United States Congress emphasize the need for regional planning agencies or health systems agencies (HSA) which would list the resources and needs of a region and develop a plan to meet its needs. These regional plans would then be incorporated into statewide plans for health administered by state health coordinating councils (SHCC). Significantly, it is proposed that both regional and state health planning groups have a majority of consumers on each board.

Common Good

For Catholic health care professionals, the first step in seeking a better organization of health care in the United States and in the world must be to free themselves from the ideology that leads Americans to analyze every social issue in terms of the American free enterprise system and the tyranny of Socialism and Communism. Unfortunately most American Catholics have received a kind of religious education which tried to refute accusations that Catholics are un-American by an effort to identify Christian social teaching with the American way of life. Such identification of any human culture with the Gospel is certain to be misleading, since the Gospel stands as a prophetic criticism of every culture, approving some of its features but correcting others.

The authentic social teaching of the Catholic Church has been very fully formulated since Leo XIII's great encyclical *Rerum Novarum* (1891) in many papal encyclicals and documents and especially by the Second Vatican Council in *The Church in the Modern World* (1965c). While this teaching contains some strong criticisms of Marxist Socialism and Communism, chiefly on three grounds — (1) its atheistic materialism, (2) its denial of the right of private property, and (3) its tendency to totalitarian government — this teaching also contains a vigorous criticism of Capitalism on the grounds (1) of its deterministic reliance on economic laws, (2) of its advocacy of unregulated competition and the profit motive, and (3) of its neglect of the Christian advocacy of the poor. Recent documents such as John XXIII's *Mater et Magistra* (1961) and Paul VI's *The Development of Peoples* (1967) have pointed out that Capitalism and Communism alike have become colonializing powers either politically or economically and are thus largely responsible for the wars and poverty which oppress the great majority of humankind (Gremillion, 1976; Ashley, 1976). Christian health care professionals, therefore, should begin their thinking about the social organization of health care from the principles of the Gospel and not from the principles of the free enterprise system any more than from those of Socialism.

Apart from ideological bias, no one economic system anymore than any one political system is simply natural, right, or Christian. Such systems are human inventions, each with some advantages and some disadvantages, to be selected according to particular historical circumstances. We need to evaluate these merits both from a theoretical point of view and from a practical, experiential point of view. In judging them ethically, we must consider both their congruity with fundamental moral and Gospel principles and their pragmatic results in a given situation. A theoretically correct system may in some circumstances result in ethical disaster, while it is sometimes necessary to tolerate theoretically wrong institutions because they are the best that can be hoped for at the moment. However, in the long run, bad principles will have bad consequences, and we must constantly strive to test our understanding of principles by experience and to bring the real situation into line with these principles once they are refined.

Catholic health care professionals, therefore, have the responsibility at the present moment to study all proposals for universal comprehensive health care and attempt to judge them in terms of theoretical principles and practical experience. Such a study is beyond the scope of this book, but it may be useful to indicate the first steps in such an ethical inquiry.

Before the United States Congress at the present time are a number of plans for national health insurance (Burns, 1973; Prussin, 1977). All of them share the following basic concepts:

1. The principle of access to health care as a fundamental human right

2. Comprehensive coverage of all types of health problems, physical and mental

3. Emphasis on positive health, that is, on prevention of disease and promotion of optimum health

4. Emphasis on provision for quality care

5. Emphasis on the education of health care professionals

6. A method of financing generally in the direction of a national trust fund built up by a progressive tax based on ability to pay and without cost sharing by the actual recipient

7. Participation by both consumers and health care professionals in administration and planning of the system

The most conservative proposal, the Fulton Bill favored by the American Medical Association (AMA), is characterized by an attempt to retain some emphasis on the responsibility of the insured to pay according to ability and an avoidance of specifics concerning consumer participation, quality standards, and methods of expanding the education of health care professionals, matters in which the AMA wants to maintain professional autonomy.

How are we to judge these objectives ethically? Two principles relevant to this judgment have been propounded previously in this book: (1) every human being does have a fundamental right to health, as acknowledged in the *Universal Declaration of Human Rights* (United Nations, 1948), article 25, because human rights are based on essential human needs; and (2) individual persons have the primary responsibility to promote their own health but because we are social beings, also have the right to seek the help of others when necessary to fulfill this responsibility and reciprocally have the duty to give the same help to others as far as they are able.

The papal encyclicals and the Second Vatican Council have repeatedly proposed a universal social principle (of which this second proposition is only an application to health care) which is called the Principle of Subsidiarity or to put it more comprehensively the Principle of the Common Good and Subsidiarity (Messner, 1965). In 1.5 we argued that the dignity of the person both requires a community and is to be found in this communal sharing, or common good. Each individual, therefore, has a need and a moral obligation to contribute to the common good and a right to share in it.

Most social evils and injustices are the result of exclusion of some persons from the common good in which they have a right to share. The ancient evil of slavery was precisely such an unjust institution wherein the slaves contributed to the common good but were not permitted to share fully in it, not only in regard to economic goods, but also in regard to spiritual goods such as education, freedom, political participation, respect, and even the right to worship the gods of the city. Thus the distribution of the common good is a fundamental demand of social justice.

Jesus, moreover, taught an ethics that clearly went beyond even this demand for distributive justice based on merit (i.e., each receives in proportion as he contributes). Jesus proclaimed the coming of the Kingdom of God (Mark 1:15) which was not (as we sometimes think) merely a heavenly kingdom, but was also the fulfillment of the Old Testament prophecies of the Reign of God on earth (Gutierrez, 1973). When Jesus said to Pilate, "My kingship is not of this world" (John 18:36), he did not mean by "world," the earth, but the present sinful order of power struggle. He was saying to Pilate, "I am not competing with you power brokers. I am building a kingdom built on a different principle: on service, not on dominion." He taught his followers to pray, "Your Kingdom come, your will be done, on earth as it is in heaven" (Matt. 6:10). The Beatitudes (Luke 6:20-22; Matt. 5:3-11) in their original form were the joyful announcement to the poor (i.e., those excluded from the common good) that at last they were to be included in that common good, not only economically, but spiritually ("the poor have the good news preached to them") (Luke 7:22). Consequently, the principle of the early Church was "from each according to his ability, to each according to his needs," a principle which Karl Marx borrowed from the Acts of the Apostles (4:32-35). Thus the Principle of the Common Good requires love and mercy, and the distribution of the common good not according to merit, but according to need. Thus the mark of all Jesus' work was his concern for the neglected, the outcast, the leper, the prostitute, the Samaritan heretic, and the pagan unbeliever.

A Christian ethics of health care distribution must be based not on merit, and certainly not on the ability to pay, but on need, because the needy are most neglected: persons who can care for themselves do not need social help. Moreover, social oppression is the chief cause of their illness — an oppression from which the more affluent members of society profit. Hence those who are helpless by reason of poverty, disease, defect, or age (the unborn or the senile) should be the first consideration of any health plan.

Yet all persons should contribute to the plan according to their *ability*. Thus the social responsibility for health care falls first on those who have the ability to heal, the health care professionals, and second on those who have the ability to pay, that is, those who have financially profited the most from society. For such affluent individuals to claim that they have made their wealth simply by their own efforts is an absurdity. They may have worked hard, but their wealth would not have been possible exclusive of the society of which they are a part. Consequently, their debt to the common good is in proportion to the wealth they have received from it.

Subsidiarity

From this notion of the common good, the notion of subsidiarity follows logically. By *subsidiarity* is meant the first responsibility in meeting human needs rests with the free and competent individual, then with the local group. Higher and higher levels of the community must assume this responsibility (1) when the lower unit cannot assume it and (2) when the lower unit refuses to assume it.

Although all persons are primarily responsibile for their own health, when they cannot assume this responsibility, either because they are too young, too old, too poor, too uneducated, or possessed of any other defect, the community at higher and higher levels must come to their aid. If a lower level neglects to fulfill the responsibility, then a higher level must correct the oversight by punishment or other remedies. Yet the higher level should never be content merely to take over responsibility, but it must work to return responsibility to a lower level. Thus we should seek to educate people in personal health care and make it possible for them to pay for such care and to hold them responsible for neglecting it. The main objection to many social reforms has been that they have not provided for this progressive decentralization. For example, the welfare system in the United States has perpetuated poverty rather than helped the dependent to become independent.

Hence any program of socialized medicine must aim at preventive medicine, at achieving a healthier and healthier population of people who can care for themselves, rather than at an ever-increasing dependence of persons on technical medical care and professional help (Freymann, 1974). As Plato observed, "A society that is always going to the doctor is a sick society" (Republic III, 405A).

Functionalism

The popes have also stressed that one of the evils of historical Capitalism and Communism alike has been the tendency of both systems to concentrate all the power of decision making in the State. Before secular Humanism became the dominant philosophy of modern society, Christian thinking was able to bring about some practical recognition that a society is not simply a two-level structure of government and citizenry, but an organic community containing many functions which are mutually interdependent (Messner, 1965).

This conception of the mutual interdependence of a community was enunciated by St. Paul in I Corinthians 12-13 and connected by him with Jesus' teaching that the greatest should become the servants of the lowest in the Kingdom of God. Hence the power to make social decisions ought to be kept as close as possible to those who experience those problems and are most strongly affected by the decisions concerning them. Only in this way can the dignity of the least members of a community be acknowledged and their interests effectively served by the greater. A paternalism which decides everything for those it claims to serve is really nothing but a form of domination and tends to become self-serving. Hence St. Paul, without directly attacking slavery, admonished the master that he should treat his slave not like a child, but like a "most dear brother" (Philemon v. 16), that is, as equal by reason of their mutual interdependence in Christ.

Hence the Principle of Subsidiarity requires us to share decision-making power not only at various vertical levels of local, state, and federal government, but also among horizontal sectors representing various functional bodies. Thus education as a basic function of society forms a body of persons, some of whom have expertness (the educators) and others of whom (the students) are trying to educate themselves through the services of the experts. Decisions about education pertain in the first place not to government but to bodies of cooperating teachers and students mutually dependent on each other. The same holds true for other basic social functions, especially for the economy, with its interdependence of management, workers, and consumers, as well as for the social organization of health care with its mutual interdependence of professional healers and health seekers. Each person in a society is related to as many such functional bodies as he or she has basic needs. The role of government is to coordinate and encourage the full development of these different organs of society, not to deprive them of their decision-making capacity.

This application of subsidiarity to the organization of society on the basis of social functions rather than on the basis of a struggle between isolated individuals defending their rights and a centralized government having all the powers of social decision in Catholic documents is usually called *corporatism*. This term is somewhat misleading for Americans for whom corporations are usually conceived as purely economic organizations. The term has also been discredited because it has been used by Fascist political parties in Europe to win Catholic support for its exact opposite, namely, totalitarianism, or total state power. We shall use instead the term *functionalism*.

Functionalism is opposed on the one hand to Communism and national Socialism (like that of Mussolini and Hitler) because they are totalitarian, concentrating all decision-making power in the hands of the State and the Military, and it is opposed on the other hand to the competitive individualism of unregulated Capitalism or free enterprise with its hidden tendency to monopolism with the resultant concentration of decision-making power in the hands of an interlocking power elite (Mills, 1956) or industrial-military complex of which President Eisenhower warned. Functionalism is not a mere theory, since it has had a powerful influence through Catholic statesmen on the formation of the European common market and of codetermination (Messner, 1965) by management and labor in Germany and other countries. Some of its implications are also evident in Latin America in the efforts of Catholic theologians and political leaders to develop a theology of liberation which is not Capitalist, Fascist, or Marxist (Gutierrez, 1973).

Politically, it might seem that functionalism would have little chance of adoption in the United States. However, certain features of some of our institutions are in fact functionalist. For example, higher education in the United States, in contrast to the statism of the lower school system, remains largely functionalist. Decisions about educational policies in our colleges and universities are made independently of government by faculties and accrediting agencies and by the right of students to choose their own schools. The student revolt of the 1960s, however, seemed to show that schools needed to admit students to a greater participation in making policies, and to a certain extent this has taken place, rendering the system still more functionalist. On the other hand, the increasing control of the government over schools by reason of their economic dependency is working strongly to destroy their functionalist character.

Similarly, after the Great Depression the growth of labor unions in this country, to a considerable degree under the influence of Catholic social thought (Messner, 1965; Abell, 1968), promised the eventual development of functionalism in the economic sphere. Unfortunately, the unions have largely neglected the social aspects of their original purpose and have been co-opted by the Capitalist market system in which they are becoming just another monopoly. Fortunately, we see some signs of a reversal of this trend in the growth of consumerism, participatory democracy, and social ecology, as well as in the increasing dissatisfaction with the resulting liberal reforms, so many of which have served only to enlarge the power of government bureaucracy. Catholics need to take advantage of this growing criticism of the so-called American way of life to propose a more personalistic and functionalist conception of society.

As regards health care, these general ethical principles of subsidiarity and functionalism have to be applied to the concrete historical situation of American medical institutions. The medical profession as it has operated in this country has been influenced by three not very consistent principles: first, there survives in medicine the ancient ideal of a profession as service which was formulated in the Hippocratic oath and reinforced by Christianity; second, there is the philosophy of secular Humanism with its strong emphasis on human rights and the duty of man to use scientific knowledge to solve human problems; and third, there is the ideology of Capitalism which has been fostered by Humanism. This Capitalist ideology is seen by many liberal secularists to be at odds with their concern for human rights and the full application of the social sciences to the planning of economic and political life, but it is defended by conservative secularists as at least preferable to the philosophy of Marxism.

As a result of these inherent contradictions, our present system of health care is now in transition it would seem from Alford's pluralist model to his centralized or regional model. Thus it is likely that some type of national health care program will be enacted, but that efforts will also be made to retain some features of pluralism that will protect the autonomy of the profession and some play of market forces to regulate consumer demand and prices. The current debate is largely about this question of mix.

In view of Christian goals a Catholic should be particularly aware of the lessons of experience in our country. The first of these is that the pluralist system did not adequately care for the poor, nor did it do much about positive health improvement. It tended to an exaggerated professional elitism, to place strong emphasis on monopolization and the profit motive, and it never produced a system of medical education that was personalistic. On the other hand, the pluralist system should be credited with promoting very rapid technological and scientific progress and with developing a great number of health care facilities equipped to give high-quality care. However, it must also be noted that this progress has led to greater expenditure of resources on the sophisticated treatment of relatively rare ailments than to better care for the health of the majority.

A centralized system is aimed at correcting some of these defects, but not in a very radical manner. Such a system will probably greatly increase bureaucratization which, as we have experienced in our welfare system, can cost a great deal and accomplish very litttle. A centralized system will provide more health care, but there is no certainty it will promote better health. Nor is a bureaucracy likely to personalize the health care it gives. Even if a sincere effort is made under this system to humanize medicine, such effort will not be guided by a Christian conception of the person, but by a secular humanist conception which, as we have so sadly experienced, may express itself not in concern for the neglected, but in their extermination by abortion or euthanasia.

It seems, therefore, that while Christians should favor a national health care program as the only practical way available to extend care to the neglected of our society, they should not have any illusions about the adequacy of such programs. To oppose national comprehensive health care in the reactionary way in which some Catholics fought the labor unions, the Child Labor Amendment, the United Nations, and the Equal Rights Amendment because such reforms are favored by secular humanists of the liberal wing only gives support to the secular humanists of the conservative wing whose views are even less compatible with Catholic social principles. Instead, Christians should support the new schemes for national comprehensive health care critically, stressing the need to incorporate into these plans as many functionalist features as possible. For example:

1. Comprehensive health care should aim primarily at the promotion of positive health, not merely at the cure of acute disease or the prolongation of life through sophisticated techniques. Therefore, it should work for (a) removal of the environmental and social causes of ill health including the commercial encouragement of unhealthy patterns of living and (b) provision of preventive health education which will give persons control over their own health.

2. Priority should be given to the problems of the most powerless, poorly informed, and least able to pay. These persons should not be cared for paternalistically, but should be admitted at once to participate in the power of decision about their own health needs.

3. Decision-making power should not be confined to a government bureaucracy, nor to autonomous professionals, but should be shared by all concerned in mutual interdependence.

4. Planning should proceed in such a way as to avoid tendencies to increase dependence upon higher levels and to promote a gradually increasing decentralization both in control and funding. However, this decentralization should not be used as an excuse for the government to neglect the monitoring of health care and the supplementation and correction of defects at lower levels of organization.

5. Planning must be a continuous process of decision making that adapts to experience and new needs, rather than a fixed plan based on projections that may be mistaken.

Christians may find support for various items of a functionalist program from different and opposed ideological camps. For example, liberals interested in ecology are convinced that environmental and social factors play the major role in poor health conditions, but conservatives also use this fact to defend the medical profession against the charge that it is responsible for these conditions. Again, the rights of health consumers are defended by liberals interested in civil rights and consumerism, but they are also defended by conservative individualists who believe that the free market is the best method of controlling health costs. Consequently, Christians should attempt to transcend ideological biases and work through a strategy of coalition to promote particular goals.

Above all, Christians should attempt to influence health education of the people and the medical education of the professionals, especially through our Catholic schools, medical schools, and teaching hospitals, toward a personalistic understanding of health and the objectives of the medical profession. We must also work to protect our Catholic institutions against the many current forces which tend to absorb them into the centralized, bureaucratic structure of our society dominated by secular Humanism. At the same time, we should approach secular humanists in a genuinely ecumenical spirit, seeking through dialogue to find grounds of agreement and cooperation.

The ethical principle underlying all such efforts to organize our society including its health care institutions in such a way as to counteract tendencies to totalitarian bureaucratism on the one hand and competitive individualism on the other can be summarily formulated in the following *Principle of the Common Good, Subsidiarity, and Functionalism*:

> A community exists to promote and share the common good among all its members "from each according to ability, to each according to need" in such a way (1) that decision making rests vertically first with the person, then with lower social levels, and horizontally with functional social units, and (2) that the higher social units intervene only to supply whatever lower units cannot supply, while working to make it easier for lower units and individual persons to achieve independent capability in the future.

6.2   LIMITS TO HEALTH CARE

If we are to make a sufficiently prophetic and radical critique of our American health system, we must give special attention to a theme which is now becoming prominent in popular discussion.

A characteristic feature of the 1960s and 1970s has been the growing criticism of the ideal of unlimited technological progress and of the modern concept of specialism in the learned disciplines and the practical professions. A "crisis of limits" is occurring in both the democratic and Marxist countries. This crisis is not easy for truebelievers in these value systems to endure, and they tend to react by claiming that the critics are reactionary opponents of progress. Actually the critics are not opposed to progress, but to the myth of progress, to an illusory concept of the nature of human progress.

Thus, Ivan Illich in his highly controversial book *Medical Nemesis* (1976) argues that Marx was correct in distinguishing between "exchange values" as a measure of welfare and "use values." Illich attempts to show that although modern industrial society has enormously increased the production of exchangeable goods (measured as the gross national product or GNP) it has in some respects been even less effective than preindustrial society in satisfying basic human needs. Nevertheless, he does not propose that we abandon scientific technology, but rather advocates that we select and develop technologies which will meet needs economically instead of increasing production of exchangeable goods at the expense of limited energy resources.

Illich chooses to study modern medicine because it is commonly cited as outstanding proof of the success of technology based on the industrial type. He attempts to deflate this claim by using two arguments. First, he argues that the success of modern medicine is based on two achievements: (1) increased life expectancy and (2) improved patient comfort in the absence of cure. The former achievement, he explains, is primarily a result of the reduction of epidemics by immunization, antibiotic drugs, and improved hygiene, that is, relatively simple technologies. The whole elaborate system of hospitalization, however, has had little effect on life expectancy and is enormously and increasingly expensive. The latter achievement, Illich insists, results in an "anesthetized culture" in which people do not know how to integrate suffering into personal growth, while in fact the quality of their life is not notably improved.

Second, he argues that modern medicine is actually producing as much poor health as it heals. These iatrogenic diseases take three forms: (1) clinical iatrogenesis produced by drugs, unnecessary surgery, and other harmful remedies administered by physicians and hospitals, (2) social iatrogenesis produced by encouraging people to become consumers of doubtful medical remedies rather than by changing the morbid social conditions that cause their ills, especially the inequitable distribution of health care, and (3) cultural iatrogenesis in the form of symbolic, psychological effects on the way persons perceive their bodily life as something meaningless in both its pleasures and suffering, as something to be possessed and used and manipulated, rather than as part of their person which has to live, grow, die, and be transcended.

The response to Illich's criticism usually has been to agree that his arguments are largely valid, but to claim they have already been recognized by the medical profession (Geiger, 1976). Illich does not deny this: in fact, he has drawn heavily on certain critics within the medical establishment. Warwick (1976) sarcastically comments that Illich himself has contributed a fourth kind of iatrogenesis, namely, "critical iatrogenesis which can be defined as a sense of unease growing out of a generalized suspicion of medicine and its practioners" (p. 572). But Illich believes these criticisms have not yet had much practical effect. He concludes that there is more hope for the future in undeveloped countries of the Third World which have the opportunity to adopt a more rational technology directed to human needs than in the advanced countries of the First and Second Worlds which will have to reverse their cultures.

Whatever the future may be, there can be no doubt that in the United States the health care profession must seriously face up to the problem of *limits*. Our problems will never be solved simply by national health care plans if (as in other systems of socialized medicine in Europe) they allow ever-mounting costs of health care such as the five hundred percent rise of per diem hospital costs for a patient since 1959. It is not surprising that a similar crisis exists in transportation or in energy in general or in population growth where the necessity of limits are admitted by all, in spite of the fact that limitation demands radical readjustments in American culture.

6.3   THE HOSPITAL AS COMMUNITY

Cure and Care

So far in this chapter we have seen that the social organization of health care in the United States is and probably will remain pluralistic, although it requires more careful planning to meet the needs of all within the limits of our resources. Now we must turn to consider the structure and function of the basic units from which this system is built. At present these units in which health care is concentrated are hospitals and medical centers dedicated primarily to the treatment of acute diseases.

On entering a great modern hospital we find ourselves in a world of its own: a strange community in which most members remain only a few days, but in which some live for months and years, and where life begins for some and ends for others. Today some critics of our system urge that we reverse the trend to concentrate health care in hospitals by developing neighborhood health centers and other facilities designed to care for ambulatory patients. Others contend this would only make things worse by fragmenting health care. J. G. Freymann (1974) believes we should work with existing hospitals but transform them into "mission oriented" institutions which would retain the advantage of a concentration of resources, but which would at the same time serve as centers of ambulatory care and preventive medicine for a wide community.

In any case, although it seems that the modern trend to hospitalize everyone who needs medical care is being gradually reversed, for the immediate future the hospital will remain the main context of health care (Freidson, 1963). It is therefore necessary to raise some questions about the ethical implications of the hospital as a human community.

According to Sigerist (1960a) the hospital evolved historically in three stages. First, the Romans established hospitals for soldiers and for work gangs of slaves for the purpose of maintaining manpower for special tasks. Second, eastern Christians instituted *xenodochia* (guesthouses) or hospitals (hotels, inns) for the poor, a development paralleled in older religions only by the Buddhists in the second century B.C. under the emperor Atoka (Glaser, 1970b). These hospitals were copied and further developed by the Muslim conquerors of portions of the Byzantine Empire, and the Muslim hospitals in turn inspired Western

Christians in the time of the Crusades to new efforts. These medieval institutions usually did not supply medical care in the strict sense, but only nursing and spiritual comfort. By the Renaissance, however, Christian hospitals were regularly visited by physicians and sometimes even became retirement homes for the rich. Third, in the eighteenth and ninteenth centuries the Christian hospitals were gradually replaced by modern public and private hospitals, generally under the inspiration of Enlightenment Humanism with its emphasis on scientific technology and the free enterprise system. Thus historically the line of development has been from an emphasis on care to one on cure.

Considerable sociological effort has been devoted to understanding this typical modern institution into which perhaps as much as eight percent of our national income is poured each year (Friedson, 1963; Rosengren, 1969; Heydebrand, 1973). It seems to be a curious mixture of several types of organization (Sloane and LeRoy, 1977).

1. It retains something of its original character as a hotel or temporary residence, with the primary function of care and custody. This purpose is most pronounced in the impaired model wherein the hospital becomes a permanent or long-term residence, approaching a total institution of the sort studied in Erving Goffman's well-known work *Asylums* (1962). As such, it is divided into the *hosts* (the administration and staff) who care for the *guests* (the patients).

2. It is also a place of cure in which the medical staff provides diagnosis and treatment for the patients. Thus it consists not only of hosts and guests, but also of *healers* and *sick*.

3. Finally, it is usually also a school in which there are *teachers* and *researchers* (overlapping roles, as in any modern university) with their *students* and *research staffs*. The students are engaged both in class work and in supervised clinical practice, and some are interns and residents in actual full-time practice.

Especially interesting is the fact that the nurses are, as it were, at the point of intersection of all these functions (Freymann, 1974). They are often themselves students in training, but they also are those who care, that is, the persons who actually carry out the host function of the hospital. At the same time nurses are an essential part of the medical staff engaged in cure, since it is they who execute many of the treatment procedures and cooperate closely with physicians in observing patients and monitoring treatments.

Today the organizational complexity of the hospital is further intensified by the fact that the hospital is becoming a governmental agency for the administration of public funds for health care. As such, it is also staffed with social workers who help patients return to the wider community. Thus the hospital today becomes one of the principal formative institutions of our society, providing a model community which is bound to affect the average American's understanding of social and personal interrelationships very profoundly. This is evidenced by the mythical power which television dramas about life in a hospital seem to exercise on the American imagination.

A Healing Community

If the modern hospital is to perform these varied functions effectively it has to solve a number of basic ethical questions. In discussing total institutions Goffmann (1962) has shown that a prison, a small village, or a monastery can never be really total, because it lacks the resources to satisfy all human needs. If it is not to foster regressive behavior in its inmates, it must find ways to be open to wider influences. The medieval monasteries found it necessary to develop a complex internal life enriched by the practice of hospitality which made them centers of communication rather than mere enclosures from the world.

Hence hospitals in the impaired model in which patients remain for long periods have two special obligations. First, they must make a constant effort to find ways in which their inmates can retain contact with the life of the outside world and can engage in a variety of stimulating and enriching experiences and occupations. Second, they must find ways to involve patients in some genuine participation in making the decisions which affect their own lives. Obviously, senile or mentally disturbed patients may have little capacity for such participation, but too often this incapacity has been fostered by patterns of institutional life which have given them no opportunity to express their preferences or to take at least some responsibility for themselves and others.

Today, largely because of the inflation of health costs, great efforts are being made to reduce the time of hospitalization for surgical patients and even for acutely ill patients, so that now the average patient residence is less than a week. What needs to be emphasized, however, is that this is not only less costly, but also better therapeutically and ethically. There is an ethical responsibility of the hospital not to disrupt the home life of patients. While the sick have the right to be relieved of many ordinary social obligations, they need to be helped to experience sickness as a part of life, not as an interruption in living.

Consequently, in spite of inconveniences to the staff, today better hospitals no longer discourage visitors, not even small children, but try to find ways to facilitate continued family contact and opportunities for the family to share in the therapeutic process. Similarly, when their condition or convalescence permits, patients should be encouraged to be of assistance to their fellow patients. The sense of isolation, abandonment, and helplessness is perhaps the most traumatic aspect of being sick, but sickness can also be an important occasion to draw people together in a shared effort of healing.

Such patient participation also requires that patients have a choice as to when they get up in the morning and retire, what they eat and wear, when they should receive visitors, and who these visitors should be. Today within necessary limits hospital care provides for such freedom, but there must also be a constant, imaginative effort to enlarge the scope of patients' activities which should be measured not by the convenience of the hospital staff, but by therapeutic and human values.

Moreover the external public should also share in making the policies by which the hospital is governed as a public institution. At some time most members of the public will have to use a hospital, and all have an interest in the kind of institution their taxes and gifts support.

In stressing the ethical significance of hospitalization as a part of life rather than as a mere interruption, we also acknowledge that hospitalization in some cases legitimately serves as a *retreat* from the destructive aspects of modern life into a quiet and healing atmosphere. Alvin Toffler in his well-known *Future Shock* (1970) shows how the pace of change in modern life demands such retreats to give people a chance to assimilate novelty. Monasteries have always provided such places of retreat for spiritual reflection, and the spa or watering place and summer resorts serve for secular retreats. The risk of using hospitals for this purpose is that such withdrawal may promote neurotic regression. However, they can also provide what Kris (1964) calls "a controlled regression in the service of the ego" apparent in the lives of many creative people, that is, an opportunity to put aside temporarily the responsibilities of active life for a process of recollection, psychodelic expansion, and reintegration of personality. However, the average noisy or even frightening and depressing hospital seldom provides such an opportunity.

The communal orientation of a hospital which we have described is primarily patient centered, but the patients will not be treated as persons if the professionals who care for them are themselves alienated by feelings that their own needs are neglected or their rights infringed. These professionals invest a great part of their lives and energy in the life of the hospital and are rightly convinced that they have special rights based on their dedication, expert knowledge, and experienced judgment.

Perhaps the most important of these professional rights is the autonomy of professional judgment. Physicians need to be free to examine their patients and to order the treatment they think best. Nurses need to feel that their responsibility for their patients is just as professional as that of physicians. How can this necessary autonomy be reconciled with the communal character of the hospital as an institution? Can the hospital administration permit physicians to use their facilities or require cooperation of nursing personnel for purposes which in the administration's judgment are either unprofessional or unethical, for example, abortion or sterilization? In chapter 9 we will discuss some of the concrete ethical questions that may arise.

However, generally speaking it is clear that prima facie professional freedom in health care insititutions, like academic freedom in universities, must be vigilantly protected. The hospital administration's duty is (1) to ascertain the competency of all professionals it admits to its staff and (2) to bring to the attention of a professional's peers any evidence or complaint about unprofessional or unethical behavior. If these peers fail to maintain standards, then the administration has no recourse but to act itself to terminate relations with the offender. The procedures to be followed in such cases should be clearly stated in the written policies and contracts of the institution.

The hospital administration not only has such disciplinary responsibilities, but it also has a positive duty to unify the multiple functions of the institution in a manner which permits both the patients and the staff to form a truly human community and not merely a "health factory." Faulty communications between physicians, nurses, auxiliaries, and administration and within these subgroups produce an atmosphere of tension very deleterious to the hospital's services which can directly affect the psychosomatic health of the patients, especially in mental hospitals. Modern administrative and communications theory provides important resources for improving such situations provided that they are used as tools to achieve ethically acceptable goals and not merely to oil an impersonal machine.

Finally, as the inflation of health care costs continues, many ethical questions arise from the economic policies of hospitals reflecting the severe pressures from which they suffer. Here two important patient rights come into question: the right to emergency care and the right to treatment once the patient is admitted. Annas (1975) shows that the courts have generally upheld the legal obligation of hospitals with emergency wards (and even of those not so equipped to the extent of their resources) to care promptly for all persons who come to them in serious need of medical attention and to continue to care for them until they are ambulatory or can safely be transferred to another hospital which is willing to receive them. He also shows that the courts are beginning to develop a doctrine on the rights of patients in so-called custodial institutions to treatment as well as to care. Christian and Humanist ethics both have accepted the teaching of the parable of the good Samaritan (Luke 10:25-37), but it is necessary in public institutions that this concern for our neighbor be given legal enforcement.

All these ethical and legal questions, which arise from the ideal of the hospital as a community of care and cure faced with the realities of modern depersonalized and competitive society, can be solved only at the price of an unremitting effort to give priority to persons over institutions and properties. Every hospital suffers from the proliferation of bureaucratic rules intended to protect the institution from exploitation by the crazy or the crafty. This red tape designed to protect the ideal purposes of the hospital soon convert it into a machine destructive of patients and staff. The chief remedy against this ever-present danger is the training of the staff to deal with borderline situations in a flexible and prudent manner and to provide a variety of methods by which self-criticism can be promoted and criticism from outside can be heard. To achieve this interplay within the staff, it is necessary to develop the staff not merely as a hierarchical structure of command responsibility, but as an interacting *health team*.

6.4   THE HEALTH TEAM

Physicians and Co-Workers

Because of the highly specialized character of modern medicine, health seekers must entrust themselves not to a single physician within the hospital, but to a *health team* (Sloane and LeRoy, 1977). The medical staff of such a team may include physicians, dentists, podiatrists, and psychologists and perhaps paramedics or medical assistants. The nursing staff will include registered nurses, practical nurses, and aides and perhaps nursing unit managers and nursing clerks. The medical departments will include physicians who are pathologists, along with many kinds of medical technologists (e.g., specialists in hematology, chemistry, microbiology, serology, histology, and cytology), other physicians who are radiologists and radiation therapists with their assistants, other technicians in encephalography and electrocardiography, and finally therapists skilled in occupation and physical therapy. They will be supplemented also by a social service department staffed by medical social work professionals, a pharmacy, a dietary department, and a health science library. In addition, there will be persons in charge of patient services such as admissions, hospital records, environmental services (housekeeping), laundry, and purchasing. The business services department involves admissions, accounting, budgeting, and credit and collection, and the buildings are cared for by a plant department.

Personnel and public relations departments are essential to secure and care for this complex body of skilled people, and the whole institution requires an elaborate administration, with its governing board and administrative staff. Finally, a health care facility makes use of the services of such outside professionals as architects, accountants, attorneys, special consultants, and sales representatives.

We have given this (incomplete) list of the various diversified professional and subprofessional roles required in a modern health care facility to make clear that any patient entering a hospital is confronted with a small army of persons who are supposed to serve the patient, but with whom the patient must deal and from whom, perhaps, the patient must protect himself or herself.

In this section we will discuss only the health team in the somewhat narrower sense of those members with whom the patient must deal very directly — the physician, the nurse, and the social worker — in order to inquire what reciprocal ethical obligations exist between the patient and these three kinds of professionals. We will then discuss the issue of the protection of the patient's rights by some type of advocate.

Traditionally the chief power of decision in any health team belongs to a licensed physician, the M.D. Supposedly licensure guarantees that physicians have the basic, integral knowledge of the human body and its essential life processes which will make it possible for them to be reasonably certain about a patient's condition and therefore able to decide (1) what emergency care is necessary and (2) what should *not* be done to the patient without further examination. Consequently, no serious step toward treating the patient can be taken without a physician's permission. Of course, in fact much emergency care is provided by first-aid persons who may have very limited training, but it is generally conceded that any patient has the right to be seen by a physician as quickly as possible (Annas, 1975).

Today the concept of the licensed medical doctor as a general practioner has been vastly altered by the growth of medical specialization. Selig Greenberg (1965) says that in 1950 only about thirty-six percent of physicians in private practice were specialists, while today about seventy percent are specialists. This growth is not clearly related to patient needs. There are too many surgeons and only about thirty percent of the required number of radiologists and psychiatrists, forty percent of anesthetists, and fifty percent of pathologists. This imbalance is largely the result of decisions by the physicians themselves who prefer a particular type of work because it is interesting, convenient, prestigious, or profitable. The possibility of a free choice of specialities is one of the features of free enterprise medicine most valued by the profession.

This rapid decline of the general practitioneer as the primary care professional has deprived patients of the advantages of having their health problems evaluated by someone who knows the patient in his or her family context over a long period and who thinks of the patient as a whole person with a continuous biography. Recently there is a trend among medical students to specialize in family medicine as a way to reconcile specialization with an interest in primary care. Otherwise, primary care is usually given by a specialist in internal medicine for adults and by a pediatrician for children.

Another approach to this problem is the diagnostic clinic in which a patient is examined in an orderly manner by a whole crew of specialists who then attempt to synthesize their findings so as to get a total understanding of the patient. Again, efforts have been made to encourage patients to have an annual checkup which can be done in a clinic and may even be largely computerized, so that the patient's health is continuously monitored and problem areas identified for further study and treatment.

None of these developments seem as yet to provide a completely satisfactory answer to the problem of how to provide the kind of primary health care which will keep the total person in clear focus while making use of all the advantages of specialized knowledge and skill.

Nurses, Social Workers, and Patient Advocates

Perhaps the key to this difficulty is to be found in a better understanding of the proper role of the nurse, which today has become very ambiguous. Originally, the nurse was the person most concerned with caring for the patient and in continuous contact with the patient. Therefore, in the patient-centered type of health care which we have been advocating in this book it would seem that the nurse is the *central* professional figure, not the physician. Primary care is the nurse's task, not that of a general practitioner, family specialist, or whatnot.

Nurses, however, have been burdened with other tasks. For long they spent much of their energy in housekeeping chores — making beds, carrying trays, and so forth. Today they have been largely relieved of these tasks by auxiliaries, but they are still much occupied with technical tasks: temperature taking, injections, medications, intravenous feeding. Moreover they are oppressed by the sexism implicit in the notion that caring is a maternal role suitable for women (Glaser, 1970b). This sexism is reflected in the fact that until recently women physicians were a small minority, while in the Soviet Union and other countries they are equal in number to men physicians. Fortunately, this trend is now reversing, and there may be as high as thirty percent of physicians within the next generation in the United States who will be women. This freeing of medicine from sexism would also be furthered if men were encouraged to enter the nursing profession in larger numbers.

Under present circumstances, however, as nursing education has advanced, able women nurses have sought administrative and teaching posts as the only way of advancement open to them. However, they would find nursing itself much more interesting if it became the real focus of health care, so that the role of the nurse, female or male, in direct contact with the patient was seen as primary care and the real source of unity in the health team. Then the nurse assigned to a given patient would become the authority having responsibility for the patient as a person who would assist the patient in making use of all the resources furnished by the health team.

This personalistic, mediating function today is often performed by the medical or psychiatric social worker. The sociological study of the medical profession led to the acknowledgment of the great importance of the social dimension in treating disease. Hence, persons trained in social process were added to healing teams. The social worker interviews patients to discover possible social factors of ethnic culture, economic status, and family structure which may have caused the disease, which may hinder treatment, or which may prevent rehabilitation. Commonly, such workers help patients as regards both their legal rights and their opportunities for public financial assistance and other matters connected with illness. They also act as liaison with the patient's family and help find ways to assure family stability in the absence of the patient from the home. Finally, social workers undertake the patient's reentry into society. In the case of psychiatric patients, this involvement is of major importance since reentry into normal life is difficult for mental patients and may lead to recommittal.

When we compare the role of the social worker with that of the nurse, we see that the social worker is chiefly concerned with patients in their normal life patterns and the nurse with patients undergoing the actual experience of sickness and healing. Consequently, these two roles are very closely connected and together constitute primary care in the strict sense of direct concern with the patient as a person. The physician's role, on the other hand, is more specialized since it is focused precisely on the diagnosis and treatment of a pathological condition or its future prevention. If this analysis is correct, it should be clear that the physician cannot be the sole decision maker in the health team. Rather the patient has the ultimate decision and is helped in this decision in the first place by the nurse and social worker who are acquainted with patients in their total personalities and life situations, in the second place by the primary care physician, and in the third place by various specialist physicians.

Recently, some hospitals are beginning also to recognize the need for *pastoral care*, not as an occasional intervention of religious ministry from outside the institution by a visiting clergyman, nor as a convenience for patients who wish religious ministration by a resident chaplain, but as a regular part of patient care, since all patients religious or secular have problems of ultimate concern which affect the success of the healing process. We will discuss this issue at length in chapter 14. Suffice it here to say that pastoral care has to be closely linked to the role of the nurse and the social worker, since it adds depth to their firsthand concern for the patient as a person.

For reasons already discussed in chapters 4 and 5, physicians will not find it easy to reconcile their proper professional autonomy with the requirements of teamwork or to relinquish the idea that they have sole decision-making power in health care while all others are merely their executive assistants. We might compare the readjustment necessary in their education and self-identity to that which Catholic priests are being forced to undergo since the Second Vatican Council. If the health team concept is to have real significance, physicians must, along with priests, come to acknowledge that they need the help of others not only in carrying out decisions, but also in making them if the people they serve are to be well served.

Recently the new profession of paramedic or medical assistant is being developed. This new role can be defined in two ways. For some, a paramedic is merely a substitute for a physician justified by the so-called doctor shortage and a medical assistant is merely a technician. Others, however, see a place for subdivision of the physician's work into several roles of a professional character, but not all demanding the full competency of a physician. In this last conception, medical assistants may share in decision-making processes and not merely in technical execution, nor are they mere emergency substitutes.

Another aspect of the health team concept is the question of the defense of patients' rights. Recently there has been much argument that patients need an *ombudsman* (Cavalier, 1970; Ravich and Rehr, 1974; Bredell, 1976) or "patient's advocate" (Annas, 1973, 1975; Annas and Healey, 1974) to support patients in their efforts to insist on adequate care (McQuillan, 1965; Freese, 1975). Annas (1973) conceives this role as an adversary one and insists that for this advocacy to have teeth the advocate must be recognized by the hospital as having (1) full access to medical records, (2) ability to call in consultants, (3) *ex officio* participation in hospital quality-of-health-care committees, (4) power to lodge complaints directly with the hospital executive committee, and (5) access to all patient support services.

Others are not ready to go this far and favor instead a patient's representative (Laetz, 1969; Emrich, 1971; Lockerby, 1973; Clapp, et al., 1975; Fry and Miller, 1975) whose role is primarily to improve communications within the health care institution (Mary Modesta, 1970). Others have experimented with patient councils (Rouse, 1971) or patient care conferences (Kravitz, 1974), all of which are devices to improve communication within the health team and between patients and the team.

It seems a mistake to confuse the notion of patients' advocate or ombudsman, which pertains to the strictly ethical dimension and is most properly a task for a lawyer, with the notion of patients' representative. The latter role seems proper to the work of the nurse, the social worker, and the pastoral care person who have to do with primary care and who mediate between the patient and the rest of the health team. They would inform patients of the availability of the advocate and call the advocate in to help all patients who believe their rights may be imperiled.

6.5   THE CATHOLIC HOSPITAL

Catholic Identity

Catholic hospitals were founded principally by religious orders of sisters and brothers to give health care especially to the neglected and in countries where Catholicism was not the chief religion as a means to ensure that the ethical and spiritual aspects of health care would be available in accordance with Catholic values. Today in the United States, the dominance of secular Humanism as a philosophy of life has so influenced and pressured the operation of such Catholic institutions that many wonder whether these institutions are any longer Catholic in any significant respect.

What characterizes a Catholic hospital? In the United States such a hospital has several obvious characteristics.

1. It has a Christian and Catholic ministry and therefore receives apostolic direction from the bishop of the diocese. Under his guidance and interpretation, it follows the *Ethical and Religious Directives for Catholic Health Care Facilities* (1971) approved by the United States Catholic Conference (the secretariat of the National Conference of Catholic Bishops), which outlines the proper spiritual care patients should receive, the duties of the hospital as a representative of the Catholic Church, and the medical procedures prohibited in Catholic health care facilities. The fact that a medicoethical rule (e.g., concerning abortion and sterilization) is contained in the *Directives* does not give it any greater doctrinal validity than it already had as a part of the ordinary teaching of the Church. Many of the ethical problems presented in this book are treated in the *Directives*, but not some of the more recent issues such as transsexual surgery and behavior control. The *Directives* were last revised in 1971, and suggestions for future revisions may be sent to the United States Catholic Conference through the bishop of the diocese.

2. A Catholic hospital is usually operated by a religious community of sisters or brothers who furnish some of the administrative and nursing staff and who have basic financial ownership and responsibility.

3. It has the name of a Catholic institution and commonly seeks charitable funding on this ground.

4. It has at least a priest chaplain (resident or nonresident) who conducts regular mass in the hospital and is responsible for sacramental administration and even pastoral counseling of the patients and staff.

5. Many of the physicians and nurses and even administrators are Catholics or must accept Catholic ethical norms. This is less and less true in many localities both because of the number of non-Catholics on the staff and because of public funding.

6. Such institutions usually are marked by various Catholic symbols,

statues, pictures, crucifixes in the rooms, evidence of some sisters and the chaplain in religious clothing, and so forth.

All of these characteristics (even the last) are more than superficial. They express the character of the hospital as a ministry of the Catholic Church, based on a conception of the interrelation of the whole person in all the biological, psychological, ethical, and spiritual dimensions dealt with in this book.

However, there is something deeper. Catholics essentially conceive of the healing ministry as an extension of the ministry of Christ (O'Rourke, 1974a; Futrell, 1977). Jesus was prophet or teacher, king or shepherd, and priest or sanctifier. The Second Vatican Council has taught that this threefold ministry should be reflected in all the works of the Church and in every member. Healing is part of the shepherding function of the Christian community, since to build this community we must be concerned with each weak member who needs restoration to vital life and participation.

Jesus healed people radically by penetrating to the spiritual core of the human personality and liberating the person from original or social sin and also from individual, personal sin, with the more superficial but real effect of healing them also psychologically and physically. A Christian hospital, therefore, is also concerned with the radical healing of those for whom it cares. The experience of sickness and healing in such a hospital should be also an experience of personal spiritual growth through suffering and redemption.

What should make a Catholic hospital a special kind of community and a model for other healing communities is that its members, both professionals and patients, are clearly aware of the presence of Christ the Healer in the midst of the community making use of his ministers — physicians, nurses, technicians, administrators, and patients in relation to each other — in his work of healing. This presence of Christ should also be celebrated ritually through the sacraments and proclaimed through the word of Scripture and of preaching, with Christ's promise of renewed life more powerful than death.

Such a religious conception of a health care institution need not weaken but should enhance its competence in all the arts and sciences of modern medicine. In a secular Humanist hospital, which is usually considered nonreligious, the vital principle is in fact the value system of secular Humanism which we described in 1.3, with its dedication to scientific progress, its concern for human rights, and its faith in the power of human reason and human cooperative effort to overcome sickness. Without that commitment to Humanist ideals, a secular hospital becomes a depersonalized machine which hurts as much as it heals. In the same way, unless a Catholic hospital gets its vitality from its own religious faith and system of values, it will become more hurtful than healing, a scandal, rather than a witness of Christ's presence in a suffering world.

Christian Identity Committees

Many hospitals today are trying to meet the growing number of bioethical problems by establishing medicomoral committees which include representatives of administration, medical staff, and ethicists or clergy. The Catholic bishops of the United States in issuing the *Ethical and Religious Directives* mentioned previously urged local bishops to promulgate these for Catholic hospitals within their dioceses and also encouraged such hospitals to set up medicomoral committees to help carry out the *Directives* practically and effectively in their institutions.

Some experience has shown, however, that such committees in Catholic institutions tend to concentrate too much on merely negative issues of a restricted sort, namely, borderline cases where there is a question of whether certain surgical procedures are forbidden by the *Ethical and Religious Directives*. Consequently, it would seem that it would be better if this committee take the broader and more positive form of a *Christian identity committee* (O'Rourke, 1974a) whose purpose would be to establish and maintain the Christian and Catholic identity of the institution, including its concern for the healing of the whole person and for medical decisions inspired and guided by a Christian hierarchy of values.

The size of such a committee would depend upon the size and nature of the health facility. It should include a balanced representation of the administrative and medical staffs including physicians, nurses, and representatives from the pastoral care and social work departments. Moreover, there should be adequate representation of the public who use the hospital. While it is important that the pastoral care department be represented, this committee should not be identified with that department since the implementation of Christian values is a responsibility of all members of the Catholic hospital, not merely of those in pastoral care. A theologian should be a member of the committee with the function of informing the whole committee on the teaching of the Catholic Church and theological developments in understanding this teaching. In selecting a theologian, it should not be assumed that just any priest or even the chaplain is competent for this role. On the other hand, the mere fact that a theologian is academically well prepared in medical ethics is not sufficent either. He must be a person deeply concerned to give the institution a clearly Catholic identity and one who also has the ability to communicate effectively with the many different groups who make up the hospital community so as to really hear and understand their difficulties.

In institutions where a considerable number of the staff or patients are not Catholics (and this is the common situation today), the ecumenical aspect of this committee is of great importance. Specific Catholic identity and ecumenism are by no means opposed goals, but great charity and an understanding of ecumenical method are essential in harmonizing them. Catholic hospitals must respect the value systems and consciences of those who are not Catholic and learn to cooperate with them in a way which permits all persons to remain loyal to their own value systems while learning to appreciate the values of others.

Such a committee should make use of consultants from outside the institution to broaden and enrich their own work. Above all close liaison should be maintained with the local church under the leadership of its bishop. While the chief executive officer of the institution or the chairperson of the board of directors will ordinarily be the official contact with the bishop, the committee should make its efforts known to the bishop, should look to his guidance in all matters that concern the *Ethical and Religious Directives*, and should work with the local church as one of its ministries in establishing the Kingdom of God.

Since most Catholic hospitals are in charge of religious communities, it is essential that the spirit of community they foster in the hospital extend to their relations with the local church and its bishop. Of course, this is a two-way street, and unfortunately the relations between the bishop of a diocese and the religious communities and their institutions within the diocese are too often uneasy, with lack of communication and suspicions on both sides. One function of a Christian identity committee would be to deal directly and openly with this structural problem, since Catholic identity requires a unity in the local and universal Church which is neither one of mere servile obedience, nor of a struggle for power, but of mutual interdependence.

Some of the questions every Catholic hospital needs to ask itself through such an identity committee are the following.

1. Jesus taught us in the parable of the good Samaritan that God's call to ministry usually comes through the presence of a neighbor in need. Who in our community needs our help to attain healing? Do we recognize their need as God's call which must be the supreme law for our institutional activities?

2. How does this institution witness to the presence of Christ in this city, county, or state by its special concern for the most neglected, the poor and the sinful, and for the dignity of life and person? How can his presence be made more evident? Do we obscure that presence by red tape, excessive financial worry, Pharisaism, or conformism to secularist values?

3. Is there any authorized way to study the needs of patients? Is there a trained person (preferably a religious sister from the nursing staff) who devotes extensive time to observing what happens to patients from the moment they enter the hospital until the time they leave? Does this person act as a patients' representative in an effective way? Is there also available a patients' advocate with legal training who can assist patients to secure their rights? Does this advocate have the freedom, access to information, and access to officers of the institution necessary to fulfill this role effectively?

4. How are employees treated in the institution? Are the principles of social justice and subsidiarity respected in their case? Is there any attempt to form Christian community? Do employees realize their importance in establishing Christian identity? How is communication among all members of the community maintained? Is there a routine way to achieve reconciliation when communication breaks down? Are

there ways and procedures to protect the rights of all employees as regards employment, assignment, working conditions, salaries, and wages? Are they dealt with paternalistically or do they have a voice which ensures them right of bargaining?

5. Is there a department of pastoral care with trained personnel and recognition as a part of the regular staff to provide both patients and staff with adequate counseling and sacramental services? Are these liturgical and sacramental services celebrated in ways that meet the needs of patients involved in the healing process?

6. Is there a good balance between the functions of care and cure in the hospital? Does the nursing staff have a focal role in the primary care of patients and in the coordinated functioning of the health team?

7. Are the potential users of the hospital represented in policy making? Are the patients involved to the degree possible in an active way in the life of the hospital community, rather than mere passive subjects of treatment?

8. Is the atmosphere of the hospital one which makes for healing and for a truly Christian appreciation of the spirituality of the person? What is done to help patients experience suffering as a maturing process? to help them keep contact with their normal life and to be prepared to reenter it?

9. Is the hospital planning and taking steps to reduce emphasis on hospitalization and to make the hospital more of a center for ambulatory care and for preventive medicine?

10. How does the Christian identity committee deal with controversial medicomoral issues? Does it have procedures to deal with difficult cases in such a way as to remain faithful to the *Ethical and Religious Directives* in a way that is pastoral rather than merely legalistic? Is there an effort to provide Christian alternatives to such forbidden practices as contraception, sterilization, and abortion? Are there provisions for ethical genetic counseling and sex instruction and therapy?

11. Is the hospital active in promoting cooperation within its own staff and with other health agencies on the basis of an ecumenical respect for the value systems of others? Does it also respect the consciences of its patients? Does it seek cooperation with other health and welfare agencies so as to promote comprehensive health care for the region?

12. Does the hospital conduct adequate educational programs to inform all members of the hospital community of the objectives, Christian value system, and areas for dialogue and exploration in such matters? Does it try to elicit the experiences and view of all in developing and refining these values and objectives?

13. Does the hospital maintain a vital relation with the local church and its bishop, priests, and other ministers? Does it consult local pastors whose parishioners are subject to its care for their cooperation? Does it relate ecumenically to other Christian churches and other local faith communities?

14. Does the institution play a civic role in promoting better health legislation and planning? Does it also inform the United States Catholic Conference through its bishops or other channels of its problems as a Catholic institution and of its recommendations for the promotion of the Catholic health ministry and for revisions of the *Ethical and Religious Directives?*

15. Does the hospital manage its financial affairs in a responsible manner in view of its primary responsibility to the poor, as well as to others? In seeking funding from either private or public sources does it ensure that it will remain free to pursue its Christian purposes without compromises that would defeat these purposes?

Where there is more than one Catholic hospital in a diocese, the local bishop may find it impossible to supervise the work of all directly.

Moreover, it may be useful to establish a diocesan Christian identity committee to assist the diocesan director in guiding the local Christian identity committees in the observance of the *Ethical and Religious Directives*. Such a committee should include representatives of all the institutions concerned, along with experienced physicians and hospital administrators, theologians especially expert in such questions, pastors acquainted with local conditions, and laypersons representative of the needs of those who use such facilities. Its functions would be the following:

1. To apply the *Ethical and Religious Directives for Catholic Health Facilities* to local situations under the directives of the bishop of the diocese

2. To serve as the proper forum for the discussion of current medico-moral problems relative to the diocesan hospitals

3. To monitor the moral implications of state and federal legislation as it affects the health care apostolate

4. To provide the bishop of the diocese with suggestions based on experience for revisions of the directives

5. To monitor the proceedings of the local hospitals' medicomoral committees and to serve as an appellant or consulting body for them

6. To direct educational activities relative to medical ethics when needed in the diocese

6.6 BIOETHICAL INSTITUTES

Concern about bioethical issues has rapidly mounted in recent years in the United States. At the level of the federal government, the Department of Health, Education, and Welfare is beginning to establish various commissions to develop ethical guidelines which will be binding on any programs of biological or ethical research which are to be funded by the federal government.

The National Conference of Catholic Bishops studies current ethical questions through several standing committees: the committees on doctrine, on human values, on moral values, and on prolife activities. Other Christian churches also issue publications on such questions, as does the World Council of Churches.

Some twenty private organizations devoted to studying bioethical issues are now in existence. Of these, the only one which deals with the whole field from an explicitly Catholic point of view is the Pope John XXIII Medical-Moral Research and Education Center sponsored by The Catholic Hospital Association in St. Louis. The Human Life

Center located at St. John's University, Collegeville, Minnesota, also deals with issues in the field of reproduction from this Catholic perspective.

One of the first and most comprehensive private institutes for bio-ethics is the Hasting Center or Institute of Society, Ethics and the Life Sciences, Hastings-on-Hudson, New York, which was founded by Daniel Callahan and other Catholic associates, but which attempts a neutral stance as regards different value systems.

Similarly, the Joseph and Rose Kennedy Institute for the Study of Human Reproduction and Bioethics was founded under Catholic auspices, but in its official literature is not committed *ex professo* to a Catholic value system. In Canada, a similar effort is the Clinical Research Institute of Montreal under the directorship of David J. Roy.

The excellent publications produced by these institutes makes it possible today for all concerned to get accurate factual information on bioethical issues and to become aware of the different positions on these issues being proposed by ethicists and theologians. Such research, however, will not have much practical use for Catholic health care facilities unless they have active committees of the sort described previously in 6.5 to educate the members of the hospital community in a concrete and practical manner.

PART III

BIOETHICAL DECISION MAKING

Chapter 7 THE LOGIC OF BIOETHICAL DECISIONS

7.1 THE LOGIC OF BIOETHICAL DEBATE

Overview

In Part I we dealt with the ethical responsibilities of persons for their own health and in Part II with the ethical responsibilities of professionals when called on to assist clients with health problems, since professionals have a responsibility both (1) to help the clients in their own decisions and (2) to make decisions themselves whether they as professionals may cooperate in clients' decisions. In Part III we will deal with some of the major areas in which such decisions are especially difficult and controversial at the present time: human experimentation, sex and reproduction, genetics, psychotherapy, and death. In order to deal with such decisions, however, we first need to discuss in this chapter and the following chapter 8 the process by which we can hope to come to some practical resolution of ethical controversies and arrive at sound decisions.

In these two chapters we speak of bioethical decisions rather than of medicomoral decisions, not because we necessarily accept the assumptions of those who prefer this term to *medical ethics* (Wallenmaier, 1975), but because it is broader in scope and includes not only problems that are ordinarily dealt with by medical professionals, but also some which are more frequently met by research biologists and psychologists dealing with human subjects.

In this chapter we will deal first with the main ethical systems which are reflected in current bioethical debates, and then we will deal with ethical thinking which roots ethical values in humane feelings (emotivist ethics, 7.2), or in the rational will of a legislator (voluntarist or duty ethics, 7.3), or in practical intelligence (means-ends or utilitarian ethics, 7.4), and finally in 7.5 we will propose what we call Prudential Personalism which attempts to synthesize all the other approaches and to found them on an analysis of the needs common to all human persons.

Competing Ethical Systems

Medical history shows that in every age medical practice has been embroiled not only in scientific controversies, but also in ethical ones. The introduction of vaccination, the use of quinine, and the administration of anesthesia all produced ethical and theological controversies (White, 1960). Health care professionals often wonder how to tread their way through such controversies which involve philosophical and religious questions beyond their own professional competence. Catholic professionals often ask why the Church does not supply them with clear-cut answers or keep out of medical matters altogether. However, there are many reasons that ethical questions are inevitably controversial.

1. Ethical questions are complex, involving many different factors such that it is possible to get different results by emphasizing different aspects of a problem.

2. Ethics deals with profound and mysterious issues of human life such that our knowledge of the values involved is incomplete and always open to further study.

3. Ethical matters cannot be completely universalized into rules because they involve the individual and individual situations, so there is always a difficulty in applying general rules to concrete cases.

4. Ethics treats questions not only of fact, but also of value. Values influence both our thought and our feelings and will. They involve an essential element of *subjectivity*, as well as an objective foundation in human experience.

5. Ethical decisions not only affect abstract questions, but also directly change our personal lives. Because such change is painful, it is difficult not to be prejudiced in ethical judgment since "no man is a good judge in his own case."

6. Ethical perceptions depend upon our concrete experience, and all persons or groups have their own history and special culture which profoundly influence their ethical outlook.

7. Fundamental to all particular ethical judgments is the religion or its equivalent philosophy of life with its *value system* to which the individual or group consciously or unconsciously adheres.

8. Besides these difficulties which arise from our human finitude are also the difficulties that have their origin in what Christians understand as human sinfulness which darkens our understanding and distorts our motivation, whether this sinfulness is the result of human history (original sin) embodied in social structures or of our individual contribution to this human condition through our acceptance of sinful institutions or our own evil initiatives (Curran, 1977a).

In view of these difficulties, how are we to develop a satisfactory and mature approach to ethical controversies? A hint of an answer can be derived from the psychological studies of Jean Piaget (1965 [1929]) and Lawrence Kohlberg (1973; Duska, 1975) which have shown that in most groups of adults there are persons at different levels of development in ethical thinking, corresponding to the phases through which a child must pass to full moral maturity. These phases can be summarized in three main steps:

1. The small child tends to make decisions on the basis of the immediate consequences of an action, of rewards and punishments.

2. The growing child begins to make decisions more and more on the basis of social approval of parents or peers. Conformity to group norms becomes paramount, and satisfactions can be delayed and suffering incurred to achieve approval of others.

3. Moral maturity is marked by an increasing internalization and independence of moral judgment. Decisions are now made on the basis of personal standards, and the standards of society become subject to criticism. The adult acts primarily for self-approval even at the cost of disapproval by the group.

It is obvious that most ethical controversies are carried on largely at the second of these levels. The debaters each proceed on the assumption that the value system of their group, whether it be that of a social class, a professional elite, or a church, is self-evident, and they make little or no effort to understand the viewpoint of opponents who live within other, competing value systems. In chapter 1 we showed that in the United States the four main value systems involved in most public debates are Humanism, Catholicism, Protestantism, and Judaism with their many subsystems. Because each of these groups rests it arguments on assumptions the others do not share, public controversies on medicomoral matters, for example, on abortion, tend to end in stalemate. However, with patience and fairness it may sometimes be possible to pursue a question to the third and mature level of ethical thinking in which it becomes possible to subject even these assumptions to examination, reinterpretation, and we hope, eventual ecumenical convergence.

Certainly, it is vital in medical ethics to outline how health care professionals who adhere to various value systems can think effectively about ethical issues in dialogue with others. The great divergence of value systems and the involvement of professionals, patients, families, hospital administrators, lawyers, and social workers require a special effort for orderly, logical thinking that can lead to the most realistic, sensitive, balanced decisions and the widest possible consensus.

In considering the development of logical modes in bioethical discussions, we will use a single example, the abortion controversy. Our purpose here is not actually to debate that issue (with which we deal in chapter 10), but to show how different modes of thinking are involved.

7.2 EMOTIVIST ETHICS

At the beginning of most discussions of an ethical issue people express felt attitudes. I am horrified at the idea of abortion and especially at the way so many people are now ready to approve what they previously regarded as a shameful crime. But you are indignant at the presumption of anyone who would force a woman to bear a child that she does not want, especially when that child will be a defective who will live a miserable life, and you are pleased that more liberal, humane views are beginning to prevail. From the outset it appears that our discussion will get nowhere. How can we discuss the obviously sincere but purely subjective feelings of another person? It is like discussing a preference for Bourbon or Scotch.

But we cannot rest content with this initial impasse. Feeling cannot be an ethical criterion which is beyond criticism, no matter how sincere it may be. People are often led by their feelings to do things that turn out to be very destructive not only to others, but also to themselves. You may feel it is all right to destroy a fetus, but what if you also feel it is all right to kill blacks or Jews? I may feel it is wrong to permit a woman to have an abortion, but what if I feel it is wrong to permit my child to be given a necessary blood transfusion?

Some modern ethicists hold that an emotivist ethics (cf. Warnock, 1960; Kerner, 1966; Urmson, 1969) of this type is the only one possible, since any discussion of values is a discussion about subjective, emotional attitudes (Ayer, 1936). Some ethicists modified this position of Ayer by asserting ought statements are not mere expressions or descriptions of emotion, but are prescriptions stating what we feel should be done, although the ground for such prescriptions still remains subjective feelings, not the knowledge of some special kind of fact (Stevenson, 1944; cf. McGrath, 1969). At first sight this reduction of moral statements to mere subjective attitudes seems unconvincing. However, there is a more plausible form of emotivism which will move our thinking a little further. Certainly not all feelings can be trusted, but we can trust our better nature, our humane feelings. The great philosopher Rousseau (1976 [1753]) argued that if people would free themselves from the prejudices acquired by bad education and the influence of a corrupt civilization and return to their natural human feelings they would make much better ethical judgments. Such is the basis of our American confidence in the common sense of the people. We believe that the common man is closer to nature and reality than is the sophisticated intellectual. We take opinion polls on many bioethical problems because we assume that what most people feel is right probably *is* right.

There is much truth in this view because it is certainly true that natural human feelings of family love, of loyalty to one's group, of sympathy for the underdog, of opposition to arrogance and tyranny, and of fairness and compassion are better guides to morality than current fads or the fanatical ideologies of armchair philosophers out of touch with basic human realities. In discussing abortion, we cannot overlook or deny the fact that most women are very reluctant to have an abortion, even when they think it right to do so. On the other hand, we cannot be insensitive to the anguish of a woman faced with bringing into the world a deformed child.

However, if we attempted to live only by our natural feelings, the progress of civilization would be impossible. Sigmund Freud in *Civilization and Its Discontents* (1930) added to Rousseau's analysis the bitter truth that civilization is an absolute necessity if we are not to be destroyed by the contradictions of our own instinctive drives. Without such civilization and the discipline it makes possible there could be no modern medical science.

Consequently, it seems necessary to accept the view of Aristotle in *The Nicomachean Ethics* (H. Veatch, 1962) who taught that emotion is to be trusted only when it has been preserved in its proper nature and yet refined, educated, and disciplined by virtue. Recently ethicists have again been insisting that good decisions are not possible merely by following rules. We need *character* if we are to consistently meet the crisis of decision (Hauerwas, 1974; Frankena, 1973). Decisions made by people who have a respect for persons, reverence for life, and compassion for suffering are likely to be good decisions, while decisions made by persons who are insensitive and lacking in sympathy are likely to be morally bad. Thus what we *do* is the outcome of what we *are* (McCabe, 1969). This is the reason why we often hear the statement "I would rather trust physicians or nurses of good character to make ethical decisions than all the experts in bioethics in the world."

This point is well taken. Ultimately, all ethical decisions do involve a degree of moral sensitivity, fairness, and compassion which are only to be found in psychologically healthy and mature people, in civilized, decent human beings. Character is all important. But what is decency? What are the standards or principles by which good characters are formed? The German physicians who carried out Hitler's evil medical experiments were men who thought of themselves, and were considered by others, as decent, ethical professionals. But they probably were not in the habit of reflecting about the ethical standards of their profession (Alexander, 1949; Shirer, 1960).

7.3   DUTY ETHICS

The Is and Ought

Thus, while granting the importance in every ethical debate of natural yet disciplined human feeling, we must move beyond feeling to ethics based on information, knowledge, reasoning, and research. Such an ethic which uses a rational procedure is called a *cognitivist* ethic. Cognitivism brings us immediately face-to-face with what has proved to be the central question of modern ethics as a discipline (Hanock, 1974; Veatch, 1973a): the problem of facts versus values or of is versus ought.

Modern science has provided us with a remarkably successful and objective method of establishing facts. Thus, if the question arises whether a woman is pregnant or whether if she is her unborn child is normal or even how to terminate this pregnancy by a procedure whose results are predictable, we know how to make tests that will ordinarily answer these questions in terms of empirically observable facts. But when we get to the questions of whether she *ought* to be pregnant, whether a defective fetus ought to be preserved, and whether her pregnancy ought to be terminated, we are no longer talking about facts which can be empirically and scientifically determined, but about values which cannot be determined by scientific methods. If values are only attitudes or feelings, as emotivist ethics maintains, then this situation is not puzzling. The facts are objective and public, but the feelings are merely someone's subjective reaction to these facts and are purely private and nondebatable.

But if ethical value is more than a matter of emotion, then the ought is also something objective and public, something we ought to be able to discuss reasonably in view of increasing agreement. How then do we get from the value-free facts with which medical science can deal to the values, oughts, and obligations with which bioethics deals (Hume, 1975 [1738])? Since G. E. Moore (1903), ethicists have claimed that we are making a "category mistake" in logic and committing "the naturalistic fallacy" when we try to pass from the *is* to the *ought*. We are mistaking what is only a cultural reality for a natural reality.

Certainly we should avoid such logical fallacies. For example, the following are factual statements (whether they are true or not is another question): Abortion is a common practice in most countries. The majority of Americans believe that abortion is ethically justified in some cases. Abortion is a relatively safe procedure. Spontaneous abortions are common. The fetus is a human person. The fetus is not a human person. Induced abortion is not a natural process. None of these true or false statements of fact tell us whether anyone ought or ought not have an abortion, and it is logically fallacious to use them as premises in a syllogism whose conclusion is an ought statement.

However, to admit that an ought statement or value judgement is different from a fact does not mean that they are unrelated. Value judgments must somehow be grounded in a knowledge of the factual situation in which we are going to act. Are not the biological facts of embryology essential to any rational decision about abortion? The question is, How are values *grounded* in facts?

The first important answer to this question was given by G. E. Moore himself and is usually called *intuitionism* (Hudson, 1967). According to Moore (1903) there is no way to pass from the facts to the ought by any logical process. No matter how detailed our description of the facts, we never discover in them any property that we can call a value. If you name such a property, it is always possible to ask the further question, but is that property good or bad? Thus if I say that a fetus is deformed, I can still ask, But should a deformed child be permitted to live? Further factual description will never answer that question. Consequently, for Moore there could be no moral discourse unless we admit that beside our rational ability to ascertain facts we also have a special *intuition* of moral principles (cf. also Ross, 1939, 1965). We intuitively recognize, for example, that cruelty is wrong.

This position, however, tends to fall back into emotivism because intuitions are private affairs hard to debate. Consequently, intuitivism usually takes the further form of an ethics of duty (deontological ethics or ethics of obligation) (Abelson and Nielsen, 1967; Frankena, 1973) which holds that morality consists in doing what is known to be right because it is *right* and for no other reason. Such an ethics does not ignore the facts, but it claims that in order for us to live as human beings we cannot merely deal with facts, but must interpret the facts in terms of moral principles which we do not derive from the facts but which help us to respond behaviorally to the facts.

Voluntarism and Legalism

The most common version of this type of ethics is what is called *voluntarism* (Bourke, 1970), which says that our ethical interpretation of the facts rests on the *will* of some lawmaker who has made the determination that some values are good and some bad, some ways of acting are moral and others immoral.

Probably most Americans tend to think of morality in terms of a code, the Ten Commandments or federal or state laws. The secular form of voluntarism identifies morality with what is *legal*. This is what is called *legalism* or *positivism* (from the term *positive*, i.e., law "posited" by the will of the sovereign). For many the Supreme Court decision settled the question of whether abortion is right or wrong. Its opponents, on the other hand, betray the same way of thinking when they label abortion a crime, that is, a breach of law.

Sociologists and anthropologists think of morality as determined not so much by written laws (which are easily changed) as by unwritten law or custom. For them, morality simply means conformity to the accepted social standards of a particular culture. They point out that in some cultures abortion is considered immoral and in others, at least in some situations, a moral duty (Bidney, 1953; Edel and Edel, 1968).

This view that there is no such thing as a universal, transcultural standard of right and wrong is moral relativism (Brandt, 1967).

The case for such positivist ethics is strong because it is certainly true that we form our moral standards only in social context with the help and guidance of the community to which we belong. No individual is capable of working out a personal system of values merely on the basis of his own limited experience and insights. Nor could we live with others if each of us lived by a merely personal ethics. Thus some kind of laws or at least customs are necessary to protect the rights of both mother and child and to educate and give direction to the ethical thinking and attitudes of all the adults involved.

Yet it is also obvious that man-made laws or accepted customs are not ultimate criteria of morality for two reasons:

1. Legal morality is always broad, crude, and unrefined. In personal living, we must supplement the law by more refined, sensitive personal standards.

2. Man-made laws and customs often become obsolete in changed circumstances and even orginally may have been destructive. Therefore, it is necessary to criticize them, refuse to obey them, or work to have them changed.

Thus those who believe the antiabortion laws were unjust worked for their liberalization, while those who favor these laws work for a constitutional amendment to make it possible to reinstate them.

Consequently, many voluntarists seek to appeal man-made laws which may be unjust to a divine law made by God, who cannot be unjust. As St. Paul said, "We ought to obey God rather than men" (Acts 5:29). But how do we know the will of God? The Jewish, Christian, and Muslim conviction is that God has revealed his will through the prophets as recorded in the Bible or Koran. Thus morality is simply defined as "obedience to the commands of God."

In the Protestant tradition, this type of voluntarism has generally predominated. While there is a great variety of Protestant ethical systems, most of them teach that since the Fall we are unable to distinguish correctly between right and wrong because we delude ourselves by a Pharisaic self-righteousness and self-justification (Brunner, 1937; Thielicke, 1969; cf. Mehl, 1971). We can be freed from this blindness only when confronted by the righteousness of God as revealed in the Word of God, especially in Jesus Christ the Incarnate Word. Even with this Biblical revelation, the will of God remains essentially mysterious to us such that we can never hope to understand why God makes such demands on us, but we can only obey Him in absolute trust.

Some recent theologians influenced by existentialism, for example, Bultmann (1958), have emphasized the notion of a radical obedience. They point out that Abraham was called by God to sacrifice his son, Isaac, in seeming contravention to the moral law. We, too, must be ready to obey the call of God in concrete situations in a way that may call us beyond any accepted norms. They are thus moving beyond a *rule* morality to an *act*, or situational, morality while remaining voluntarists. Protestant ethics also emphasizes that even when we know God's will we cannot fulfill it except by the *grace* of God which frees us from a perfectionist anxiety about the Law to put our trust in God who is able to overcome our failures.

Catholic theologians such as William of Ockham and Suarez (Coppleston, 1963) have also developed voluntaristic systems, but generally Catholics have not favored this approach because the emphasis on blind submission to God's will does not seem to do justice to the Biblical doctrine that we are created in the image and likeness of God. True, this image has been profoundly distorted by human sin, so that without God's revelation we could never come to a correct idea of our true nature or our divine destiny to be raised to friendship with God, nor without the grace given us in Christ would we ever be able to achieve that goal. But it is also true that the gifts of human intelligence and freedom given to us by God in our creation, in which this image and likeness first of all consist, remain a part of our nature even in its fallen state.

After we are reborn through grace, these gifts are again freed to enable us not only to obey God blindly, but to obey Him intelligently and freely. God's will remains in many ways mysterious, yet it is not an arbitrary will, but God's wisdom which he shares with us so that, by his grace, we can cooperate with his plans for our lives. Thus, Catholic moral theology strives to go beyond voluntarism to an ethics that insists that God wants us to understand his wise purposes and to use our own intelligence and experience in executing them (Böckle, 1968; Häring, 1968b). Thus we might read Jesus' parable of the talents (Matt. 25:14-23) as indicating that when God commands us as his servants to carry out a task He also demands some creativity on our part in obeying these commands. Voluntarism does not seem to take this creativity into account.

Moral Autonomy

The inability of Catholics and Protestants to resolve these and other theological issues led ethical thinkers of the Enlightenment in the eighteenth century to present a purely rational ethics not based on revelation which would be more consistent with their new religion of secular Humanism. Rousseau's emotivism was one such system, but there was also a new form of voluntarism proposed by Immanuel Kant (Schroeder, 1940; Teale, 1975). Kant was a voluntarist in the sense that he accepted the idea, derived from his pietist Protestant background, that morality is a matter of legislation, but he believed human beings must legislate for themselves. Morality cannot be heteronomous (a law from outside) from society, nor from a God beyond our understanding (theonomy) (Tillich, 1967), but must be autonomous, each person legislating for himself. We must be confident that if we each legislate for ourselves reasonably God will ratify and sanction our decisions.

It might seem that this self-legislation would lead to the crudest form of emotivism, but Kant insisted that we must legislate not emotionally but rationally (hence his system is sometimes called ethical rationalism), and Kant argued that this type of legislation requires that our moral norms be completely free of any mere self-serving or self-interest (hence his system is also called moral purism or altruism). All moral norms or maxims must take the form of the categorical imperative: Act so that the rule of your action can be the norm for all men equally.

This rule, of course, offers no actual ethical content, but it does contain the form of pure disinterestedness or universalizability which any moral rule must have to be truly moral (Frankena, 1973). For Kant the content of such rules has to be supplied from a consideration of the consequences, as judged by our feelings (as thought Rousseau, whom Kant admired) and experience. Thus Kant argued, "It is our duty never to lie, no matter what the consequences" because if everyone lied the mutual trust on which society is founded would become impossible. I cannot expect you to tell the truth to me unless I tell the truth to you.

Kant's theory in its original form is commonly rejected today as unrealistic. It is doubtful that psychologically speaking this pure disinterestedness is even possible as a normal human attitude, nor is it clear that by this method we can really arrive at concrete yet unexceptional rules. However, numerous modern ethicists have tried to revise Kant's duty ethics in a more acceptable form. A very popular version is that of John Rawls (1971) which attempts to found morality on an implied contract by which human persons agree to protect each others' rights or that of William K. Frankena (1973) who proposes two principles, those of beneficence and justice, to which all other moral rules can be reduced and which in case of conflict must be reconciled with each other as well as is possible. Frankena justifies these rules much as Kant would by arguing that only if we legislate such norms for ourselves will a human, social life be possible. Paul Ramsey (1962, 1965), one of our most distinguished bioethicists, has effectively used this approach in opposing abortion.

These various forms of voluntaristic reasoning are evident today in bioethical debates, but all seem inadequate. Thus in the abortion debate the appeal to the will of God revealed in the Bible runs up against the fact that there is no text in either the Old Testament or the New Testament which speaks unambiguously about the problem (Noonan, 1970b). Are we to conclude, therefore, that if God has not spoken on the issue abortion is permissible (Cerling, 1971)? There are many other actions not explicitly forbidden in the Scriptures that almost all Christians condemn (e.g., slavery). A voluntarist, therefore, must take the view that the Bible often speaks only of general principles of morality which we must then apply to particular cases and new problems. But by what logic is this application made? Nor is the appeal to human legislation, whether of the heteronomous kind or of the Kantian autonomous kind, sufficent. The laws of the state may be unjust, while Kantian philosophers, in spite of their very ingenious efforts, have not succeeded in showing how we can pass from the *form* of a universal moral rule as just or beneficient to deciding what is truly just or beneficent without introducing a different type of logic.

Voluntaristic ethics, if it is to get down to concrete cases, must make use of the human capacity not only to obey, but also to reason. Even if God has revealed his will, we must apply these commandments intelligently to actual situations. Even if we have the power to legislate for ourselves by reason, this use of reason cannot be merely abstract, but must concern itself with the facts of life. Thus, the abortion debate must move beyond discussions of law and of abstract justice to a discussion of human individual and social needs and the alternative ways of meeting these needs.

7.4   CONSEQUENTIALIST MEANS-ENDS ETHICS

Means and Ends

If ethical debate comes to a dead end when we merely appeal to personal emotional attitudes or to laws which rest on the will of God or man, we are forced to move on to what are commonly called natural law arguments (Fuchs, 1963; Curran, 1977). There is much misunderstanding of what this term *natural law* (which is admittedly confusing) means. It does not mean that morality rests on self-evident rules which are naturally known to everyone. It is not self-evident that abortion is always wrong or sometimes right. Such an argument would be emotivist or intuitionist. What is distinctive about natural law ethics is that it is based on generalization from human experience, rather than on reference to subjective attitudes (Messner, 1965; Simon, 1965; Armstrong, 1966; McQuarrie, 1970) or to a legislated rule. Thus, when we argue that war is wrong because experience shows that in a war nobody really wins, we are using the logic of natural law. In the abortion debate the con arguments about the human rights of a fetus are natural law arguments, but so are the pro arguments about the rights of the mother and the misery of the unwanted child.

Such a logic is said to be a naturalist ethics because it contends that we can pass from values to facts, from the is to the ought in terms of the factual consequences of this or that action. An action is morally good if in fact it tends to produce good consequences and wrong if it tends to produce bad consequences. Obviously, this argument would be circular unless we can determine whether the consequences are good or bad.

This determination is made by contending that human activity is undertaken to fulfill human needs. Some of these needs are generated by our culture and therefore are neither universal nor undebatable. Others are self-chosen, and they too cannot serve as the basis of moral rules since they may be self-destructive. But there are other needs which are natural in the sense that they are genetically inherent in every member of the human species and are the source of the development and the survival of our species in the evolutionary struggle. Moral behavior, therefore, is the kind of action whose consequence is the satisfaction of these natural needs. For example, natural law ethics requires every individual to eat the right amount and quality of food and to act socially so that all members of the community can also be well fed.

Such a means-ends ethics, in contrast to an ethics of duty, is also called teleological from the Greek word *telos*, "goal" or "end." Its logic is that of arguing in terms of ends and means, that is, of needs and the consequences of actions intended to satisfy these needs. It says that an action is moral if three conditions are fulfilled:

1. The act must be certifiable by human experience and reason to be an effective way of achieving some human goal.
2. The intended goal must be a basic human need.
3. The Principle of Totality (2.4) must be followed so that proper priority and complementarity of the hierarchy of human needs is observed.

The first of these conditions is fulfilled in every rational human act, but is violated when we act irrationally, foolishly, impulsively. For example, abortion is a foolish means of contraception, and irresponsible parenthood a foolish way of being prolife.

The second condition is needed in order to distinguish moral behavior from actions which are technically good but not morally good. Thus a physician may perform a medically skillful abortion which nevertheless cannot be ethically justified. For it to be ethically justified, we need to consider not only the goal of the medical procedure, but also whether this goal is consistent with basic human needs. Thus good medical procedure in assisting a woman to bear a child is ethically unquestionable because the need to reproduce is inherent in the human structure, but it is not clear how deliberate abortion meets such a need.

However, the third condition is also necessary because (again, as we have seen in 2.4) we have to assign priorities to the hierarchy of human needs and to harmonize them. Thus it is possible that the need to reproduce must be subordinated to some higher psychological or social need, in which case a valid argument for abortion may be proposed. On the other hand, valid arguments might also be drawn from this same principle on the grounds that the need and right of the child to life are more fundamental than the mother's need and right for greater freedom.

Kinds of Means-Ends Ethics

Means-ends ethics (teleological or naturalist ethics) has several varieties, in some of which the needs of a human person are considered to be purely *individual*. This is called egoism, or what Ayn Rand (1964), a current advocate, calls "the new selfishness" and others call "libertarianism." At first, this view is shocking and the very opposite of Kant's ethics which was based on the idea that any self-interested action is immoral by definition. However, Kant's puristic duty ethics is less credible than egoism. Certainly all of us have the responsibility (3.4) to care for our own needs and interests. We cannot demand that others do everything for us, nor are we justified in criticizing others because they take care of themselves. Even Jesus Christ in giving us the Great Commandment which sounds so altruistic — "Love God and your neighbor as yourself" — indicated that we must also love ourselves. The efforts of some theologians who defend duty ethics to explain away that "as yourself" have not been very successful (cf. Outka, 1972).

In 1.2 we showed that self-love is not necessarily selfishness. Genuine self-love not only is consistent with the love of others, but also demands that we love others, because our deepest human need requires those spiritual goods which can be best enjoyed in community. To seek our own personal good is not to remain selfishly individualistic but is to learn to share in communal life. Such sharing is what makes us images of God, because God Himself is a communal Trinity of Father, Son, and Holy Spirit who share one being and life and who generously share this being and life with us through our creation and redemption.

Thus egoism is inadequate, not because it approves self-love, but because it proposes an incomplete view of human needs. Thus in the abortion debate we cannot argue merely in terms of the woman's *private* convenience. We must take into account her need as a member of society to protect the rights of all human beings (of course, this accounting does not settle the question of whether the fetus *is* a human being). Catholic theology has never rejected the notion that self-love is legitimate. In fact, it condemned as heretical the theory of pure love which some quietists proposed, according to which true saints should become indifferent to their own happiness (Conzemius, 1970).

Few ethicists have accepted egoism; rather, they have opposed Kantian duty ethics by a utilitarianism based on the notion of the greatest good for the greatest number (Smart and Williams, 1973; Harman, 1977). In its current forms, utilitarianism is often called consequentialism and is probably the most favored ethics in modern United States society wherein Humanism dominates. Any teleological ethics is based on evaluating the consequences of an action as a means to an end, but as we will see, there are different ways of estimating these consequences. Utilitarian consequentialism makes this estimate by a calculation of positive gains and negative losses in a quantitative manner, enumerating these gains and losses as comparable items. Its model is that of an economic exchange in which we can calculate gains and losses in terms of a uniform monetary measure. No wonder that such an ethics, with its cost-and-benefit analysis, is very understandable and acceptable in American society where we are very used to thinking in this kind of computerizable logic! Some people identify this type of logic with reason itself.

One form of this ethics is act utilitarianism, exemplified by the works of Joseph Fletcher, one of the pioneers of current bioethics (1966, 1967; Barr, 1970), and has been widely influential under the title of situation ethics. Fletcher's approach is intelligible when we realize that he is a Protestant theologian in reaction to the duty ethics prominent in the Protestant tradition, to which many Catholic conservatives also seem to have committed themselves. For Fletcher there is only one absolute moral rule, that of love (*agape* in New Testament Greek). We must always do what is loving. Fletcher settles abortion cases, not by saying that abortion is always wrong or always permissible, but by judging the consequences of having or not having an abortion for this particular woman in this particular situation in view of "loving action."

But what is loving action? It has generally been pointed out by Fletcher's critics (P. Ramsey, 1965; Cox, 1968; Outka, 1968; Cunningham, 1970; King, 1970; Spring, 1970) that in his actual solution of cases Fletcher has been forced gradually to develop various generalizations and rules. Furthermore, he asserts without proving (1) that the rule of love is a universal rule (egoism does not admit this) and (2) that no other rules are universal. His only argument for this second assumption is that with sufficient ingenuity we always imagine a hardship case in which it seems difficult to apply the usual rule. But this argument only proves that ethical decisions are difficult. The same objection can be brought against the rule of love which is certainly very difficult to apply in many cases.

Consequently, most utilitarians reject pure situationism (Brandt, 1959; cf. P. Ramsey, 1965) and advocate some form of rule utilitarianism (as Fletcher seems to do in practice) whereby we must make our cost-and-benefit calculations on the basis of experience formulated in normative generalizations, that is, moral rules.

Whether any rule admits of exception cannot be decided a priori. In dealing with scientific facts, we long ago learned that the formulation of any natural physical law is only approximate and must be refined (e.g., Einstein's refinement of Newton's gravitational laws). Moreover, a prediction based on natural physical law is always merely probable because in the concrete instance another law may modify the outcome (e.g., the law of gravitation is offset by the law of electromagnetic attraction when we use a magnet to lift a piece of metal). Why is it surprising then that our formulation of moral natural laws (which have a basis in natural facts) needs to be refined as our knowledge of human needs and situations increases or that there may be a conflict of laws in concrete cases? Many rule utilitarians make this point by saying that moral rules have only a prima facie obligation (Ross, 1939); that is, we assume that they bind us unless we find sufficient reason to make an exception. Thus many ethicists today would consider that mothers are bound prima facie by the rule that in general the consequences of carrying the unborn child to term are more desirable than is an abortion, but that in some cases special circumstances shift the cost-and-benefit balance in favor of an abortion.

Ethical debate based on utilitarianism, however, also tends to end in an impasse. To many it seems based on a very superficial, overly economic view of the needs of human persons and human communities. It makes its calculations of cost-and-benefit consequences by treating human values as quantitatively comparable *items*, without taking adequate account of the unified, hierarchical, interdependent structure of the human person or the person's relation to a community sharing higher values, which we have discussed in chapter 1. Some utilitarians (Mill, 1962 [1863]) have tried to introduce a qualitative element into their system, but to do so consistently demands an essentially different type of ethics, which we will next propose.

7.5 PRUDENTIAL PERSONALISM

Criteria of Morality

Much of current ethical debate, especially medicomoral debate and that over human sexuality, polarizes into what seems an irreconcilable dichotomy between an ethics of duty with its absolute moral norms and consequentialism with its cost-and-benefit calculus. After reviewing the current situation in Catholic moral theology and referring to similar reviews by Charles E. Curran (1975a), Bruno Schüller (1973, 1974) and Richard A. McCormick (1977) rightly conclude that if Catholic moral theology is to respect its own tradition it must avoid both extremes.

As Bernard Häring (1966; Vereecke, 1962) has shown, the basic reason that Catholic moral theology finds itself in this quandry is that after the Council of Trent the textbooks used in seminaries replaced the means-ends ethics of the medieval theologians which emphasized the development of the virtues coordinated by Christian love and prudence with a duty ethics emphasizing the Commandments. Protestant theologians during this period also generally taught a duty ethics to which Kant finally gave a philosophical systematization. This widespread theological trend reflected the attitudes of secular society which in the Age of Reason stressed the need for centralized sovereign authority acting through codified laws and clear lines of command.

However, at the end of the nineteenth century the Thomistic revival in Catholic theology and the antirationalistic reaction in Protestant theology began a trend back toward a means-ends ethics which is clearly evident in the documents of the Second Vatican Council (1965c) which taught that the "objective criteria" of moral right and wrong are based on "the nature of the human person and human action" (*Church in the Modern World*, n. 51).

Charles E. Curran(1977a) has argued that such an ethics is a "mixed form" rather than a pure duty ethics or a means-ends ethics. It would agree with duty ethics that objective criteria of morality cannot be reduced exclusively to the consequences of an action as a means-ends ethics asserts, but it would agree with a means-ends ethics that these criteria must include such consequences. Curran calls this third model "ethics of relationality and responsibility" (cf. H. Niebuhr, 1963; Jonsen, 1968). We cannot claim complete control over our lives (as means-ends ethics seems to assume), nor can we reduce our responsibilities to obedience to general norms (as duty ethics assumes). Rather we have to respond to the persons and events which confront us in life in ways that maximize human values, making creative use of the resources available to us. Curran believes that such an ethics is more in keeping with a Christian understanding of our dependence on the grace of God and our encounters with other persons than a duty ethics with its danger of legalism or a means-ends ethics with its danger of illusions about our rational control over our lives.

As we understand Curran, however, it seems to us that his ethics of relationality and responsibility should be classified not as a mixed form, but rather as a personalist form of means-ends ethics. We too would insist that any modern Christian ethics must stress the fact that the "ends" of human action are always *persons* and the community of interrelated persons responding to each other. At the center of this community is a Tri-Personal God with whom the initiative always belongs and on whose grace we completely depend to make any fully human response. Yet to respond to persons is to direct our actions to the good of persons, and this always is a matter of free choice of means to ends, of acts that relate us to persons or alienate us from them.

We have already argued that a duty ethics is inadequate because it only traces the criteria of morality back to the will of some lawmaker, whether that lawmaker be God, the government, or the autonomous individual. We must still ask, Why is the will of the lawmaker itself righteous? The ultimate answer to this query must be given in terms of the practical wisdom or *prudence* by which the legislator makes wise rules for the benefit of those who are to obey. As soon as we begin to ask about "benefit for someone," we are constructing a means-ends ethics which measures the rightness or wrongness of human action by its helpful or harmful consequences, that is, as an effective means to the goals of human life (the satisfaction of human needs).

We accept this means-ends type of ethics wholeheartedly and we use the term *prudential* because it indicates the practical, goal-seeking character (Pieper, 1966) and even the situational or contextual character of this ethics. For a prudential ethics morality ultimately is not a matter of obeying abstract rules, but of intelligently seeking appropriate, concrete behavior by which to achieve human personal goals. However, we do not deny the value of laws or rules (cf. 8.1-3), but only contend that what makes such laws obligatory is their helpfulness in guiding prudential decisions to successful goal achievement.

Obviously, however, this still leaves the question, What goals are morally right for a human being? As we have seen the Second Vatican Council answered this by saying that these goals are determined by "the nature of the human person and human action." Theologically, this can only mean that the ultimate measure of morality is the pattern of Jesus Christ in whom alone what it is to be fully human has been revealed to us, undistorted by sin.

The United States bishops in their joint pastoral letter *To Live in Christ Jesus* (1976) have written:

> All of us seek happiness: life, peace, joy, a wholeness and wholesomeness of being. The happiness we seek and for which we are fashioned is given to us in Jesus, God's supreme gift of love . . . God reveals to us in Jesus who we are and how we are to live. Yet He has made us free, able and obliged to decide how we shall respond to our calling. We must make concrete in the particular circumstances of our lives what the call to holiness and the commandment of love require. This is not easy. We know, too, that decisions may not be arbitrary, for "good" and "bad," "right" and "wrong" are not simply what we choose to make them. And so God gives us His guidance in manifold forms. (p. 8)

Thus a means-ends ethics which goes no further than consequentialism, utilitarianism, or situationism is inadequate not because it judges actions in terms of their consequences, but because it fails to evaluate these consequences in the light of a correct understanding of authentic human goals. These goals are determined not by the customs of a particular culture, nor by individual preference, but by "the nature of the human person." Hence we speak of the ethics we advocate as "personalism" because it evaluates human goals and the means to these goals in terms of the self-actualization or fulfillment of the human person in community.

Historians of ethics usually characterize this approach to morality as an ethics of self-realization and cite Plato, Aristotle, Hegel, Royce, and even Dewey as typical proponents (Jones, 1969). We accept this classification provided that two points are kept clear: (1) the ethics we propose is not based on intuitionism or idealism of any sort, since its principles are derived from human, historical experience, especially the experience of perfect human actualization in the historical Jesus and (less perfectly) in his true disciples throughout the history of the Christian community, and (2) nor is this ethics of self-realization to be understood as individualism or egoism, but as essentially communitarian, in accordance with the notion of person developed in chapter 1.

A Prudential Personalism, therefore, proposes we judge the rightness or wrongness of human actions by asking, "How does this action in its context contribute to the growth of persons in community?" Hence the consequences of any human act must be evaluated not in terms of immediate pains and pleasures, nor even in terms of other immediate qualitative values, but must all be referred to the actualization of the human person in relation to other persons. Because consequentialists and utilitarians fail to provide such a conception of full human personhood as the goal of every human action, but content themselves with more superficial values, they end with an ethics of expediency in which the end justifies the means, that is, *any* means. Following consequentialism or utilitarianism, we risk wasting our lives in the pursuit of unsatisfying and often inconsistent goals which ultimately leave our deepest human needs frustrated.

Obviously, to construct a Prudential Personalism we are forced back to questions about the inherent finality of the human person and of the subordinate finalities of all those functions which integrate the human person as a complex whole. These inherent finalities are not themselves something we can choose, since we cannot choose to be human. By God's gift we *are* human. We can only choose how to realize that humanity in its fullness by morally good action or frustrate its fulfillment by bad action. Moreover, our growth and fulfillment as human persons has a twofold aspect: on the one hand our growth is a response to the vocation which God gives to each of us in our unique existence (Rahner, 1961), and on the other hand, it is our response to the common essential humanity that unites us to others in the human community.

However, it is not necessary to work out a complete metaphysics of the human person before we can begin to construct a personalist ethics. As Mortimer Adler has well argued (1970), it is sufficient to begin with a commonsense notion of what it is to be human. Of course, the more we can enrich and deepen this understanding, both through the behavioral sciences and through theological reflection on the life of Christ, the more adequate and refined will be our moral judgments.

Thus a Prudential Personalism provides a logic of moral decision that takes the following form:

1. We need to be as clear as we can about the goal of human life set by the Creator for human beings in common and for *this* human being in his or her uniqueness. We have to achieve this self-understanding by making use of all the kinds of information of our conscience which we described in 3.4.

2. We soon discover that this effort at self-understanding does not result in a single principle (such as Fletcher's "act lovingly"), but in an indefinite number of principles reflecting the complex, multi-dimensional constitution of the human person (1.4). Therefore, the Principle of Totality and Integrity (2.4) comes into play as we attempt to assign priorities among these various basic goals and realize their interdependence. Out of this reflection comes our system of values, which we need to formulate in the moral rules which help us to make prudent choices.

3. In terms of this value system expressed in moral rules (which are open to development as we grow in self-understanding) we strive to inform our consciences concerning particular moral choices (3.4) in a prudent manner, that is, by keeping in mind both our goals with their relative priorities and the concrete circumstances, risks, and fore-seen special consequences of a particular act. Such a moral logic is, therefore, "prudential" in its practical, intelligent effort to reach our goals, and it is "personalist" in that it works not for superficial goals but for the total realization of the inherent needs of the human person in community.

Facts and Values

To return to our example of an abortion decision, a duty ethicist faced with such a case will ask if there are rules requiring or forbiding abortion in such cases. If no rule is discovered, the duty ethicist tells us to feel free to do what seems convenient. If there is a conflict of rules, the duty ethicist will seek another rule for their resolution or fall back on the rule of do the lesser evil.

A utilitarian or consequentialist faced with the same case will consider the probable consequences of having or not having the abortion and will attempt to judge whether it will be of greater or less benefit to the persons concerned, evaluating benefit in terms of subjective satisfaction, or in terms of what appears desirable or undesirable, but without seeking to ground such evaluations in any teleology *inherent* in the persons concerned. Abortion will thus be judged in terms of the subjective sufferings or relief of the mother, the possible sufferings of an unwanted or defective child, the various advantages to society, and so forth.

A Prudential Personalist will try to take into account all the aforesaid consequences, but will evaluate them in terms of what they mean for the self-realization of the persons involved and of the community of persons of which they are a part. Thus, it must first be determined whether the fetus is a person, and then the various consequences of abortion or of bearing the child must be evaluated in what they mean to the self-actualization of both the mother and the child and of the community of which they are a part in terms of an understanding of the finalities inherent in human persons both as unique individuals and as part of the total human community.

When we speak of inherent finalities in the human person, we are brought back to the modern ethicists' puzzlement about how to get from facts to values, from the is to the ought. As Henry Veatch (1971) has shown, this problem had its origin in the mechanistic view of the world favored by many modern scientists. If man is a machine produced by the blind forces of evolution, what sense can there be in speaking of any inherent goals or purposes in the human person? Human goals or purposes in such a view are simply a matter of individual choice, or they are imposed on us by the laws and customs of the culture in which we have been raised.

However, we can gladly accept the discoveries of modern science including the evolutionary origin of man without accepting the mechanistic interpretation of these facts, or denying either our common sense or our Christian conviction that we human persons have been created for a purpose and that this purpose is manifest in our genetically determined physical and psychological constitution as individuals and as part of the human species. This dynamic structure of our human nature with its innate needs is a part of the order of facts which can be determined empirically by the life sciences and interpreted philosophically to provide us with a unified view of what it is to be human. Such an empirically grounded view furnishes the basis for an ethics that goes beyond cultural relativism. Thus, whenever in this book we refer to basic human needs or to human nature, we have in mind a philosophical account of the human person which takes into full account the findings of modern biology and psychology and which is in keeping with what the health care professionals know about the human body and psyche.

When human needs are viewed not merely as static facts, but as goals to be achieved, they become values, that is, goods to be desired and sought. Thus it is a biological fact that we need to eat in order to live, but when we ourselves perceive this necessity and begin to make free choices about how we can best fulfill this need in various circumstances, human intelligence, freedom, and creativity enter into the biological process of nutrition and it takes on a truly human, ethical meaning.   Considered in their totality as a system of needs, these genetically inherent requirements of life become genuinely obligatory oughts because we need to be ourselves and to use our freedom to achieve self-realization.

This need for self-realization is itself a fact of human biology and psychology. Indeed, it is the central unifying feature of what it is to be a human person, an embodied intelligent freedom. We act morally when we perceive that fact and freely respond to its practical challenge; we act immorally when we refuse to respond realistically to this challenge and yield ourselves to disorganized and inconsistent impulses. As McDonagh (1972, 1975) has argued, moral living is an openness to a call and a stewardship of a gift. The gift is our human personhood and the call is the purpose inherent in that personhood.

Thus when we discuss such an issue as abortion, an adequate logic of ethics forces us to go beyond mere utilitarianism and to ask such questions as, For what purpose are we gifted with sexuality? Is the unborn child a gift of God and for what purpose has He created it? For what purpose are we social beings who care for the helpless and also for women in the crisis of pregnancy? For what purpose are we gifted with the intelligence and skill of medical art: to further life or to destroy it?

Health care professionals cannot shrug off such questions as philosophical or theological problems outside their field. It is true that they have received a predominantly scientific education which may have led them to be suspicious of any philosophical effort to read values into facts.   When philosophers speak about the human person, a scientifically educated person may prefer to talk about the human organism, reducing everything directly to observable facts systematized by some kind of mathematical or quasimathematical theory. However, no matter how foreign to their regular way of thinking it may be for scientists to reflect on the value implications of biological or psychological facts, such reflection is inescapable if there is to be harmony between medical ethical decisions and medical science.

On the other hand, some philosophers and theologians are intensely uncomfortable with any effort to root ethics in biological or psychological structures.   They are afraid that this will result in a fixed and static conception of human nature, and they would prefer to relate ethics to history and the humanities rather than to the sciences. To this view we would respond that the evolutionary view of man, at both the biological and the anthropological levels, is in no way contrary to the Prudential Personalism we have outlined here. We do not have in mind some kind of timeless human nature, but simply the historically existing human species which is made up of unique individuals all with their own biography but which nevertheless do really form a community based on certain common needs which are not the product of culture but rather its source. For the Christian this historical community is centered in Jesus of Nazareth, God's Word revealed in perfect humanity.

7.6   SUMMARY

Ethical decisions are always made within some value system, and in American society there is a plurality of such systems. Therefore, we need to be fully conscious of our own value system and to enter into dialogue with others to reduce conflict and to find some area of consensus. Thus in bioethical matters we need a logic which will help us make decisions which are consistent with our Christian system of values, but which will also enable us to recognize analogies between our system of values and those of others.

One such logic (emotivism) solves ethical questions by references to emotional preferences and can serve as the basis of dialogue if we can distinguish between sincere and humane and decent feelings and those which are their opposites. Another logic (voluntarism or duty ethics) solves ethical questions by reference to the will of God, to recognized laws or customs, or to personal principles of behavior. This also can serve as a basis of dialogue if we can find authorities we recognize in common or moral principles with which we ourselves can agree perhaps for our own reasons. Another line of reasoning (consequentialism, utilitarianism, or situationism) attempts to find a solution which seems to bring the most satisfaction and the least hurt to all in the concrete situation. This type of thinking is very practical and realistic and must certainly form an important element in every public discussion in a pluralistic society. However, it may very well result in proposals which some members of the community will reject as unprincipled, merely expedient, shortsighted, and immoral.

In order to resolve the impasse which thus arises between those in a community who take their stand on absolute principles or authoritative laws and those who argue for pragmatic solutions, Catholic moral theology has attempted to find a middle course, which we have formulated as a Prudential Personalism. Such an approach attempts to think in terms of the consequences of any action for the good of the persons and the community involved, but it evaluates these consequences in terms of needs and purposes which have been established not by subjective preference, nor merely by abstract laws, but by the constitution of the human person in its individual and communal dynamism.

CHAPTER 8

NORMS OF CHRISTIAN DECISION IN BIOETHICS

8.1   NORMS OF CONSCIENCE ENLIGHTENED BY CHRISTIAN FATIH

8.1-1   Is There a Christian Ethics?

Today the question is debated whether there is a distinctly Christian ethics (McQuarrie, 1970; Rigali, 1971; Curran, 1975; Gustafson, 1975a). The moral values of the New Testament are also found in other religions and philosophies of life. In 1.3 we illustrated this fact by referring to the list of such values in the *Universal Declaration of Human Rights* to which all the nations of the world, whatever their ideologies, have subscribed. Yet, as we also argued in 1.3, two value systems may agree on a list of important values, yet differ markedly in their *hierarchy* of values. Thus we would expect that a Christian ethics would be characterized primarily by the priority it gives to certain values and the reasons it gives for these priorities. A Christian reflecting on the human values listed in the *Universal Declaration* will give them certain emphases and meanings in the light of the Gospel of Jesus Christ which are specifically Christian.

The great disciple of Jesus, St. Paul, summarized these Christian priorities as *faith*, *hope*, and *charity* (Rom. 13). Moreover, Paul makes clear that for him all these primary values take their full meaning from the conviction that the full life of the human person will be achieved only through a personal union with God in eternal life through incorporation in the risen Christ. A secular Humanist, a Marxist, a Muslim, and a Buddhist would all agree that faith, hope, and love are important human values, but they would differ in the emphases they give these among all values, and they would not understand them in this Christological way. Thus faith, hope, and love are common to many value systems but only in an analogical, not a univocal, sense.

To stress this analogy of common ethical terms, however, is not to deny that these terms may refer to experiences which are common to persons who use them in different senses. Analogical terms may refer to quite diverse experiences, or they may refer to one and the same experience understood in somewhat different ways in function of different systems of thought. For example, the term *love* may be used by one person to refer to an experience of sexual love and by another to refer to an experience of love for the poor. The experiences are quite different; the term is the same, but it is used analogically. On the other hand, when *love* is used by a Christian, a Buddhist, and a Humanist to refer to sexual love, the experience for all may be very much the same, and yet the term is still used analogically because of the very different ways in which each of these three interpret that experience in the context of their different views of life and different value systems.

Consequently, although Christians may be aware that when they use such terms as *faith*, *hope*, and *love* they use them with a special meaning that is only analogical to the way these terms are used by non-Christians, this need not entail that the Christian believes that non-Christians do not *experience the realities* to which these terms refer just as the Christian does. Some Christians, of course, think that non-Christians have no experience of grace nor of the true God who reveals Himself by grace, but Catholic theology has always admitted that non-Christians might be living by grace quite as really and perhaps even more intensely than Christians; that is, they experience the same realities as Christians, but they do not name them in the same way, or even when they do name them in the same way, nevertheless do not understand them in the same way. Since the Second Vatican Council, moreover, many Catholic theologians admit that grace may act not only on those of other religions, but that it may also act *through* these religions in different symbols and languages. Christians do not claim a monopoly on the true God or his grace, but only that the gracious God has made Himself most fully, explicity, and intimately know to humanity in Jesus Christ.

By love the Christian understands first of all that charity or *agape* which God has for us and which by grace He gives us as a power to love Him more than ourselves and our neighbor as ourselves. Jesus taught that the Great Commandment of Love, understood in this sense, sums up all other ethical rules (Mark 12:28-34; Matt. 22:34-40; Spicq, 1963; Furnish, 1972; Outka, 1972). This Christian love, however, is not a mere feeling as an emotivist might think, but is based on Christian faith, an enlightenment by the revealed and Incarnate Word, Jesus Christ, who tells us who God is and what our relation to Him and to our neighbor must be. Thus Christian faith moves us from an emotivist to a cognitivist level of ethical understanding, since faith is not merely a blind trust, but is also a genuine understanding of God's purpose for us, an imperfect but real share in God's wisdom. Hence Christian faith moves us beyond a duty ethics of mere obedience to God's will to a means-ends level of intelligent creative purpose and free choice.

Moreover, our relation to God and neighbor is not something simply fixed, but it is teleological, in a process of actualization which will not be complete until we reach an ultimate intimacy with the Triune God beyond this present life. Until we reach this goal, we also need Christian hope by which we do not trust in our own powers, but in the promises and grace of God manifested in the death and resurrection of Christ in order to achieve our individual and communal goals. Thus a "theology of hope" (Moltmann, 1967) or of "liberation" (Gutierrez, 1973) gives to Christian ethics an open, creative outlook analogous to the progressivism of pragmatism or the revolutionary hope of Marxism (Kamenka, 1972).

These three Pauline terms *faith*, *hope*, and *love* can serve as a way of classifying and developing a set of ethical principles for Prudential Personalism in a specifically Christian sense, which we will then apply to bioethical questions. These principles are expressed in terms which are common to most ethical systems in the analogical way just explained.

Some would call these principles philosophical as contrasted to those of a theological ethics (moral theology, Christian ethics). However, the terms *philosophical* and *theological* are themselves distinguishable only in function of some world view, so that this distinction has to be made in different ways in different world views. Hence, it is preferable to consider these principles and the terms in which they are expressed simply as analogically common to most ethical systems whether these systems are characterized as philosophical or theological. We will then give them a specifically Christian interpretation, leaving others to interpret them analogically according to their own thought systems. A Christian, for example, a Thomist, can also give them a philosophical interpretation in terms of the way the relation of philosophy to theology and of natural reason to revelation are understood in such a Christian theology (Bourke, 1951).

8.1-2   What Is an Ethical Principle?

In speaking of principles we are by no means opting for what McCormick (1977) has called a "deductive ethics" in contrast to a historical, existential ethics. Quite the contrary. We do not accept the notion of the duty or intuitionist ethics that we can establish a priori principles from which practical, ethical rules can be deduced in the manner of an axiomatic system.

By *principles* we mean general ethical rules derived from human experience and constantly tested and refined in experience. We cannot deduce conclusions from them, but we can use them to guide our intelligent analysis of concrete ethical situations. Actual ethical decision (cf. 3.4) depends not merely upon abstract reasoning, but upon *prudence* in which several other factors are also involved. At the same time, we would not agree with consequentialists that these principles are merely statistical generalizations or prima facie rules (Ross, 1965) because they are grounded in our understanding of what it is to be a human person and what it is to be a human person redeemed by Christ. Such understanding is not final or complete. It can be deepened and refined by historical experience, research, prayer, Christian living, conflict, and dialogue with other world views, but it is a genuine intellectual insight into these experiences which has a permanent and universal validity for the whole human race, as is evident from the *Universal Declaration of Human Rights* (1.3).

When bioethical debate is shallow and fruitless, it is usually because such simple, basic insights are ignored or minimized, with no effort to understand them as they appear at least analogically in the opponent's value system. By using them we can make our ethical decisions more sensitive to deep human needs, as we can ecumenically transcend some of the impasses that today divide persons of different world views (Tavard, 1973).

The first five principles or norms (some of which have been discussed previously) which we group together pertain to the formation of a prudent conscience (cf. 3.4). Since conscience is a kind of intelligent decision making, it is directly cognitive, a kind of *knowing*. Christians are acutely aware that our sin and the sinful structures of the world in which we live have blinded our human self-understanding (Rom. 1:18-32). Furthermore, God has not only called us in Christ to be freed from this blindness, but has also invited us to share in his own glory and transcendent wisdom (Rom. 5:1-3; 11:33-36). This enlightenment of our human conscience is the work of Christ's Holy Spirit through the gift of faith. Hence the Christian understanding of these principles, analogically common to many different ethical systems, interprets them in view of the Christian model of what it is to be human, a model found perfectly realized only in Jesus Christ. Only to the degree that we use this model of Christ is it possible for us to discriminate adequately between moral good and evil (Schnackenburg, 1965; Gustafson, 1976).

8.1-3 Principle of Prudent Conscience

The distinguished French biologist Jacques Monod in his book *Chance and Necessity* (1971; cf. Lewis, 1974) argues that there really is only one moral value — scientific truth — since any ethics not based on realism and facing the facts is an immoral form of self-delusion. Monod's notion of truth is too narrow and reductionistic (since the scientific method is only one way of arriving at truth), but he was quite correct in saying that the need to know the truth is the deepest need of human nature on which all morality depends. If we do not know what our real needs are, we cannot develop a means-ends ethics. This does not mean that the only value of truth is its practical use as a guide to living: truth is also something enjoyable in itself, as even the pragmatic John Dewey admitted in *Art as Experience* (1959 [1934]).

This value of truth, both practical and as something enjoyable in itself, has been emphasized in the *Universal Declaration of Human Rights* (United Nations, 1948):

> *Article 18:* Everyone has the right to freedom of thought, conscience and religion; this right includes freedom to change his religion or belief, and freedom, either alone or in community with others and in public or private, to manifest his religion or belief in teaching, practice, worship and observance.

> *Article 19:* Everyone has the right to freedom of opinion and expression; this right includes freedom to hold opinions without interference and to seek, receive and impart information and ideas through any media and regardless of frontiers.

> *Article 26:* (1) Everyone has the right to education. Education shall be free, at least in the elementary and fundamental stages. Elementary education shall be compulsory. Technical and professional education shall be made generally available and higher education shall be equally accessible to all on the basis of merit.

> (2) Education shall be directed to the full development of the human personality and to the strengthening of respect for human rights and fundamental freedoms. It shall promote understanding, tolerance and friendship among all nations, racial or religious groups, and shall further the activities of the United Nations for the maintenance of peace.

> (3) Parents have a prior right to choose the kind of education that shall be given to their children.

Christian moral theology also has insisted on the fundamental character of truth for all other values. The deepest and most profound truth accessible to us is the truth of Christian *faith*, which alone can give us true freedom. This truth of faith is found in Jesus Christ and his teaching and life. Catholic Christianity, however, has always believed that this faith by no means exempts the Christian from also seeking truth through human reason and science. Critics are inclined to say, "You Catholics talk a lot about reason and natural law in ethical matters, but when it comes right down to it, you really rely only on the dogmas of the Church. Your use of reason is merely a rationalization of what you believe by blind faith." The only answer we can give to that is to acknowledge our responsibility as Christians to be honest and faithful *both* to the light of faith and the light of reason and to make the intellectual effort to bring these two sources of knowledge into an authentic harmony with each other. To sacrifice one to the other is itself unethical because it betrays the truth, whatever its source.

However, Christians are not really in a different situation in this matter than are adherents of other religions, including Marxism and Humanism. As we showed in 1.3, all human beings have some kind of religion or equivalent philosophy of life, a world view and a system of values which rests ultimately on certain basic convictions which are not accepted by adherents to a different system. Thus Jacques Monod, as a secular Humanist, had a basic conviction in the power of science which many others would not accept without qualification (Polyani, 1964).

This conviction was the foundation of his philosophy of life. Christian faith rests on other basic convictions. In a pluralistic world we ought to respect these fundamental differences and be willing to work through ecumenical dialogue to achieve a greater consensus. All of us ought to be willing to argue for our basic convictions, but we have no need to apologize for them. The Christian world view is unquestionably one of the major ethical systems of human history which has earned a right to be heard in any ethical discussion.

This commitment to truth is expressed in the *Principle of Prudent Conscience* which was developed at length in 3.4. Here we need only to repeat the formulation given there.

> In every free decision involving an ethical question, we are morally obliged:
>
> 1. To inform ourselves as fully as possible in our practical situation as to both the facts and the ethical norms.
>
> 2. To form a morally certain judgment of conscience on the basis of this information.
>
> 3. To act according to this informed conscience.
>
> 4. To accept responsibility for our actions whether conscientious or not.

We will show in chapter 9 that the *Principle of Informed Consent* which plays a very important role in many bioethical discussions today is simply a corollary of the *Principle of Prudent Conscience*. It is obvious that if all human persons must act according to their own informed conscience, then it is unethical for me to ask *other* persons to cooperate with me or to permit me to act on them unless I share with them the revelant information required for each of us to decide whether such an act is licit. Thus, I cannot ask for their consent unless I have helped them have an informed conscience. To do so would be to deny their human dignity and moral responsibility.

The specifically Christian understanding of this Principle of Prudent Conscience derives from the kind of information required to act like a Christian (Rudin, 1964). Christians need whatever human information is available from personal and social experience and from the sciences, but in view of the Christian goal of life, they must also turn to the Word of God in Christ for the model. Christ is known to us both in his historical reality and in his actual presence in the world today only in the Christian community, its Scriptures, its Tradition, its official pastors in their teaching role, and its Sacraments as they are experienced in the actual life and prayer of individual Christians. Consequently, all these sources of information must be sought and listened to if this principle is to have a full Christian application (Pieper, 1966; May, 1975).

8.1-4 Principle of Moral Discrimination

Moral Life and Death

We are moral beings because we thoughtfully and freely choose what we do or do not do in view of the life goal to which we are committed. Of course, most of us have a rather vague understanding of what that central purpose in our lives may be, and we often act impulsively and inconsistently so that the plan and unity of our lives is obscure. Jesus spoke of us as "wandering sheep" (Mark 6:34; Luke 15:4-7) because our lives seem without purpose or plan. Yet in every person's life, if we observe carefully, the fundamental commitment is evident, shaping every important decision. Thus we say of a physician or nurse, "There is someone who really cares about people and it shows in everything he does in both his private and professional life" or "That one may be an expert professional, but is a selfish person who is always acting for personal advancement or money." This fundamental commitment (or "fundamental option" as many moralists call it today [cf. Hart, 1970; E. Cooper,1972])is the foundation of all morality. Jesus said, "It is what comes out of a man that makes him unclean; for it is from within, from men's hearts, that evil intentions emerge" (Mark 7:21). Morality is thus first of all a matter of our fundamental commitment or *generic intention*, that is, the general intention which gives unity and pattern to our whole life.

The Bible indicates in many places (e.g., Psalms 1; Deut. 30:15-20; Prov. 1 to 9; Rom. 8:1-13) that ultimately there are only two life commitments open to us: the two ways are "wisdom" and "folly." Edna McDonagh (1975) has recently characterized these as the "open way" and the "closed way." We are committed to the open way when we are ready to accept the truth whenever it confronts us and to seek to understand ourselves and all of reality more and more truly and then to act in accordance with truth, constantly widening and deepening our love of all the persons and things that make up the universe.

Whoever honestly pursues this open way is moving toward the light, because it is God who is drawing that person to Himself. The closed way is what the Scriptures frequently refer to as "idolatry," commitment to a false god, who is the god of darkness and hatred, and who turns out to be simply a symbol of the false self as it contracts on itself, feeds on itself, locked up in the prison of its own prejudices, illusions, and hatreds, and seeks to dominate and use all other persons and things for itself. Although this evil way is focused on the idol of the self, this is not the true human self, but a corrupted self. Those who seek the open way seem to lose themselves, but they find their true self made by God for Himself (Mark 8:35).

Thus physicians and nurses committed to the open way of life are always growing as persons and professionals, always widening their interests and concerns, always fulfilling themselves by giving to others and receiving from others with humility and gratitude. But physicians and nurses committed to a closed way of life are always contracting more and more into a selfish world, preoccupied with status and power, hedged in by prejudice, pride, and fear of competition and deadened by pessimism, cynicism, and apathy.

The term *mortal sin* so familiar to Catholics really refers to this commitment to a closed, selfish, idolatrous life. The choice of such a life is not made, at least ordinarily, without a long preceding process of alienation from God and neighbor. Little by little through a thousand acts of petty selfishness, indifference to others, superficial thinking, indifference, vanity, and deception do persons finally come to the breaking point at which they decide to serve themselves rather than to serve God and neighbor. Jesus said, "No one can serve two masters. He will either hate the first and love the second, or treat the first with respect and the second with scorn. You cannot be the slave both of God and of money" (Matt. 6:24). For "money" here we can substitute any idol, that is, the closed self.

Actions which do not do serious harm to ourselves or others (but which nevertheless are harmful and which if we do not try to remedy them may soon turn into a pattern of behavior that forms the process leading up to mortal sin) are called *venial sins*. Morally speaking, they are utterly different from mortal sin because they do not change the fundamental orientation of our lives as does mortal sin, but they confuse and weaken our movement toward our true goal and can finally end in a mortally sinful break with that commitment. We might compare them to the many little quarrels, insensitivities, and neglects which are part of the married lives of most people. If a couple admits these faults and tries to remedy them by positive acts of love, such acts and omissions may not harm the marriage very much, but if they are passed over, they gradually cool love, widening the distance and lack of communication between the couple until at last the marriage is broken by rejection and the death of love.

Thus falling into moral sin is a long process, but it is also a crucial event. The breaking point comes when a person breaks off the commitment to openness toward God and withdraws into the closed self. Such an act of mortal sin can take place either *explicitly* by a deliberate turning away from our true goal in life, from God or at least from that search for the Ultimate Good, or it can take place *implicitly* when we choose to do something which we know to be seriously contradictory to that commitment. "If any one says: 'My love is fixed on God, and hates his brother', he is a liar" (I John 4:20). We cannot be open to God, to light, to love, to truth, and at the same time do serious harm either to our neighbor or to our true self. Thus, mortal sins are acts which explicitly turn us from our true end, from the open way of life, or which do so implicitly by contradicting that way of life and what it implies. Health care professionals who claim to be religious or respectable, but who knowingly and deliberately seriously neglect or misuse professional skill or status so that others are harmed or the professionals' own development as persons is seriously impaired commit mortal sin and make commitments to idolatrous goals in life.

However, because we often act unthinkingly or when too much influenced by emotion or from lack of needed information, we may act with good intention and yet do a great deal of harm. Although, as we have seen, our goodwill or *subjective* intention is the very root of morality, yet goodwill is not sufficient to get us to our goal unless it includes the effort to make our actions *objectively* effective. A physician who wants to heal a patient, but who keeps making mistakes in diagnosis and treatment, deserves credit for goodwill, but the patient will not be any the better for it. Moreover, unless physicians make an effort to correct their mistakes, they cannot really claim to have goodwill at all. Thus, our morally good actions are first of all to be judged on our good *intention*, but they must also be judged objectively. All the good intentions in the world do not save ourselves or others from the bad consequences of objectively wrong actions (E. D'Arcy, 1963) nor from the responsibility of repairing these wrongs which stand in our way and the way of others in achieving our true human goals. Hence moral rightness or wrongness is constituted by the *relation* between a particular action and this true goal of human living as this relation is perceived and freely intended by a human person.

This relation, however, is not simple, but is conditioned in several ways. First, we do not simply intend to reach our goal by a general intention. That goal can only be reached by taking definite steps. As the saying goes, If you will the end, you must also will the means. It is not enough to intend to love God, unless as St. James says this love expresses itself in concrete acts of care for our neighbor (James 2:14-17). Hence, each particular act specifies our remote and general intention by a proximate and specific intention which we call the moral object or purpose of the act. Note that this proximate intention is not other than our general intention, but is a further, concrete determination of it. I love God by bandaging this patient's wound.

Second, it must be noticed that a moral object has both a form and a content. The moral form of the act of bandaging wounds is my intention to serve patients in their effort to regain health through a particular healing procedure; the content of the act, however, is the therapeutic procedure itself considered as a process of cleansing, medicating, bandaging, and so forth. It is at this point that medical facts and moral values come together to form a single act which is at the same time a physical, biological, and psychological process and yet also a moral act invested with human meaning. It is a medical act, but it is also a moral act which we express by the term *care*, which implies not merely technical skill, but also human personal concern for the patient.

How is it that facts and values can meet in this way? Obviously, it is because in the act of health care taken in its biological and psychological aspects there are already values (actions which are harmful or beneficial to the human organism). The bandaging process is helpful to the human organism because it furthers the natural processes within the organism itself toward health and optimal functioning. There may also be negative values (disvalues) since the bandage may impede circulation, and so forth. However, if on the whole the bandaging is helpful to nature, then a professional faced with the decision of whether to bandage or not to bandage can ethically decide to do so. When this decision is made in view of the patient's good and the professional's commitment to caring for the patient, then this merely biological and technical act, simple as it is, becomes a moral act with a moral object. Thus, in any moral object we can distinguish the content of the act (technically referred to as the physical or ontic or premoral or nonmoral object) and the specific moral purpose which makes the physical act into a moral act.

Third, we must notice that specific moral acts are always performed in a context or situation, for example, the act of bandaging is commonly performed by a nurse in a hospital or clinic during daytime hours. As long as the situation is an ordinary or normal one, it does not modify the moral character of an action. However, sometimes there may be unusual features of the situation which are morally significant, for example, if the nurse bandages the wound of a fugitive criminal, she may find herself an accomplice of his crime. Hence, in determining the morality of an action once we know what the specific moral object is, we need then to ask if there are any special circumstances which might modify the moral significance of the action. These circumstances can be of place, of time, or of person (as in the example just cited). They can also be a matter of *intention* when in addition to the specific intention of the act the agent has some additional and special motive, for example, if the nurse bandages the patient not only to help the patient, but also to teach an aide how to perform the procedure. Such an intention is a *circumstantial* intention.

Note that we have now used the term *intention* in three different senses: (1) our general intention of our life's goal (fundamental option), (2) our specific intention of this particular act as a means to that goal (moral object with its nonmoral content), and (3) possible additional motives (circumstantial intentions).

The special circumstances of an action which is of itself morally wrong can make it worse, for example, the fact that a nurse neglects a child patient is probably more irresponsible than if an adult is the one neglected. If the action is good, circumstances can make it better, for example, a nurse deserves more credit for attention to a difficult patient. But can circumstances make a bad act good? Catholic moral theology has traditionally held that if a moral object in its own specific intention is morally wrong (intrinsically evil) it can then not be made morally good by any special circumstance. For example, killing a suffering patient, because the act kills an innocent person, can never be morally justified, no matter what the special circumstances of the patient (age, member of one's family, degree of suffering, etc.) nor the good intention of the agent (e.g., intention to end the patient's pain). However, recently question has been raised whether this traditional teaching requires revision.

Exceptionless Moral Norms

One important effort at such a revision of traditional Catholic teaching on moral discrimination has been proposed by Josef Fuchs (1971) of the Gregorian University in Rome, based on the original work of Peter Knauer (1967) and further developed by Bruno Schüller (1973, 1974). This theory developed by German theologians has been further clarified in the United States by Richard McCormick (1973a, 1973b, 1975, 1976, 1977) and applied practically by many American authors writing in the field of medical ethics (Maguire, 1974; Dedek, 1975; Curran, 1977a; Kosnik, 1977; Boyle, 1977). Hence it requires careful but necessarily brief analysis here. Current controversies among Catholic moralists largely reflect different evaluations of Fuchs's views, some being strongly critical (Grisez, 1970b; Connery, 1973; Quay, 1975; May, 1975, 1977a, 1977b).

Fuchs points out that any revision of moral theology true to Catholic Tradition must avoid subjectivism, that is, must not judge the morality of an action merely on the basis of the good intention of the agent. On the other hand, in an effort to be objective traditional moral theology too often tried to decide the morality of an action solely on the basis of the moral object, that is, on the nature of the action considered in the abstract apart from the context of the agent's intention and the circumstances. Fuchs, therefore, argues it would be more truly objective to judge the morality of an act by taking into consideration the moral object, intention, and circumstances *simultaneously*.

Fuchs's position implies that no act considered in its intrinsic nature solely according to its moral object can be judged "intrinsically evil" (*malum per se*). Hence, he logically concludes we must abandon the classical notion of "absolute moral norms," since all moral rules may admit of exception given some special combination of object, circumstances, and intention. Fuchs says that practically speaking he cannot imagine how it could ever be morally justifiable to torture an innocent child, but he would admit theoretically that even this act might be morally good under some very peculiar circumstances and for some special purpose. Nevertheless, he rejects moral relativism, because there are moral rules which hold "for the most part."

If, following Fuchs's argument, we undertake to judge the morality of acts by the moral object only when it is taken conjointly with the circumstances and intention, we have to deal with the fact that most moral acts in the concrete are morally ambiguous, since they involve both good and bad elements — pros and cons, benefits and costs. It might seem, therefore, that we are often forced to "do evil that good may come of it." However, those who hold Fuchs's position (e.g., Janssens, 1972) argue that this difficulty can be solved by carefully distinguishing between the premoral or ontic content of the human act and its moral meaning. The content of an act may include premoral disvalues as well as values, yet formally speaking the act as a whole can be morally good (as we also admit; see 8.1-2).

Since an act may contain both values and disvalues, how do we decide whether it is morally good or evil as a whole? Fuchs and his followers believe this question can be reduced to the application of a single principle which they call the principle of proportion or of preference, according to which an act is morally good if the proportion of values it implies exceeds the disvalues, taking into account simultaneously the nature of the act, the circumstances, and the intention of the agent.

What is to be thought of this methodology of moral discernment? It is very attractive in its apparent simplicity and realism. However, while we agree that a revision of traditional Catholic moral theology is long overdue and we welcome all contributions by theologians to this common task, we do not believe that the principle of proportion provides a satisfactory foundation for such a revision. Here we can only state briefly two chief difficulties.

First, it seems that this theory does not provide grounds by which Christian ethics can escape ethnocentrism and maintain a prophetic countercultural witness in obedience to God rather than to men (Acts 5:29). Undoubtedly human morality is historically and culturally conditioned. However, in seeking a true moral judgment we also seek to transcend (however difficult this may be) the enthnocentrism of our personal and cultural situation precisely because culture is not something given to us human beings, but is something which we have the responsibility to create and re-form. Consequently, we are always required to judge and reformulate the moral standards of our culture against some higher, deeper, more universal standard. The Christian appeals to the Gospel for this transcultural, transhistorical standard.

However, the Gospel itself confirms, even as it surpasses, the order of creation or nature, the natural law as this is rightly understood in the light of the Gospel. This law is confirmed in the Ten Commandments of the Old Testament, confirmed and perfected by Jesus in the Sermon on the Mount, and appealed to by St. Paul in Romans 1 in judgment on merely human moral standards.

Nor can we reduce this natural law simply to the power of human reason to take into account all factors of a moral situation, as Fuchs (1971) now seems to reinterpret the traditional Thomistic teaching. For Aquinas to say that natural law is human reason includes the affirmation that our human reason rightly used can discover a purposeful order in the world prior to any willed human purpose. Our willed human purposes must conform to this natural order if they are to be fully human and ethical. We can discover these natural purposes in the innate needs of our human persons, in their common biological and psychological structures, and in the fundamental social relations upon which the survival of our human community depends.

Thus, when we seek to revise the moral norms of a particular culture in light of the universal demands of the Gospel and the order of Creation, we attempt to make these norms participate in the *absolute* character of these demands as founding rights and obligations which have no exception because they apply to all human persons and all societies. Even when conflicts appear to arise between these rights, we proceed to seek a resolution of such conflicts with confidence that such a resolution is a practical goal, even when frequently we lack the wisdom to find it. Hence, it is necessary to maintain that some kinds of human acts are *direct* violations of such basic rights and therefore *intrinsically* unethical — means which contradict the ends to which they are ordered — and thus are always contrary to reason, nature, and the Gospel. To build up a moral system in which on principle every moral norm may have an exception, as Fuchs does, seems to be tantamount to saying that prior to human culture there is no determinant order of nature which must be respected by human culture.

Nevertheless, to insist, as we do, on the potential significance of human acts in their intrinsic physical and psychological structures does not force us to accept biologism (cf. Curran, 1975, 1977a), because we do not consider this premoral structure or order of nature as the actual formal determinant of morality, but only as its material condition. Human intentions, creativity, and culture can transform given biological relations in unpredictable ways, just as no one can predict what an artist can make out of a block of stone. However, a good artist respects his material, and so does a moral human being respect his or her biologically given body and psyche, both as intrinsically forming the human person and as essentially relative to other human persons in the family and society. Indeed, we must even respect our own native culture, but only to the degree it perfects, not contradicts, the order of the Gospel and of nature.

A *second* difficulty about Fuchs's theory is that the principle of proportion does not really provide a practical, nonarbitrary way to determine the morality of concrete acts. Its proponents point out that in traditional moral theology also proportion between good and evil consequences was considered a determinant of morality (cf. 8.1-5). However, the older theologians used proportion in this sense only with the presupposition of a hierarchy of values based on *intrinsic* morality by which it was possible to measure the relative importance of various values and disvalues. Once we abandon intrinsic morality and make the principle of proportion the primary determinant, it is no longer clear how such an evaluation can be made. Thus, the new method, in spite of its rejection of utilitarianism, makes itself vulnerable to all the objections raised against utilitarianism by duty ethics (Frankena, 1973; Brock, 1973). This difficulty appears clearly in practice when we read how McCormick (1973b) argues for "virtually exceptionless" norms such as that forbidding euthanasia because the evils involved seem to outweigh any likely goods, while Maguire (1974a) sees no difficulty in admitting that in some cases euthanasia is justified because the good outweighs the evil.

Why then has Fuchs's system gained so many adherents? Concretely, it seems to be because many theologians were disillusioned with the way natural law arguments were used in the contraception controversy (cf. 10.1) and are looking for a new approach which will respond more realistically to all aspects of a concrete moral situation. However, the fact that some of the absolute norms of classical moral theology appear today insufficiently grounded does not prove there are no such norms, nor that none are known, but only that they require better formulation as we continue our search for a more profound understanding of the mystery of the human person in community. Further, as Henry Veatch (1971) has shown, since the rise of modern science ethicists have been overpowered by the mechanistic explanation of the world according to which nature including our human bodily nature lacks all inherent teleology or finality. Hence it would seem that values cannot be grounded in the order of nature but only in the order of culture. Consequently, most modern ethical theories refer these values not to nature but to the historical development of culture, as Fuchs does. However, there is good reason to think that in this last quarter of the twentieth century scientism is on the wane, and that a Christian ethics for the future should not be built on scientistic assumptions. We believe that the personalist-communitarian view of human nature which we have sketched in chapters 1 and 2 is entirely consistent with the achievements of modern natural and behavioral science once this is freed of its idealistic and mechanistic interpretations.

In pointing out these inadequacies of the approach of Fuchs and others to the task of revising Catholic moral theology, we do not mean to reject the important contribution moralists of this school are making to medical ethics. By their emphasis on analyzing all dimensions of moral conflicts and their effort to weigh all the consequences of an action, they are contributing to the transformation of the moral theologies of the manuals from a legalistic duty ethics to a means-ends ethics in the form of a personalistic ethics of responsibility (Curran, 1977a). In chapter 7 we advocated the same transformation, but we believe it should be made in accordance with the natural law tradition, not in contravention of it.

We also believe that it is important for health care professionals to contribute to this restoration of a sense of the natural order in Catholic thinking, precisely because they have the opportunity to realize how science well understood uncovers the natural order in the human person and how the medical art cooperates with "the wisdom of the body" (Cannon, 1939).

Moral Discrimination

How then do we discriminate between moral and immoral actions? We have to ask ourselves and others two basic questions:

1. Does it *directly* alienate me from my authentic life goal of loving God above all and my neighbor as myself?

2. Does it *indirectly* alienate me from that goal by neglecting or rejecting some intermediate goal necessary to attain that ultimate goal?

If either is the case, then the action is mortally evil. If it is evil but falls short of such radical rejection either (1) because the action is not serious in the injury it does or (2) because I do not consent to it fully and deliberately, then the action is venial, that is, it hinders full movement toward the goal but is not contradictory to it.

Determining whether any given human act is essentially contradictory to the true ends of human living as to be intrinsically evil is of course not a simple process. We should never be quick to conclude, that any act is mortally evil or to generalize our judgment in the form of absolute norms. But the possibility that such a norm prevails is real, and in some cases it is obviously realized. Furthermore, when such absolute norms have become an accepted part of the standards of our culture or of the ordinary teaching of our Church, we ought to consider them prima facie binding in conscience unless careful study shows they need modification or clarification.

This is the same caution that is observed by the sanely conservative physician who knows that professional responsibility to the patient requires the use of well-tested treatments and not merely experimental ones. Those who are willing to base their lives or to counsel others to base their lives on some new morality must justify such modification of traditional norms with strong arguments. At the same time, we also fail in our obligation to inform our conscience when we close our eyes to new suggestions about how to improve our previous moral understanding. Being blind to new thought may be a sin against the light and the Spirit, a deadly sin indeed.

We can now formulate the *Principle of Moral Discrimination* as follows:

1. A deliberate act, freely consented to, is mortally sinful if it breaks our life commitment to God directly or indirectly by doing serious harm to human persons (one's self included) who are his children.

2. Whether an act is sinful or ethical can be determined:
   a. By first considering if it can be an appropriate means to the love of God and neighbor, or whether its intrinsic teleology renders it contradictory to such a purpose.
   b. By then considering the circumstances including any circumstantial intention which may make an indifferent act a good means to this love of God and neighbor, a good means better, or an evil means either more or less evil, but which cannot make an intrinsically evil act (i.e., a means contradictory to the end) simply morally good.

The specifically Christian understanding of this principle derives from the revelation in Christ that the goal of human life is to share in the life of Father, Son, and Holy Spirit (Matt. 11:25-30; Luke 10:22; I John 1:3). Every moral choice must be guided by our longing to reach this goal, which absolutely excludes mortal sin, that is, acts which would turn us away from that goal directly, whether directed toward God or neighbor. All our intelligent freedom must be used to facilitate this journey to God for ourselves and others. In this pursuit, we must use our own creativity to the fullest, but we must also respect the creative wisdom of God which has made us what we are and which guides us providentially in the concrete circumstances of our lives. In this we imitate Jesus who remained faithful in all his actions to the call his Father gave him, even in the historical situation of his times and under the shadow of the cross.

8.1-5 Principle of Double Effect

We have already noted that a good moral act may involve not only values, but also disvalues. Certainly we are often puzzled by the undesirable side effects of actions we feel morally obliged to do. The moralists of the principle of proportion school discussed in the last section use this principle to handle all such cases. For them, an action is morally good when the agent acts so as to maximize values and minimize disvalues (Van der Poel, 1968; Curran, 1975). Some frequently speak of the necessity of choosing the "lesser evil" in the many moral dilemmas which we find in our lives today. They are not proposing that we do moral evil, but rather that we are morally obliged to choose the alternative which involves the lesser disvalues (premoral evils).

We have explained why we think such considerations, although not invalid, are insufficient moral guides. We must not only avoid causing more harm than good by an action, but we must also refuse to do something that is intrinsically wrong, even if in some circumstances it seems that this action may lead to greater good than evil, or that refusing to do it may lead to greater evil than good. Our confidence is that ultimately intrinsically wrong actions, because they give a wrong basic orientation to our course of action, will in the long run lead to greater evil than good, no matter how attractive and beneficial they may appear in the short run.   For example, a lie undermines the trust on which a good relation between human beings rests and thus corrupts the whole relation with at least the risk of harmful long-range consequences.

It might seem, therefore, that we should never perform any action from which we foresee evil results, but should insist on performing only those actions which have good consequences. Otherwise, it would seem that we are responsible for the evil and have at least partially done evil as a means to a good end. However, this position of moral purism or rigorism (or tutiorism, i.e., doing only what is morally safe) is no sounder than the principle of the lesser evil because it makes action almost impossible in a world wherein even the best actions do in fact have some evil results. Since refusal to act is itself often a neglect of duty, this kind of purism actually leads to sins of omission or withdrawal from our responsibilities.

Consequently, moralists have developed the *Principle of Double Effect* as a rule by which the extremes of consequentialism and moral purism can be avoided (Mangan, 1949; Ghoos, 1951). It can be expressed as follows:

> When an action has foreseen consequences that are both good and evil, we can and should permit it if the following conditions (Connell, 1968) are met:
>
> 1. The object of the act is not intrinsically evil. (This condition avoids consequentialism and is simply the Principle of Moral Discrimination, 8.1-2).
>
> 2. The intention of the agent is to achieve the good effects and to avoid the evil as far as possible. (This condition avoids purism since it recognizes that we can intend the good while recognizing that we are indirectly responsible for some evil.)
>
> 3. The good effects are equal or greater than the ill effects.
>
> 4. The good effect follows from the action at least as immediately as the evil effect.

The purpose of this final requirement is to exclude the use of an evil means to achieve a good end since such action would also violate the first requirement. This final condition is not always easy to apply. Because of these difficulties, there have been several recent attempts to reformulate the principle. The suggestion which seems to the writers of this book the most persuasive is made by Germain Grisez (1970a, 1970b, 1974). Grisez (1974) points out:

> . . . The ambiguity of ambiguous actions can be of two kinds. In one type the destructive aspect of the action is the means by which the positive aspect is realized. In the second the two aspects are really inseparably

linked in one action; the positive aspect does not produce the destructive, nor does the destructive produce the positive; the act embraces both results directly. (p. 140)

He cites as an example of the first the old practice of castrating boy sopranos for the purpose of producing beautiful music. In this case the act of mutilation is one act (a means) intended for the sake of another distinct act (making music). This is doing evil for a good purpose, because the intention of the first act is to mutilate (an evil), although the intention of the second act is to make music (a good). On the other hand, the second kind of ambiguous action is illustrated by castration of a boy to prevent the spread of cancer. In this case there is only one indivisible act intended, namely, an act of healing (good) which, however, contains two effects (one good, one bad) inseparably connected. The essential ethical difference between the two cases is that in the second the *evil* need not be intended but only permitted, while in the first case the agent *must* intend the evil (otherwise the act would never be performed), although the agent intends it only as a means and not an end.

It might seem that Grisez's suggestion is itself ambiguous in application, since it requires us to decide when an act is really indivisible. However, Grisez shows that although in given cases the answer is not always obvious it can be worked out in objective manner by analyzing the actual free choices which are open to an agent. The advantage of this new formulation is that it no longer forces us to consider only the order of physical causality in an act (i.e., whether in an operation the mutilation of the body or the healing follows directly from the surgical incision), but takes this physical order along with the moral intention which gives unity to all the physical elements of the act.

Charles E. Curran (1975) has also recently reviewed the various new views on double effect and grants that Grisez's formulation has much to commend it. However, he prefers the route taken by the principle of proportion theorists who have reduced the Principle of Double Effect, first, to "commensurate reason" (Knauer, 1967) and, then, to the principle of proportion. We on the contrary believe the Principle of Double Effect should be retained, but its importance should not be exaggerated. It is only a corollary of the more fundamental Principle of Moral Discrimination as a rule which comes into play as a way of discovering whether an act which is clearly good in intention is in fact an excuse for the use of morally evil means. When a prudent examination of a course of action does not reveal this lack of integrity, we have every right to take the benefit of the doubt and judge on the basis of the good and practical intention. Thus in medical ethics we would begin with the assumption that if the professional intends the good of the patient and undertakes the most effective therapy known medically to achieve this good that the procedure is ethical *unless* there are clear reasons to show that this involves *demonstrably* evil means. The Principle of Double Effect either in its old form or in its reformulation by Grisez suggests some tests we can apply, but ultimately the discrimination remains prudential, a prudence which ordinarily needs reinforcement by professional and community consensus or legitimate moral authority.

The specifically Christian understanding of this principle of double effect arises from our Biblical understanding of the origin of evil in the world which differs markedly from the Buddhist idea that evil is illusion or the secular Humanist idea that evil is an inevitable part of evolutionary progress (Bowker, 1970). Christians believe that we as the community of the human race, and in some measure as individuals, have rebelled against God's loving will for us and chosen to "know good and evil" (Gen. 3:4), that is, to live in an ambiguous world where good and evil are mixed confusedly. To find a straight path through such a world is impossible without the guidance of Christ and the Holy Spirit he has sent us, but it also requires us to use our intelligence to the fullest to separate what is essentially good and accidentally evil from what is essentially evil and accidentally good. Jesus calls on us to be "cunning as serpents, yet harmless as doves" (Matt. 10:16) and rebuked the witless imprudence of some of his followers (Luke 16:8).

8.1-6 Principle of Legitimate Cooperation

From what has been said, it follows that we must be careful not to cooperate in or promote the actions of others when these acts are immoral (Healy, 1956; Kelly, 1958). Obviously, it is immoral to cooperate with an evil action by intending it one's self, for example, to furnish a relative with the means of suicide because one wishes to be rid of the burden, although one would never actually murder the relative directly. To actually intend the evil purpose is *formal cooperation*, no matter how small one's share in the actual physical execution. Advising, counseling, promoting, or condoning an evil action, even when sometimes done merely by being silent when one has a duty to speak up or express an opinion, is formal cooperation because such actions signify agreement with evil.

Material cooperation, on the other hand, is any kind of cooperation in which one does *not intend* the evil effects, but only the good. When such material cooperation is immediate (e.g., physicians who assist in abortion which they personally disapprove but with which they cooperate because the woman requests their technical assistance), it amounts to the same as formal cooperation since it is a direct contribution to an evil act in which the cooperator shares the responsibility for the act (Merkelbach, 1959). On the other hand, mediate material cooperation which can be proximate or remote is under certain conditions sometimes justified and even necessary. These conditions are as follows (McFadden, 1967).

First, the more remote the cooperation, the easier it is to justify. For example, the manufacture of morphine is remote from drug abuse since morphine also has important and legitimate medical uses. But the sale of morphine is closer to actual abuse and must be carefully regulated to ensure that it is put only to legitimate uses.

Second, the good achieved by the cooperation must outweigh the contribution of the cooperator to the evil and the degree of evil. Thus persons whose livelihood depends upon a job (because it is impossible or difficult to get another similar job) are justified in working for certain institutions (or hospitals) wherein abortion is performed provided they disapprove and do not immediately cooperate with an abortion.

Thus in such institutions there are many different degrees of cooperative proximity, ranging from the nurses whose cooperation is very proximate to the janitor of the building whose cooperation is very remote; yet all have the moral responsibility of deciding if there is sufficient reason to justify their material cooperation with the destruction of the innocent, just as the same responsibility rests on participants in a war effort in which obliteration bombing of noncombatants is regularly employed.

This justification exists (1) because the cooperation is not formal (the person does not want the abortion and would try to prevent it if possible), (2) because the material cooperation is mediate since most of the person's work does not contribute to the abortion (except if the institution is an abortion clinic wherein all or most of the work is abortion related), and (3) because the loss of job is a very serious matter.

Third, the evil effects of scandal, that is, the bad example that can be set, must be weighed. Even the appearance of cooperation with evil helps this evil to continue. The Christian has a serious duty to take a stand against evil and to share in it as little as possible. Thus Christians should take as active a part as is practically possible in protesting against evils in institutions in which they work or from which they benefit. Catholic hospitals in particular have the responsibility to consider the kind of example they set in a community even by appearing to condone evils (cf. chapter 9 for more specific norms of cooperation in regard to abortion).

If we refused even remote material cooperation in the affairs of a community, we would also sin by *omission* since doing good also would become impossible (Curran, 1975; O'Rourke, 1976). A Christian purist would be unable to act as a citizen or to share in any institution because every government, human institution, and even organized religion commits some evil and unjust acts. By belonging to such an organization, we somewhat cooperate with these evils. Yet we have a moral obligation to belong to social institutions since only through them can legitimate human needs be served.

Charles E. Curran (1975) has shown how the Second Vatican Council in the *Declaration on Religious Liberty* (1965b) advanced Catholic moral thinking by permitting a degree of cooperation by Catholics with non-Catholics in their religious activities which moralists had previously considered unjustifiable. In part the council grounded this on a more benign view of the religious truth found in such practices, but also on the respect due to the consciences of others, even when these others may be in error. Thus, we may sometimes cooperate with other *persons* out of respect for their right to act according to their conscience, even when we cannot in good conscience ourselves cooperate with their *acts as such*. Curran points out that if this type of cooperation is permitted in so sacred a matter as religious worship it must also be permissible in lesser matters such as many of those of which medical ethics treats. We would agree with this important observation, but would emphasize that it would not justify immediate cooperation in intrinsically wrong acts (e.g., suicide), especially when they involve the rights of a third party (e.g., abortion), any more than such cooperation would be permitted in religious matters (e.g., polygamy, ritual murder).

The Committee on Doctrine of the National Conference of Catholic Bishops (NCCB) recently (Nov. 22, 1977) issued a commentary concerning the possibility of using material cooperation in the matter of direct sterilization. Because of the sensitive nature of such judgments, the document states clearly that any decision in this regard must be made in dialogue with the local bishop.

Thus, we can formulate the *Principle of Legitimate Cooperation* as follows:

> It is always unethical to cooperate formally with an immoral act (i.e., to intend the evil act itself), but it may be an ethical duty to cooperate materially with an evil act (i.e., without intending the evil act itself) when only in this way can a greater evil be prevented, provided (1) that the cooperation is not immediate and (2) that the degree of cooperation and the danger of scandal are taken into account in judging this proportion.

8.1-7 Principle of Professional Communication

Obviously we cannot really arrive at truth simply by individual effort. No single person has all the information needed for good decisions, nor can truth be arrived at except by a social effort. Every human institution, particularly every modern health care institution, is an enormously complex system of *information*. The moment a patient enters, a process of taking a history, of performing tests, of filling out records, of keeping charts, and so forth, begins. Furthermore, an endless amount of research contained in the medical library and in the brains of a network of technologists and specialists begins to be applied to the process of diagnosis and prescription for the patient's treatment. Moreover, because the institution is an administrative network of cooperating personnel, there is the problem of interpersonal relations among the staff and the patients themselves.

This whole network is essentially dependent on good *communication*, which is impossible without (1) trust, (2) contact among the people who have information, (3) clear articulation and expression of information, and (4) continuous feedback by which failures in communication can be corrected. Modern communication theory has shown that this work of communication depends first upon good emotional relations among the communicators since emotional conflict is a powerful barrier to communication and brings into play all sorts of uncontrollable, unconscious factors. It thus becomes a serious moral duty in every institution to promote an emotional openness among both the staff and the patients.

Since we have discussed the application of the *Principle of Professional Communication* in detail in 5.2, we need only repeat the principle here.

Health care professionals have the responsibility:

1. To strive to establish and preserve trust at both the emotional and rational levels,

2. To share the information they possess which is legitimately needed by others in order to have an informed conscience,

3. To refrain from lying or giving misinformation,

4. To keep secret information which is not legitimately needed by others, but which if revealed might either harm the patient or others or destroy trust.

The Christian specification of this principle arises from the Christian understanding of trust and forgiveness. Jesus, in the case of Nicodemus (John 3:1-21), the Samaritan woman (4:1-42), and the adulterous woman (8:1-11) and elsewhere, is represented as dealing with individuals in a way that established their trust and their confidence in its full acceptance of them even in their sinfulness. The Church in its sacrament of reconciliation has established the confessional seal of total confidentiality so that people might feel free to unburden themselves not merely of physical and psychological problems but of their real guilt. For the Christian, therefore, professional confidentiality is not only professional; it expresses respect for the dignity of the human being whom only God has a right to judge (Matt. 7:1-5).

8.2 NORMS OF CHRISTIAN LOVE

Motivation

We have just listed the norms that relate directly to our knowing, reasoning, and judging processes in decision making. We next come to the norms that relate more to our affective *motivation* since motivation powerfully influences judgment for good or ill. Such motivation has both a structural or relational aspect and a dynamic or processive aspect. The structural aspect has to do with the interpersonal relations which bind persons together in community, and the ethical norms which govern these relations can rightly be called norms of love, as distinguished from the norms of conscience which we have just discussed.

By *love* we mean not only a kind of feeling, but also the practical *will* which leads us to be concerned about another person and that person's true needs. Furthermore, it motivates us to help that other person fulfill these needs by sharing with her the values we ourselves enjoy.

In any Christian ethics, the fundamental truth is that there is a Triune God and that "God is love" (John 4:8). God loves us not because He has first needed our love, but because his love for us has made us lovable:

> God's love was revealed in our midst in this way: he sent his only Son to the world that we might have life through him. Love, then, consists in this: not that we have loved God, but that he has loved us and has sent his Son as an offering for our sins . . . If we love one another, God dwells in us and his love is brought to perfection in us. (I John 4:9-10, 12)

The great theologians have all taught that the essence of the Christian life is the sharing by grace in this love of God by which we love Him and one another by the very same love by which He has created and redeemed us (Gilleman, 1961; Pieper, 1974). God's love is thus a life-giving and healing activity, and the health care ministry is a work of love by which we cooperate with God in giving life and healing sickness. God's love can never be a merely sentimental love because it is built on faith and on all truth that we derive from human reason and science. Therefore, the health care professional's love must be a love informed by the best available medical knowledge and skill.

Christian professionals know that God has loved them first, and that whatever love professionals have is a share in this divine love, which must be shared in turn with others, not by a minimal performance of duties, but as a generous concern and realistic care for those in need. However, under the pressures of daily work with its frustrations, this vision and realization of God's personal love as the source and motivation of that work can become very dim and can fade into a deadly routine. Jesus, the great physician, found the pressure of the sick so great that he, too, had to retire into a desert place to pray and to regain hope and strength:

> The whole town came crowding around the door, and he cured many who were suffering from diseases of one kind or another . . . In the morning, long before dawn, he got up and left the house, and went off to a lonely place and prayed there. (Mark 1:33, 35)

Three particular norms help to define the content of Christian love: (1) we must value every person as a unique, irreplaceable member of the human community (Principle of Human Dignity in Community); (2) we must encourage every person to play a role in the common life and fully share its fruits (Principle of Common Good, Subsidiarity, and Functionalism); and (3) we must assist all persons to realize their full potential (Principle of Totality and Integrity). In previous chapters we have developed these three principles. Here we will restate them with some reflections on their specifically Christian understanding.

8.2-1 Principle of Human Dignity in Community

Although today the unique value of every human being is affirmed by all religions and philosophies of life and the inalienable rights of the person are guaranteed by the constitutions of most governments, yet these rights are silently contradicted by three trends which seem to characterize contemporary life: (1) persons are swallowed up in totalitarian, bureaucratic institutions; (2) persons who are unnecessary for the efficient operations of these institutions — women, the very young, the very old, the uneducated, the defective — are treated as non-persons; (3) even successful persons find their happiness not in sharing their lives with others but in private, individualistic satisfactions.

In 1.5 we tried to show how the right understanding of human personhood and our essentially social nature can help us overcome this contradiction. We conclude with the following formulation of the *Principle of Human Dignity in Community*:

> All ethical decisions (including those involved in health care) must aim at human dignity, that is, the maximum, integrated satisfaction of the innate and cultural needs of every human person including his or her biological, psychological, ethical, and spiritual needs as a member of the world community and national communities which exist for this purpose only.

The Christian specification of this principle comes from what Jesus Christ added to our understanding of ourselves as created by God in his own image to share his eternal Triune life in our total person as bodily and resurrected beings. The community in question, therefore, is not only this temporal human community, but also the Kingdom of God into which even the least and most unworthy human beings are called.

8.2-2 Principle of the Common Good, Subsidiary, and Functionalism

The Principle of Human Dignity in Community requires that we also establish the various levels of responsibility within the community. In chapter 3 we argue that the primary responsibility for health rests with the individual concerned and that the whole work of health care professionals must be conceived as a cooperative service to individuals in their personal search for health. At the same time, no individual is self-sufficient in this search and can achieve health only with the help of the community. Consequently, it is also essential to give attention to the *Principle of the Common Good, Subsidiarity, and Functionalism* which we discussed and formulated in 6.2 as follows:

> A community exists to promote and share the common good among all its members "from each according to ability, to each according to need" in such a way (1) that decision making rests vertically first with the person, then with the lower social levels, and horizontally with functional social units, and (2) that the higher social units intervene only to supply whatever the lower units cannot supply, while working to make it easier for lower units and individual persons to achieve independent capability in the future.

The Christian specification of this principle is given by St. Paul in I Corinthians (12-13) where he shows that the Christian understanding of the person based on Jesus' concern for "the little ones," "the least brethren" (Mark 9:33-37) must be the principle that governs the Church, conceived as the Body of Christ, ensouled by the Holy Spirit, which is the model for the coming Kingdom of God. The conception of social authority as service rather than domination (Mark 10:41-45) is at the heart of the Gospel.

8.2-3 Principle of Totality and Integrity

This principle was also previously discussed in detail in 2.4 and can be repeated here:

> The good of the whole person, correlative to the common good of the community, should be the measure of the use, care, and preservation of its partial functions such that lower functions may be sacrificed to higher functions only for the better functioning of the whole, compensating as far as possible for the proper value of each sacrificed function and never destroying the basic capacities that are definitive of human personhood except when necessary to preserve life itself.

There is a certain analogy between this principle and the Principle of Subsidiarity, but only an analogy. Both reflect the fact that the community and the person are complex systems in which there is a mutual interdependence of the whole and its parts. They differ radically, however, because the human person is a natural, primary unit in which the parts depend completely on the whole and exist for its sake. On the contrary, the community is a system made up of primary units, that is, human persons, and exists for their sake, not merely as isolated individuals, but as sharers in a common, profoundly interrelated life. If we fallaciously turn this analogy into an univocal concept, we fall into the error of totalitarianism which sacrifices the person to the communal state.

The great importance of this principle for medical ethics is that it establishes a norm for setting priorities when one human value must be subordinate to another. In chapter 2 we worked out this hierarchy of values in terms of the biological, psychological, ethical, and spiritual dimensions of human personality. There, we tried to show that the spiritual and ethical values have higher priority than the psychological and biological values, but that such priority must not be understood *dualistically* as if the lower can simply be sacrificed to the higher values. Rather, we argued, in the human person there is a mutual interdependence of the body and the soul, the lower and the higher, as expressed in this Principle of Totality and Integrity.

This principle is rightly classified as one of the norms of love because it expresses the sense in which each of us must have a proper love of *self*, without which the love of others is impossible and is a mere sentimental altruism. Its specific Christian character arises from the Incarnation in which the Word of God became flesh, lived a bodily life, died, and was resurrected in the body transformed in glory. Consequently, Christian anthropology, while admitting both a certain polarity in the human person because of our commonality with the animal and earthly world and our spiritual intelligence, freedom, and openness to God, yet opposes any kind of dualism which would deny the dignity of Christ's human body, our resurrection, and the fact that we are "temples of the Holy Spirit" (I Cor. 3:16). This principle is well expressed by the writer of Ephesians (5:21-33) when he makes the analogy between Christ's love for us, a man's love for his wife, and our love for our own bodies.

8.3 NORMS OF GROWTH STRENGTHENED BY CHRISTIAN HOPE

Growth

Having discussed the norms of faith and love, we must now consider what theologians call the *eschatological* (looking to the end of the world) aspect of ethics. The human person and the human community are not structures of static relations, but are dynamic — living, growing, developing, and evolving. This is why we have opted for a teleological, goal-directed, means-ends ethics. Furthermore, our human goals are not always clearly envisioned in advance. As we progress toward our goals, these goals themselves undergo a new look. They open out ahead of us like the horizon of a landscape through which we travel. John Dewey (1948 [1920]) made an important contribution to ethics by stressing this dynamic character of human goals, which is vividly felt in American culture. Sometimes Christian thinkers have not taken this dynamism of our life fully into account in their ethical discussions, yet we find that Jesus centered his teaching in the theme of the Kingdom of God, a goal so mysterious that Jesus could express it only in terms of parables.

Recently, Christian theologians such as Jürgen Moltmann, Johannes B. Metz, and Wolfhart Pannenburg (Capps, 1970) have begun the construction of "theologies of hope" to bring out the many ways in which the Gospel is not merely a message about the superiority of heaven to earth, but a call to transform the earth as we journey heavenward. In this way they are finding areas of agreement with Humanism and Marxism which also emphasize that to be human is to work for the future. Certainly Christian faith sees in every earthly event (even if that event is a crucifixion) a promise, an opportunity to be used, an invitation by a God of the future to share in building the future. In health care this sense of hope is the source of all healing, so that to be a health care professional is constantly to affirm the possibility of turning suffering into a victory over disease and death.

We will now formulate three norms which express certain aspects of this hope-filled dynamism of Christian ethics: the Principle of Growth Through Suffering, the Principle of Personalized Sexuality, and the Principle of Stewardship and Creativity.

8.3-1 Principle of Growth Through Suffering

Happiness and Suffering

In any teleological ethics, the ultimate criterion of morality is *happiness*. An action is morally good because it leads to happiness. However, sometimes people fail to take into account that in the actual conditions of human existence not all that appears to be happiness is really so. The only authentic happiness is one which satisfies the whole person in his or her deepest and most ultimate needs and does so permanently. Thus it is quite possible for persons to think they are happy because they have achieved goals that are partial, superficial, and unstable. Thus on television we witness the extravagant joy of winners in giveaway contests, knowing that in fact such happiness will quickly fade and prove to have been utterly fake. Thus it is also possible for persons to have really achieved goals that are encompassing, profound, and lasting and yet to be in a state of great suffering because circumstances do not yet permit the full experience of satisfaction. Thus a great writer who has completed a masterpiece or a scientist who has achieved the discovery of a lifetime or a statesman who has successfully carried through a great reform may feel exhausted, torn by inner conflict, and depressed. Yet such persons are to be envied because ultimately they know they have reached the goal of their whole life.

Thus from an ethical point of view it is essential to realize that we cannot measure true human happiness merely by pleasure, comfort, or freedom from anxiety, tension, and guilt. Normally pleasure, comfort, and peace are the *consequences* and the *signs* of the achievement of authentic human goals and the fulfillment of true human needs, and hence they are good and desirable. But they are secondary signs and not the proof or measure of real human achievement.

This is the reason why a hedonistic ethics is unrealistic. The person who judges a marriage, for example, by the satisfactory orgasms which he or she has had or by the lack of discomfort or tension in the marriage is making a serious mistake (cf. Masters and Johnson, 1976). These are normal signs of a satisfactory marriage relation and can be ethically desired and enjoyed, but they do not constitute the true core of a successful marriage whose goal we will argue in 8.3-2 requires the integration of pleasure with love and family living. Sometimes complete hedonistic satisfaction can exist in a marriage which is profoundly inadequate. Sometimes such satisfaction is defective, at least temporarily, in a truly sound marriage.

Medical people should recognize the truth of this principle. They know that pain is commonly a sign of something wrong in the body and comfort a sign of health, but that they are not fundamental. Pain is often an accompaniment of a healing process or even of necessary exercise. Pleasure and comfort may mask a serious disease. Thus physicians use pain and comfort as preliminary *signs* which lead to further investigation, but they know that such signs are not themselves healthy functioning nor proof of it. The psychiatrist knows the same thing. Patients may claim to be happy and comfortable, but unconsciously they may have deep psychological ills. On the other hand, anxiety and crisis may be a part of a healing or growth process. Yet psychological comfort and freedom from anxiety can be *signs* of increasing health and as such are to be respected.

Relevant to ethical questions, therefore, we need to look at the *deeper* and more *total* needs and not to measure good and bad merely in terms of pleasure and pain. Short-range goals, that is, immediate satisfactions, have to yield ethically to long-range goals. Since the 1960s this concept has been criticized by some on the grounds that an ethics which is always delaying human satisfaction to the future while requiring sacrifices in the present is a pie-in-the-sky ethics and that emphasis also has to be given to the "now," to the need for pleasure and satisfaction in life.

In reply, we must admit "Man cannot live bodily without pleasure," as Aquinas said (1976 ed.; cf. C. Williams, 1974). Pleasure is necessary for physical and mental health, for self-understanding (Milhaven, 1976), and for the maintenance of determination and courage for long-run goals. Short-range pleasures and comforts must be present to a moderate degree and strains and pains cannot be endured too long. Thus *leisure recreation* (the restoration of human powers through rest and satisfaction) is an essential need of human life, and *contemplation* ought to become a predominate quality of life (Pieper, 1964). A work ethic by which life is simply striving for a far-off, never-attained goal is a bad ethic (Adler, 1970). Authentic fulfillment is not to be found by the maximization of sensual pleasure (as hedonism insists), but rather by intensifying deeper spiritual pleasures along with moderate sensual pleasures. Thus a good marriage depends not so much upon increasing concern for the techniques of successful orgasm as it does upon a shift from a relation based on sensual satisfaction to one based on deeper and more lasting satisfactions, on real community of interests and friendship. The effort to make sensual pleasure infinite is misplaced since it aims at an impossible goal and is bound to be frustrated. The only infinite goods are of the spiritual order. Sensual pleasure at best is a recreation which prepares us for continued effort to gain these spiritual goods or is simply a spontaneous, effortless, and unsought consequence of the achievement of higher goals.

Nor is it true that even spiritual goods have to be left to the next life. Christian experience is that interior peace and spiritual joy can be achieved, if not perfectly, yet really and substantially here and now.

The health care profession, therefore, although its task is to relieve pain and restore health, ought not to regard pain and suffering as the greatest of evils. Rather it has to help the patient use times of suffering as means of total personal growth. Yet this requires us to face the mystery of suffering and death honestly.

There are many ways in which people suffer. In a certain sense, there are as many ways of suffering as there are specialities within the field of health care. But we can limit the types by categorizing suffering as physical or psychic. Though each and every physical or psychic suffering does not lead to death, suffering and death are connected intimately. Suffering, whether physical or psychic, is a violation or subversion of a person's bodily integrity or psychic stability. Death is the ultimate and complete violation or subversion of the human person.

The man with cancer, the child with leukemia, the woman with cardiac difficulties all suffer from serious and impairing illness. But the physical or psychic impairment is only part of the problem. Lurking behind each of these illnesses, influencing the reaction of all persons to their sickness, is the question, Will this cause death? Am I going to die soon? To treat people as though their illness has no connection with death is to treat diseases or symptoms, rather than treat the whole person. Sensitive and aware health care professionals will help their patients face death, as they seek to help them regain their health. Many perceptive students of life in America tell us that much of our physical illness and mental anguish is the result of our inability to face death (E. Becker, 1973; Gatch, 1969; Mack, 1973). Not only for the sake of their patients then, but for their own sake as well, Christians in the field of health care will do well to ponder and understand the meaning of suffering and death. In a very real way, one cannot help another face sickness and death unless one has faced death in one's own life (Kübler-Ross, 1969). Certainly, it is possible to prescribe medicine and to make diagnoses and to perform medical procedures upon a person, but one is not able to cure a person, to heal in the proper sense of the word, unless he or she has some grasp of the meaning of suffering and death and the way in which they are a vital part of our human life.

Mystery of Death

From time immemorial, human beings have viewed suffering and death and asked Why? (D'Arcy, 1936). Why would a loving God allow people to suffer (Agress, 1974)? Why could God allow a child to be born with Down's syndrome? allow the father of a large family to undergo a mental breakdown? allow a mother to be taken from her growing family when others, aging or without children, are left untouched? People both wise and callow have questioned the meaning of suffering and death since the beginning of time (Bowker, 1970). In the Judeo-Christian Tradition, some insight has been gained over the centuries concerning these concomitants of human existence. Some of the knowledge and understanding is found in the Scripture; much of it is in oral tradition of churches and families. Yet, let us admit that suffering and death are mysteries — mysteries that we will never unravel clearly and completely in this life — because they are bound up in the intimate life and love of God (Lepp, 1968; Jungel, 1974). Admitting that suffering and death are mysteries which we cannot solve fully in this life may seem to be a denial or delimitation of the human desire and power to know the truth. Actually, it is not a denial of human potential and aspiration, rather it is an admission that human beings are incapable of knowing everything, and that God plays a very important part in the life of any individual person or any group of persons.

To say that suffering and death are mysteries does not take them out of the realm of human investigation, nor does it mean that we should stand in helpless awe of sickness and death (C. Lewis, 1943). After all, some of the great moments in human history are the result of man's efforts and success in conquering illness and disease. However, there is a point beyond which human beings cannot go. We shall never eliminate all suffering, and we know that each one of us must die. These ultimate truths are testimony to the power of our Creator, with whom we cooperate in the genesis and continuation of the human race, but who in the last analysis is the ruler of the world, the Lord of the Universe.

Given the power and prestige of the health care professions, acknowledging the importance of God in human life, the mystery of his presence as evidenced through suffering and death, is an important step in humanizing that profession. To accept limitations is to accept one's humanity (Ferrater Mora, 1965). Health care professionals who assume a position of unlimited power in the process of healing have an outlook that is unrealistic. They think upon themselves as the persons who cure, rather than realizing that it is God who cures and the health care professionals who cooperate in this work by using the forces of nature.

"Death was not God's doing; he takes no pleasure in the extinction of the living. To be — for this he created all" (Wis. 1:13-14). "God had not wished to include suffering and death in man's destiny" (Pius XII, 1944, p. 57; cf. also Farrer, 1961; Hick, 1966). Whence, then, came suffering and death? St. Paul says, "Through one man sin entered the world and with sin death, death thus coming to all men inasmuch as all sinned" (Rom. 5:12). This original sin was essentially a sin of pride, the will to be like God not by using God's gifts to come closer to God in community, but to use these gifts to set up the human individual in self-centered domination of the world apart from God (Oraison, 1964). It is this misuse of God's gifts from the beginning of our human race to this day which has prevented us from overcoming the natural causes of suffering and death and introduced into the world countless unnatural causes and transformed natural death, which might have been a joyful completion of this life and a serene passage into a greater life, into a blind, terrifying mystery.

However, although we have turned our back on God, He has not turned from us, but has offered us forgiveness and restoration. Yet in his mercy, He cannot deny our human freedom but has called us to return to Him, not simply by restoring us to our innocent beginnings, but by a long history which is a time of struggle and learning from experience, an experience in which suffering is inevitable. For the Christian, however, and for all who travel the same road in less clear ways, God has revealed in Christ the direction of our journey and the power of grace by which it can be traveled (O'Meara, 1975). In baptism, according to St. Paul (Rom. 6:1-11) through the Cross of Christ we have died and been reborn in a new creation which will be completed in the resurrection of the body in eternal life. We live now in such unity with Christ that all the events of our lives take on meaning from his life and death. Consequently, both the joy and the suffering of this life have a Christian meaning: its joys are signs of the hope for ever-lasting life in his Kingdom which is already present here on earth in promise and its sorrows are a sharing in his Cross through which a victorious ressurection is to be achieved.

Jesus came to conquer suffering and death. In what sense can we say that he succeeded? We still get sick, we continue to suffer, and death is inevitable. He conquered sickness, suffering, and death in the sense that he gave them a new meaning, a new power. By believing in Jesus as our savior, by joining our suffering and death to his, we overcome the evil aspect of suffering and death. Through his sacrifice, we are able to conquer the evil that is associated with suffering and death (Lyonnet, 1970). Though the results of original and actual sin are still present in our lives, they no longer dominate our lives and they no longer serve as punishment. Rather, suffering and death are trans-formed into the very actions which help us fulfill our destiny (Pieper, 1969).

In our era, the potential transformation through death has been investigated more thoroughly than in ages past. At one time death was defined as separation of body and soul. While this definition is true, it is no longer an adequate definition of death. In their attempts to specify more clearly what it means to die, modern theologians have concentrated upon death as a personal act of a human being (Rahner, 1965) — an act which terminates earthly existence, but which also fulfills it. Hence, the person is not merely passive in the face of death, and death is different for the just and the sinner. In the view of Karl Rahner, a view accepted and developed by many theologians, death is an active consummation brought about by all persons, themselves, a maturing self-realization which embodies what each person has made of himself or herself during life. Death becomes a ratification of life, not merely an inevitable process (Boros, 1965). It is an event, an action in which the person is intimately involved. Dying with Christ is an adventure, a consequence of, but not a penalty for, sin. This, of course, is a new approach to death, thoroughly in keeping with the Christian Tradition. Indeed, this view of death seems to describe more clearly the experience of Christ, who offered his life, rather than have it taken from him, who culminated his love and generosity in the final act of obedience to the Father: "It is consummated" (John 19:30). Not only pastoral care personnel, but also those in other fields of the healing profession, will enrich their own lives and the lives of their patients if they are able to communicate this notion of death.

In our Christian viewpoint of things, then, we look upon suffering and death in two distinct ways. On the one hand, it is evil because it is the result of sin; on the other hand, it is a liberating and grace-filled experience if the proper motivation is present (Pittenger, 1973). These two ways are not contradictory; rather, they are complementary. Suffering and death, joined to the suffering and death of Jesus, represent not dissolution but growth, not punishment but fulfillment, not sadness but joy. God allows suffering and death to enable us to live with Christ now and forever.

This mystery, because it is a mystery, can never be adequately formulated in words, but for purposes of ethical discussion we can express it as a *Principle of Growth Through Suffering* as follows:

> As pleasure is a truly human need only when it is the consequence of the satisfaction of the authentic needs of the total human person, so suffering and even bodily death when endured with courage can be the source of personal growth in private and communal living.

8.3-2 Principle of Personalized Sexuality

Sexual Values

Throughout the history of ethics there has been a tendency to treat human sexuality as if it were simply an animal function requiring to be restrained lest it turn human beings into brutes. Modern ethics is insistent that sexuality as much as any other human function be specifically humanized or personalized. Human beings should make love humanly, just as surely as they should think humanly.

Because it is specifically human, our sexual life has its free decisions and therefore its ethical dilemmas. They might have been considered under norms of love, but more properly they belong to the norms of hope because sexual love in a very special way looks toward the future, since the survival of the human community, as well as the maturation and fulfillment of the individual, depends upon it.

However, in our pluralistic society sexuality is understood very differently in various value systems. Consequently, it will be necessary to discuss the values of sexuality at considerable length before formulating these values in a principle that may be of assistance in illuminating the many and complex bioethical issues to be discussed in chapter 10.

Human sexuality is not merely one aspect of the human person, but a dimension affecting every other aspect of personality (Goergen, 1975). It is a complex of many values, but these values can be summarized in four chief categories. First, sex is a search for *sensual* pleasure and satisfaction, releasing physical and psychic tensions (C. Williams, 1974; Milhaven, 1976; Manning, 1972). Second, sex is a search for the completion of the human person through an intimate personal union of *love* expressed by bodily union. Ordinarily, it is also conceived as complementation of the male and female by one another so that each achieves a more complete humanity. Third, sex is a necessity for the *procreation* of children and their education in the family so as to expand the human community and guarantee its future beyond the death of individual members. Fourth, sex is a *religious* mystery, somehow revealing the cosmic order. These values are commonly recognized in all the great religions and philosophies of life and are protected and developed in every viable human culture.

In our modern culture dominated by Humanism these values are generally thought to be combined in sexuality simply by the accident of the purposeless process of biological evolution. Hence we human beings are free to combine or separate these different values according to our own purposes. Therefore, for Humanists, it seems entirely reasonable sometimes to use sex purely for the sake of pleasure apart from any relation to love or family, sometimes to use it for love without any reference to family, and sometimes to use it to reproduce (e.g., by artificial insemination) without any reference to love or pleasure. For Humanists, moreover, if sex can be said to have a religious value, it is because romantic love and sexual ecstasy are often considered the highest happiness in our passing life, without which human experience is incomplete (Rubin, 1970). Consequently, for many Humanists sexual morality can be reduced to two fundamental norms: (1) social norms which hinder human freedom to achieve these sexual values in ways the individual desires, as long as no other person is harmed, are unjust (Menninger, 1938, 1942; Marcuse, 1974), and (2) sexual behavior (at least among consenting adults) is entirely a private matter to be determined by personal choice.

The traditional Christian value system differs from Humanism not in denying these values (as some Humanists suppose), but chiefly on two positive points. First, these values of sexuality are ethically *inseparable* by human choice, because their combination is not the result of mere evolution, but of God's wise provision for our human good. Second, the religious value of sex is that it provides an experience of love which teaches us the meaning of other kinds of love, especially the love between God and the human community. Hence sex is only a relative good subordinated to greater values, so that individuals may freely choose celibacy for the sake of such higher values without thereby forfeiting personal fulfillment.

In this book we cannot document these Christian views in Scripture and Tradition, but only refer readers to such studies as those of Grelot (1964), Thielicke (1964), Schnackenburg (1965), Kosnick (1977), and Sapp (1977) on the Scriptural foundations and of Schillebeeckx (1965) and Noonan (1965) on the Catholic Tradition. These studies show that the Scriptures present many themes concerning sexuality from many points of view rather than in the form of a systematic teaching. However, making full allowance for this fact and for the historical developments within the Scripture, we believe that it is clear that in the Bible the four values of *pleasure, love, family,* and *sacramentality* which we have described are always treated as intrinsically related and inseparable, and that sexual behavior which separates them is always disapproved. Furthermore, it is clear in the long tradition of the Church that it was this Biblical teaching, and not merely the influences of Greek philosophy or other religious traditions, which guided the Church in its constant affirmation that the God-given purpose of sexuality is permanent fidelity in marriage and family and that celibacy is an ethically good way of life.

These two fundamental teachings are precisely those affirmed by Jesus himself in the texts forbidding divorce (Mark 10:2-12; Matt. 19:39; 5:31-32; Luke 16:18; I Cor. 7:10) in which Jesus appeals to the order of creation, and those in which Jesus calls on his disciples to leave all things to follow him (Matt. 19:29 and parallels) in the celibate life he himself lived (I Cor. 7). The religious or sacramental meaning of sexuality is most clearly expressed in Ephesians (5:22-33) where the writer takes up the Old Testament symbol of Yahweh as the husband of the Chosen People and building on Jesus' own references to himself as the Bridegroom (Mark 2:10-20) transforms this into a symbol of the love between Christ and his community. Thus human married love becomes an analogue through which we learn how God loves us and what our response to Him through love of our neighbor should be.

Undoubtedly this Christian ideal seems to many a very unrealistic and therefore harmful ethics. In the last twenty years, empirical studies on human sexual behavior (Kinsey, 1948, 1953; Masters and Johnson, 1966, 1970; Weinberg, 1976; *Journal of Sexual Research*; *Sexual Behavior*; Kosnick, 1977) have given extensive evidence (if anybody doubted it) that most human beings come far short of the Christian ideal of sexual integration. It seems that before marriage, the great majority of Americans engage in masturbation and casual sexual encounters including homosexual ones. It is estimated that at least five percent of the population are exclusively homosexual in orientation (Marshall and Suggs, 1971). A high percentage of marriages end in divorce and extramarital sex is often concurrent with marriage. Furthermore, many children are unwanted or abused and even more suffer serious psychological damage from conflicts between parents. At the same time, contraceptive practice seems to predominate in American sexual life and is backed up with the widespread practice of abortion, so that the United States birthrate is approaching the zero-growth level.

The pressure of this sexual revolution and the worldwide concern about the population explosion press especially hard on the Catholic couple who are deeply committed to the Christian life and are loyal to the Church. At one time, a large family was an economic asset because the children contributed to the family living. Today in the United States, it is a heavy debit, particularly since modern health care ensures the survival of most children, and modern education requires long and expensive years of dependency on the parents. At the same time, the mother of the family has been educated to expect a life as an autonomous person to which constant pregnancy and child care may be a continual frustration. With the mobility of American life, the breakup of the extended family, and the difficulty of obtaining inexpensive help, the mother of today may feel oppressed by a continual burden of child care. The father on the other hand, forced by economic conditions to be away from home a large part of the day, is under growing pressure to provide for his family. The result, as evidenced by the divorce rate, is greatly weakened family stability and great psychological strain on the parents (Schur, 1966).

In the face of this social situation which makes the raising of a large family very difficult for many couples there is an insistence on the part of the Church that sexual love be personalized, that it be a profound love relation. Yet the Church continues to insist that such relations be confined to the legally enforced institution of marriage. The result is that many Catholic couples have testified that some means of family limitation is imperative, but that either prolonged or periodic abstinence has imperiled their marriage and thus imperiled proper care for their children (Birmingham, 1964a).

At the same time, Catholic couples have hanging over them the fear of mortal sin, that is, separation from God and denial of the right to receive the sacraments if they resort to forbidden sexual practices. Even if in their own consciences they feel themselves justified, they still have the burden of guilt feelings resulting from the conflict between their own consciences and the authoritative teaching of the Church. Thus it appears that the Catholic is being asked by the pastors of the Church to reconcile the demands of strict negative rules against extramarital relations or contraception within marriage and at the same time to achieve positive values of married love, fidelity, and responsibility to give the children an excellent education. Granted that heroism is sometimes required of the Christian, is it reasonable to expect such heroism of the average person through the many years of daily family living? And if these pressures are heroic for the normal man and woman, what about those who suffer from various forms of physical or psychological weakness or abnormality? Nor is this situation exclusive to Catholics. While Protestant Christians may be more permissive about contraceptive practices, they generally also propose to their people a rigorous ideal excluding extramarital sex (Thielicke, 1964; cf. Roy, 1974). Is it any wonder then that traditional Christian ideals of sexuality seem unrealistic not only to many Humanists, but also to many Christians?

However, realism depends on one's vision of reality — one's world view and value system. Humanism has dominated the growth of modern society in the last two hundred years and, naturally enough, has used scientific research and technology to promote its own perception of reality and to implement its own values. The stable family has not been a major objective of this society, as it would be for a social order shaped by a Christian vision. It is not surprising, therefore, that more and more the Christian understanding and living of sexuality as essentially *family living* today appears outmoded and impracticable. However, the theology of liberation (Gutierrez, 1973) is beginning to make us aware that minority groups (and active Christians are a minority in the modern world) must no longer allow the powerful to define reality for the weak. Consequently, rather than simply conforming to dominant views of what practical, realistic sexual life should be, Christians must work for changes in social structures that will make it practical and realistic to live the Biblical ideal of family life.

Moreover, it may very well be that for the future the Christian ideal of marriage and family may prove more realistic than our present sexual revolution. When we turn to the data of anthropological and behavioral science (Kosnick, 1977), we discover that amidst the vast variety of sexual customs in the human race two features stand out as universal: (1) every human culture that has endured regulates sexual behavior by social norms, as diverse as these norms are in some respects, and (2) the primary social function of these norms is to protect the basic family unit as the chief means of educating the children on whom the future of the community depends. It is not surprising, therefore, that the sexual morality of the Old Testament which arose from the experience of an oppressed people is directed to this same goal of strengthening family life. Jesus accepted this Old Testament emphasis, intensified it, personalized it, yet relativized it by his example of celibacy for the Kingdom.

Of course, today, many believe that because in our times we have technological capabilities far beyond those possessed by former cultures we must use these technologies to promote a Humanist system of values, particularly a Humanist view of sexuality (Francoeur, 1970, 1972). Technology, however, can be used to promote Christian values just as well as to promote Humanist values. In 1.3 we argued that in a pluralistic, global society it is imperative that all human communities work together to widen their consensus on ethical questions. Hence, Christians should not seek to impose their sexual ideals on others, but they should not accept the sexual ideals of others without question. At the same time, it means that within the Christian community there has to be great understanding and compassion for those who find it very difficult to live by Christian ideals in a world so complex and torn by so many crosscurrents.

Personalized Sexuality

A first step toward any better pastoral approach to sexuality is an improved theology of marriage. Beginning with the work of Herbert Doms (1939) and culminating in the Second Vatican Council (1965b) and Paul VI's encyclical *Humanae Vitae* (1968a; Congregation for Doctrine, 1976) a new formulation of the theology of marriage has taken on authoritative status in the Catholic Church. The former language which spoke of the value of procreation as the *primary end* of marriage has been abandoned, and the meaning of marriage is now said to be *love*, but love of a special kind. The characteristics of this love are that it is *human, total, faithful (and exclusive)*, and *fruitful*. The terms *human* and *total* indicate that it involves the whole human personality and thus includes the values of bodily pleasure along with the other aspects of male-female love.   The term *faithful and exclusive* indicates that this love is permanent and monogamous, and the term *fruitful* indicates that it is normally completed by children. This conception of sexuality, therefore, describes *human* sexuality in its specific character as human and not merely animal, although it includes human animality.   The council and Paul VI emphasize this by indicating that in speaking of procreation what is referred to is not irresponsible or fatalistic procreation, but "responsible parenthood," that is, a couple produces children precisely to express their love for each other and their concern for society, and hence is limited to those children for which the couple with the proper assistance of the community can care for and educate properly.

Such a conception of sexuality can be said to be personalized because it attempts to use sex for truly interpersonal purposes. Thus it excludes bestiality and autoeroticism as truly human uses of sex because they seek sexual satisfaction separated from the expression of love for another.   This separation of pleasure from a truly human purpose (as we explained in 8.3) leads to an addictive or compulsive pattern of behavior which restricts human freedom and makes it more difficult to form interpersonal relations (Brockman, 1972; Delhaye, 1976). Personalized sexuality also excludes sexual relations outside the permanent commitment of marriage because they are contrary to its character of a total giving of the person.   Finally it questions homosexual unions because the love so expressed lacks that complementarity of male and female related to the fruitfulness of marriage. In all these forms of sexual relations the full meaning of sexuality is essentially frustrated and its integrated values separated.

Of course, it can be argued that if for some reason persons cannot achieve all the values of sexuality why may they not at least achieve those which are possible to them, for example, why cannot lonely old people satisfy themselves by masturbation or homosexuals by a loving relation with another of their own sex? Certainly it is sometimes justifiable for married people to realize some of the values of marriage when responsible parenthood or accidental sterility makes it impossible to have children.   In this case, however, the love which they express to each other is an integral love, containing as its source all the other values of the marriage, even if these values cannot be effectively realized. But in the sexual practices in which there is a separation of essential values either this love is lacking (as in autoeroticism) or from the outset it lacks the full meaning of sexual love.   Thus premarital love is not a total giving in a permanent commitment, while homosexual love may indeed be a permanent commitment in friendship, but it lacks that male-female complementarity which is essential to the specific character of sexual love with its intrinsic relation to the family.

The pastoral care of persons struggling with all these problems is beyond the scope of this book, but to be consistent with the Scriptures and the Tradition of the Christian community we believe they must be guided by this integrated complex of values, which we can formulate in the following *Principle of Personalized Sexuality*:

> The use of human sexuality must be in keeping with its intrinsic specifically human teleology which is (1) the loving, pleasurable, bodily expression of the complementary union of a male and a female person and (2) the perpetuation and expansion of this personal communion through the family they beget and educate.

Its specifically Christian interpretation can be summed up simply by repeating that its religious symbolism is to witness in this passing world of birth and death to the fidelity of love between Christ and his people, a love whose transcendent and everlasting character is also especially symbolized and witnessed by Christian celibacy.

8.3-3   Principle of Stewardship and Creativity

Cocreators

The hope that leads human beings to endure the inevitable pain of human existence and to overcome our sentence to death by the perpetuation of the human community also leads us to struggle with our environment.   Profoundly the author of Genesis 3 symbolizes the evil of death by the expulsion from the Garden, the burden of sexism by the curse on Eve, and the burden of our struggle with the environment by the curse on Adam.   These are the fundamental realities of our human situation, yet Scripture tells us they are not what God wanted for us.   He has given us the power of intelligence, restored by grace in Christ, the new Adam, by which we deal with these problems.   Yet, although we may deal with these evils well or badly, we cannot escape the struggle and still remain human (Heilbrunner, 1974; Haigherty, 1962).

In 3.3 we dealt at length with this Principle of Stewardship and Creativity which has become even more important in our times as a guide to the use of modern medical technology (Fromm, 1974), and here we repeat it:

1. We are ethically obliged to use our natural environment and our multidimensional human nature as precious gifts, with profound respect for their intrinsic teleology.

2. We are also obliged to use our creativity as an equally precious gift to improve our environment and our nature, with a caution set by the limits of our actual knowledge and by the risk of destroying that same creativity.

The specifically Christian character of this principle derives from the fact that in the risen Christ we already have the pledge that the Kingdom of God will eventually be built and from the coming of his Holy Spirit we have the power to share in this building of the Kingdom and the redemption and re-creation of the world. The Gospel does not encourage us simply to wait until the Lord returns, indifferent to the world's fate as Marxists and Humanists accuse us of doing. Rather, we are called to play a historical role in the liberation of the human race from poverty, disease, and oppression with the assistance of the power of God.

8.4 SUMMARY

To sum up this discussion of the principles which govern bioethical decisions from a Christian point of view, we can say:

1. Faith requires us to act with an informed conscience, which requires the intellectual effort of moral discrimination between right and wrong even in complex cases wherein moral actions involve evil side effects or material cooperation. It also requires a relation of trust between persons (especially between professional and client) in which there is an honest exchange of the information necessary for an informed conscience.

2. Hope requires us to accept growth through suffering, to continue the human community through the institution of the family, and to fulfill in a creative manner our stewardship of our own nature and the world God has given us.

3. Love requires a profound respect for human dignity no matter what the condition of the person. It also requires a proper love of one's self and a responsibility for one's own health. Finally, it requires us to work for and share in the common good. We must accept the social responsibility of promoting the distribution of health care for all.

PART IV

DIFFICULT BIOETHICAL DECISIONS

CHAPTER 9 MEDICAL LIMITS: ABORTION, TRIAGE, AND EXPERIMENTATION

9.1 DECIDING WHO IS THE HUMAN SUBJECT OF MEDICAL ACTION

Self-Identity

Chapters 3 and 4 showed that a profession has limits which are set not merely by professional expertness but by the fundamental *purpose* of the profession. To act outside these limits in a way extraneous or contradictory to this basic purpose is to act unprofessionally and unethically. It was also argued that the purpose of the health care profession is to serve human persons (who are more agents than patients) to achieve physical and psychological health as dimensions of human wholeness.

Hence there are two basic ethical decisions that must be made before a health care professional starts any medical procedure: (1) Who is the human person (or persons) I am serving? (2) What can I do that will benefit this person's (or these persons') health? This chapter will explore some of the ethical difficulties involved in answering these apparently simple questions.

As to the first question, we have seen in chapter 6 that the health care profession is ultimately responsible to serve the health of *all* human persons, including future generations. However, in concrete situations, this responsibility is limited and these limits must be determined. Granted that the profession must play an active role in social and political decisions about health care for all — granted also that there are Good Samaritan responsibilities in many emergency situations — yet ordinarily the professional assumes responsibility for *this* patient when she enters the physician's office or comes to the admissions department in a hospital. It is at this point that a limited contract is implicitly or explicitly set up between the person with health needs and the professional who serves these needs.

Ordinarily the professional can easily recognize the patient, but just who is the patient when the doctor is confronted by a pregnant woman, or a body whose heart is beating but whose brain exhibits only a flat electroencephalogram, or a criminal who is in excellent health but who has agreed to be the subject of a medical experiment which may make him very ill? Is the pregnant woman one person or two? Is the body a person or not? Is the experimental subject someone who has health needs?

Some would question whether the medical profession deals only with human persons. What of veterinary medicine? What of "the rights of animals" urged by antivivisectionists? or even of the total biosphere urged by ecologists? We must admit that there are serious ethical questions about cruelty to animals and depredation of the environment (Singer, 1975). Undoubtedly a lack of reverence for life or its sanctity opens the way to ruthlessness toward human persons (P. Ramsey, 1967; Callahan, 1969b; B. Scott, 1972; B. Brody, 1973, 1975). Yet it is also true that if we blur the distinction between our respect for human rights and our respect for subhuman nature, we may end by minimizing the value of both. Some argue that, after all, experimentation on animal subjects and on human subjects is only a matter of difference of degree. For reasons elaborated in chapters 1 and 2, in this book it is assumed that the health care profession deals with human persons whose rights are of a different order of value than the respect due to other forms of life, although that respect is of genuine ethical importance.

Today there also are some who argue that the terms *human being* and *human person* are not identical nor coextensive (Becker, 1975; Engelhardt, 1974). *Human being* seems to be a biological term, equivalent to "member of the human species" for which there are definite empirical criteria, just as for *elephant* or *pigeon*, while the term *human person* seems to be a legal, philosophical, or theological term with value implications relative to a particular culture or social system. How is the health care profession going to deal with this issue honestly without at the same time getting bogged down in philosophical debates beyond its competence (Milhaven, 1970; Noonan, 1973; Bok, 1974a)?

It seems to us the medical profession should work toward consensus on this issue first of all on the basis of what it knows best, namely, biology and psychology, plus its own professional *self-understanding* ("Toward A Definition", 1975). While such considerations may need to be completed by legal, philosophical, or theological reflections, these reflections must take into full account and be consistent with direct professional experience. It would be a gross evasion of responsibility to follow the example of the Nazi physicians and leave it to others to determine which human beings are persons and which nonpersons (Alexander, 1949).

If we proceed in this manner, the issue is not quite so obscure as some pretend (Nardone, 1973). First of all, in deciding who is a human person health care professionals should begin with the basic certitude that they — doctors, nurses, and medical researchers — are not only human beings but human persons! Our understanding of what it is to be a person must begin from such self-understanding. It cannot be merely external and behavioristic, nor can it rest simply on cultural or semantic conventions (Callahan, 1973c).

The long controversy over behaviorism in psychology has established that although in scientific research we should always strive to make definitions operational in order to maximize objectivity we cannot ever completely eliminate from psychology the element of *empathy*. In understanding psychological phenomena the observer must first study himself in order to be objective about his own observations and inter- pretations.   This is only another application of the basic epistemological principle made familiar to us in physics by the theory of relativity according to which the observer can never stand completely outside what he observes.   His observation is part of the processes which he is observing.

Consequently, medical professionals must always try to understand themselves in relation to patients with empathy and compassion.   In trying to understand the sick person and the process of healing, we must all make use of our own experience of what it is for us to be sick or well (Nolen, 1976; Denes, 1976).   This is essential for sound ethical decision also, as is clear from the fact that almost all great ethical teachers have agreed that the Golden Rule, Do unto others as you would have them do unto you, is basic to any humanistic ethics.

How does the doctor, nurse, or medical researcher know she is a human person and not a computer, a piece of medical apparatus, a corpse, a bit of tissue, or even an experimental animal?   The basic reasons, as we have argued in chapters 1 and 3, are that the professional experiences herself (1) as an intelligent person capable of abstract reason and free decision and (2) as a member of a human community with which she shares a common life of thought, feeling, and moral action. We also suggested in 4.3 that modern medical education sometimes tends to obscure rather than to develop this human self-awareness in the medical student.   Perhaps this accounts in part for the current con- fusion about this issue of personhood.

Granted this fundamental self-awareness of personality, health care professionals have to integrate this with their biological and psychological knowledge, beginning with their own bodies.   Why is *my* body a human body which gives me membership in the human species?   To ask this question is to become aware at once that a definition of human person- hood must necessarily define a type of being which is not static and fixed but essentially a being in *process*, a being *becoming*.   I cannot define myself as a fixed, timeless object, but I must include the notion of my *biography* or life history in the definition.

It is no accident that the usual first step in all medical practice is (and has been since the time of Greek medicine) the taking of the patient's history.   A body cannot be called a human person without taking into account its past and also the future open to it.   A corpse is no longer a person because it has no capacity for a human future.   An unfertilized ovum, a sperm, or any isolated body cell also is not a person because of itself it has no inherent capacity to become an organism with a human future.

Thus philosophers are correct who insist a definition of a human person cannot be merely "substantialist" (Donceel, 1970a, 1970b, 1975; Callahan, 1970b; Engelhardt, 1974, 1975b). It must be processive. However, it is an error to conclude from this that in a process universe all processes are merely gradual changes like a rise in temperature or an increase in size or velocity. Such a conclusion is a radical distortion of process philosophy as developed by Hegel, Marx, Bergson, Whitehead, Dewey, and Teilhard de Chardin (Ruff, 1968, 1970). As Alfred North Whitehead (1957 [1929]) so vigorously emphasized, the essence of any process view of reality must allow for genuine *novelty* in the world. In the complex processes of becoming new, entities emerge which are continuous with the past *materially* but discontinuous with it in actuality and activity (Ashley, 1973). Process is not always a mere reshuffling of what was already there or its intensification or adulteration, but the emergence of new realities radically distinct from those which previously existed.

Therefore an appeal to the process way of looking at reality, so congenial to the scientific mind, does not eliminate the problem of identifying novelty and origination. We still need to ask exactly when in the long process of biological reproduction is the critical point at which a new organism, which did not exist before, comes into existence so that where there was one organism, there are now two, or where there were two, there is now a unique third. Anyone who has studied under the microscope the complex way in which one-celled organisms reproduce by fission know that long and elaborate processes precede and follow the moment of separation, but no observer can doubt there is a critical point.

Biography

Thus a definition of the human person must not merely be synchronic but diachronic. It must be biographical (McClendon, 1974). Unless it is the same identical human person who enters the hospital and leaves somewhat healthier — unless sickness and healing are processes that take place as episodes in the life of a person with a continuous identity — and unless coming alive and dying are not merely arbitrary divisions, the whole work of health care becomes meaningless.

Now the biography of any human person also includes remarkable morphological and functional changes. The difference in morphology and behavior of the newborn infant, the preadolescent, the mature adult, and the senile are not as startling as the differences between a caterpillar and a butterfly, but they are remarkable indeed. Yet the practicing physician is not in doubt that he is the same person as the medical student whose trials and learning experiences he so well remembers, and as the young boy who first dreamed of being a doctor, or as the infant whom he cannot recollect but whose scars and immunities he still bears in his adult body and understands as part of his own medical history. Nor does he doubt that the child whose prenatal existence he first confirmed, whom he helped deliver, and whose health he has assisted to adulthood and beyond is the same identical person. Perhaps the growth of specialization in health care somewhat obscures this view of the patient as a man or woman with a long life history, but it certainly does not put it in doubt.

Thus a medical definition of human personhood begins with the notion of the person as a conscious, intelligent, free adult, but it must include the entire biography of the unique organism whose personhood is fully self-conscious and fully evident in morphology and behavior only at certain periods of that biography. This means that even if we define personhood behavioristically we must take into account not only *actual*, here-and-now performance, but also the capacity or *potentiality* for behavior.

The term *potentiality* has many senses in current usage and it is necessary, even at the cost of pedantry, to distinguish some of them, since confused uses of the term are at the bottom of many current arguments about the origin of the human person (Ashley, 1973; Wade, 1975). First of all, we speak of any kind of stuff or material as having the potentiality of being made or formed into an unlimited number of very different kinds of things. In this sense, the subatomic particles are potentially all the things that make up the universe, and we can say that the gaseous nebula from which our galaxy originally came was potentially the human race. Potentiality in this sense of mere "stuff" is something *passive*, as clay in the hand of the sculptor.

But there are other senses in which potentiality is conceived *actively* as the power to mold and develop passively potential material. Thus the sculptor has the active potentiality (i.e., capability) to form clay into a variety of figures. It is this active sense of potentiality which is especially useful in understanding living organisms. At any given moment of its biography an organism has both a structure and a variety of functions. These functions are active potentialities which depend upon the existence of the structure as an actuality; for example, a bird has the power to fly only when its wing structures have been actually developed. But what is more important is that basic to all the functions of an organism is the potentiality for self-development, that is, to elaborate its own structures and thus to acquire more diversified functions. This capacity for self-development is the function that gives unity to all the others and guarantees the biographical identity of the organism.

Obviously this potentiality for self-development, like any function, presupposes some kind of organic structure, but it is necessarily a minimal structure since on its relatively simple basis the organism is able to elaborate itself into its adult complexity. Modern embryology has shown clearly that this minimal or initial structure must be understood in an epigenetic, and not in a preformist, way (Gilchrist, 1968). This means that in the original, simplest structure we do not have a miniature model of the completed, elaborated structure, but we do have the information necessary to develop it. It is entirely inadequate to think of the genetic endowment of an organism as a small mock-up of the adult. Even to call it a blueprint is misleading because no blueprint can even reproduce itself, let alone produce a building. Rather, we must say that a developing organism contains the potentiality for active self-development, a potentiality based on a minimal actual structure, yet containing all the information necessary to produce a maximum actual structure.

Thus the zygote or fertilized ovum of sexually reproducing species is not a "blob of protoplasm": it is a complete, unified structure, although that structure is very simple compared to that of the adult into which it will develop itself. This simple structure somehow contains all the information and all the active potentiality of self-development necessary to live its whole biography of interaction with its environment. It is this minimal structure which makes it actually a member of a definite species. The zygote of a cat, biologically speaking, is not potentially a cat; it is actually a member of the cat species with the potentiality of becoming a perfectly self-developed cat. Of course, only the adult cat can carry out all the various functions of cat life because only at maturity is the cat structure elaborated and diversified to the point that it has all the active potentialities of cat life, but from the beginning the cat zygote had the basic active potentiality to develop all these structures and the functions following on them.

If we apply these distinctions to the case of the origin of the human person, we see at once that it is a mistake to argue that if the fetus is a human being potentially then so are the ovum and sperm. Biologically, the ovum and sperm are not complete organisms, nor does either possess the genetic information necessary for self-development into a human being because they are haploid (i.e., they have only half the requisite set of chromosomes and genes).

Thus it seems difficult indeed for a scientifically educated health care professional to doubt that he or she has been the same person with a continuous biography since that unique zygote began to develop itself into this adult who can look back over this personal history and acknowledge it as his or her own. Nevertheless, there are some scientific objections which can be raised against this biologically well-established conclusion.

Puzzles

First, there is the claim (Häring, 1976) that perhaps fifty percent of all zygotes perish at an early stage of development (although a recent study indicates this may be actually less than fifteen percent [Hilgers, 1977]). Does that mean that so many members of our human race came into existence and perished so soon? In answer to this difficulty, two points should be made. (1) Through most of human history, at least fifty percent of all infants perished in infancy. Therefore, if this argument proves anything, it proves that infants are no more persons that fetuses. (2) There is evidence that the complex process of fertilization frequently fails to be successfully completed (Diamond, 1975). Probably many of these zygotes are only apparently such and would not be complete organisms or human persons according to our definition.

A second objection, which has much influenced certain Catholic theologians (Wassmer, 1968; LeJeune, 1969; Cavanaugh, 1970; Dedek, 1972; Curran, 1975; Häring, 1976), rests on the notion that after fertilization is completed there still remains a period (perhaps as long as two or three weeks) when the unique identity of the organism still remains indeterminate. The evidence offered for this is that during this time the zygote sometimes divides to produce twins or even multiple offsprings. Furthermore, it has been shown in experiments with some animal fetuses *in vitro* that at this stage the twins can be recombined to form a single organism capable of subsequent normal development, although Hilgers (1977) gives reasons why this is unlikely in human embryology.

How is this phenomenon to be interpreted biologically? It makes no biological sense to say that up to the time of twinning there was simply a mass of cells, rather than a single human organism. If that were the case, how account for the normal development of the zygote up to the point of twinning? And how does the event of twinning produce two or more organisms out of what is not an organism? What agent brings this event about? A much more probable explanation would be the following (Ashley, 1976a).

It seems to be true that every diploid cell of the body has the basic potentiality to develop into a complete individual. Hence, in the future it may be possible to clone or reproduce human beings asexually not from germ cells but from any body cell (Watson, 1971). This potentiality is inhibited in embryological development by the process of somatic cell differentiation into various fixed types and remains actualizable only in germ cells. It is not strange, therefore, that at a very early stage of development some cells of an embryo may become detached and develop independently into a twin, or that the embryo may divide into two equal parts, each of which may develop as two new organisms of the same genetic composition. Such events do not prove that previously no human being existed, but only that this existing human being has given rise to a clone asexually or has ceased to exist and given rise to new twins by asexual fission. This occurence, like any process of multiple birth in the human species, is an accident of development which results from some genetic defect or evironmental accident.

Other objections are raised by those who argue that the fetus is only a part of the mother's body (Mannes, 1967; Wahlberg, 1971; Lader, 1973) or that it is similar to a tumor, or who argue that the embryo is not a distinct organism until implantation in the uterine wall or until the fetus is viable independently of the uterus prematurely or by normal delivery (cf. Wasserstrom, 1975). Such arguments ignore two basic biological facts. (1) The zygote has a new genetic composition different from any part of the mother's body. Nor is this difference merely due to some mutational defect (as perhaps is the case in some tumors), but is due to a unique combination of genes which gives the zygote the potentiality of development into a complete adult. (2) The embryo does not depend upon the mother for further genetic information or guidance in development, but merely for nourishment and shelter. The newborn infant still depends upon the mother for nourishment and protection. Finally, every organism, even the adult human person, always remains dependent upon an appropriate environment. In this respect, the adult and the embryo differ only in degree.

A final biological argument is that of delayed hominization which goes back to Aristotle, which has greatly influenced Catholic thought because of its adoption by the medieval theologians Albert the Great and Thomas Aquinas and which has been recently revived by Joseph Donceel (1970, 1970a), Plé (1971), Häring (1973), and Eike-Henner W. Kluge (1975). Aristotle argued that until an organism has developed to the point that it has a central organ with the minimal structure required for psychological functions it should be considered a vegetative, rather than an animal, being. For Aristotle, this "central organ" is the heart. Donceel and Kluge argue that in modern biology it is the central nervous system and especially the cerebrum. Since the cerebrum is observable in the fetus only toward the end of the third month, this would mean that prior to this stage the embryo or fetus is not even an animal organism and *a fortiori* not human.

The weakness of this argument (Ashley, 1976) is that it defines a priori the minimal structure necessary for the organism to be a human person in the sense we have already explained, that is, an organism which actually has the potentiality to develop itself into a human adult capable of intelligent and free activity. We now know, as Aristotle and Aquinas did not, that prior to the appearance of the brain and the central organ of the fetus there is a sequence of primordial centers of development in the embryo going back continuously to the nucleus of the zygote which has contained from the beginning all the information and active potentiality necessary to eventually develop the brain and bring it to the stage of adult functioning. Thus, while it is true that the developing fetus first exhibits vegetative (physiological) and animal (psychological and motor) functions and finally (long after birth) specifically human functions, it possesses from conception the active potentiality to develop all these functional abilities. It is the minimal structure necessary for this active potentiality of self-development which (even on the basis of Aristotle's and Aquinas's philosophical principles) is required for an organism to be actually a human person, not the brain structures necessary for adult psychological activities.

Thus a health care professional beginning with a self-understanding of personal identity and attempting to trace this back to its origins by the light of biological science can scarcely doubt that the critical point is at completed conception. Nevertheless, this conviction will be attacked by some on legal, philosophical, or theological grounds. Western legal tradition (for reasons we will explore in 9.2) has always been ambiguous on this question (J. Smith, 1967; Callahan, 1970b; Grisez, 1970a; Louisell and Noonan, 1970; De Marco, 1974).

Advocacy of Personhood

These legal doubts have led some recent philosophers to argue that personhood as the subject of rights cannot be determined merely by biological criteria, but must be defined by social consensus. While such consensus should not rest on merely arbitrary criteria like those proposed by racists, it can never be absolute, since only adults capable of actually functioning as free citizens are unequivocally persons. The advocates of such views generally argue for a dividing line late in fetal development, or birth, or even one or two years of infancy and propose also excluding seriously defective children from personhood (Leijen, 1970; Joseph Fletcher, 1972 [cf. Childress, 1974], 1974a, 1974b; Mead, 1973; Engelhardt, 1973a, 1973b, 1974, 1975; R. M. Green, 1974).

This book is not the place to answer these types of arguments in detail. It will suffice to point out the dubious assumptions on which they are based. The legal arguments assume a legal positivism according to which human rights are the result of law, rather than the basis against which the justice of the laws is to be measured. Even those who appeal to the venerable tradition of Jewish religious law must ask whether the tradition on this point is the final word, or whether in light of modern science and modern views of human dignity and equality, a stricter view on the origin of human personhood, is more conformed to the fundamental ethical principles of Judaism (Rosner, 1972; Feldman, 1974; "Judaism," 1975; Fox, 1975; Jakobovits, 1975; Trendler, 1975).

The philosophical arguments seem to rest on the idealistic assumption that ethical values are simply human constructs relative to a particular culture. If our definition of the human person and hence of human rights is merely man-made, then how is it possible to criticize the laws as unjust or a culture as inhumane? There must be an appeal to criteria which transcend man-made laws and values. This is why in the United States we have always appealed to the "inalienable rights of man," as does the *Universal Declaration of Human Rights* of the United Nations (1948).

This need for a prophetic criticism of man-made laws and customs has always been the basis of the Christian theological insistence that the definition of personhood should be broad and should extend to the unborn (Noonan, 1970a; Williams, 1970; Nelson, 1973; Outler, 1973; G. Scott, 1974).

Thus it would seem that health care professionals should begin with the attitude of giving the benefit of the doubt, or what Seymour Siegel (1975) has called "a bias for life" in behalf of the developing human organism and respect its rights as a human person. As a group of professionals who have the clearest notion of the biological criteria of human personhood, they have a responsibility to defend these rights socially and politically against possible doubts on the part of other professions less biologically knowledgeable and to explain them clearly to the laity who are likely to judge more by appearances and popular impressions than by scientific fact. Health care professionals should be just as ready to protest a lack of respect for the unborn as they should to oppose the biological fallacies of racism or antifeminism.

We have next to ask whether this giving the benefit of the doubt to the personhood of the fetus is so absolute that we must treat every living body that might be human as having human rights. Can any trauma short of death destroy personhood? Can any defect, genetic or traumatic, in the fetus be so severe as to constitute an adequate criterion that the fetus is not or perhaps never was a person?

We have already admitted that there may be many cases in which the process of fertilization was so abnormal that no true zygote is ever formed and a spontaneous abortion results. It has also long been recognized that women may give birth to masses of tissue without recognizable human form which have probably resulted from an abnormal pregnancy (O'Donnell, 1976). The most difficult case, however, is that of an anencephalic fetus which is viable and may live for some years and which is morphologically a normal human child except that it lacks the higher brain centers.

In such cases, we must remember the casuistic rule, Presumptions yield to facts. Hence, it would be overscrupulous to attribute personhood and human rights to a defective fetus if we could establish with a high degree of scientific probability that it is so radically defective genetically or in the course of development has suffered so severe a trauma that it lacks the active potentiality to develop the brain structures necessary for at least some minimal activity of human thought and freedom. As we have just argued, it is this active potentiality which constitutes human personhood and makes the normal embryo or fetus actually a human person. It follows also that the adult who has received a brain injury which definitely destroys those brain centers (which science cannot yet clearly identify, cf. 13.2) necessary for such a minimal activity of human thought and freedom would perhaps no longer be a living person.

However, we must not be hasty in thus dropping the benefit of the doubt in actual cases. As long as we are dealing with the fetus or the infant, we are dealing with an organism whose active potentialities are still known to us only by examining the actual structures, genetic or partially developed. An observer of an infant rendered abnormal by thalidomide taken by its mother during her pregnancy might suppose that it has a radical genetic defect, yet such a child certainly possesses the genetic information for normal development. Moreover, even when we know that a defect really is genetic in origin, is it not possible that what was lacking was not the information to build a normal brain, but simply the information necessary for certain physiological activities necessary to nourish the brain in its normal development? In that case, should we say that the embryo lacked the potentiality to develop a normal brain? or rather that it lacked the potentiality for normal digestion or circulation, functions which do not directly define human personhood?

On the other hand, in the case of the adult with a severe brain injury, it is much more obvious when certain structures necessary for intelligent, free activity have been definitively destroyed. With this destruction also goes the active potentiality to develop such structures, since in the adult the brain cannot regenerate itself. Yet even in this case, we must recall that our knowledge of the localization of brain function still remains very ambiguous.

From this it follows that there is need for more research on the minimal structures necessary for human personhood. At present, the attitude of health care professionals should be conservative, favoring the personhood of the human organism from conception to the time that brain death can be securely established. In light of this basic attitude, we are now ready to discuss in practical, ethical terms whether abortion and euthanasia can be seen as serving the rights of the human person concerned, or whether they violate this person's rights for the benefit of another. If this latter is the case, then such actions lie outside the limits of the health care professional.

9.2   ABORTION

Traditional Views

Abortion is the termination of a pregnancy with resulting death of the human fetus. Abortion may occur spontaneously, in which case it is usually called a miscarriage, or it may be caused deliberately and then it is called an induced or procured abortion. Catholic theologians also distinguish between those procured abortions which are *direct* and those which are *indirect*. A direct abortion is one in which the direct, immediate intention of the procedure is to destroy the human fetus at any stage after conception or to expel it when it is not viable. In our society most procured abortions are direct in nature. An indirect abortion is one in which the direct, immediate intention of the procedure is to treat the mother, but in which the death of the fetus is an incidental and secondary result which would have been avoided if it had been possible. Two examples of indirect abortion are surgery for ectopic pregnancy and surgery for a cancerous uterus when the woman is pregnant (United States Catholic Conference, *Ethical and Religious Directives*, 1971, nn. 13, 16).

Today it is generally conceded by Catholic theologians that such indirect abortion may be justified by the principle of double effect (8.1-3; Bouscaren, 1944; O'Donnell, 1976) (1) because the act, itself, is directly for the purpose of treating the mother and hence ethical; (2) because the mother and physician do not have any evil circumstantial intention, that is, they would save the child if they could; (3) because the death of the child is not the *means* by which the mother is treated, but only a result of the treatment (i.e., it is not a cause but an effect of the act); and (4) because there is a proportionate reason if the treatment is necessary to save the life of the mother, especially when we consider that the child is doomed anyway.

The real area of difficulty, therefore, concerns *direct* abortion, of which many millions are now performed each year in the world. On this subject there is an age-old controversy. Although in all human cultures people have valued, loved, and protected their children and it has been recognized as one of the most basic of ethical responsibilities, direct abortion has also been widely practiced. A study of primitive cultures (Devereux, 1955) shows that the motivation for abortion in these cultures is highly varied including not only pragmatic reasons, but also religious and symbolic reasons arising from unconscious urges, such as hostility to male domination. This was also true of the ancient civilizations, although here economic and demographic factors came more and more to prevail, so that in the Greco-Roman world in which Christianity arose abortion and infanticide in some places produced rates of reproduction below the zero-growth level (Noonan, 1967). For these cultures, it can be generally said that abortion and infanticide were not strictly distinguished. In Roman culture, for example, an infant did not have legal status until accepted by the *pater familias*. Hence the tradition that the illegitimate are in effect nonpersons.

In contrast to these views is the attitude in the Jewish Scriptures. For the Jews all human life has as its author the One God whose creative power produces the child in the mother's womb and brings it step-by-step to full life. The parents play only an instrumental role in this creative process, so that from the beginning there is a direct, personal I-Thou relation between the Creator and the human being whom He is creating, just as truly as He created Adam. Several of the Prophets of Israel express the profound religious conviction that it was God who formed them in their mother's womb for a special purpose (Fazziola, 1975). These texts led to later theological speculations among the more mystical or philosophical Jewish thinkers on the time of the "infusion of the human soul," speculations which joined with Greek philosophical tendencies that also tended to enhance the respect for the dignity of the unborn (Feldman, 1974). In any case, Orthodox Jews are convinced that when the child of a Jewish mother becomes a "living soul" it is destined for the Kingdom of God, although this membership in the Chosen People requires to be sealed after birth by circumcision for the male. Thus death in the womb does not exclude salvation.

However, Jewish thought in practical ethics has been dominated by the legislation of the Torah which in time was elaborated by the system of rabbinical interpretation which became normative for post-Biblical Judaism. The Torah inculcates a high respect for human life, and the rabbis insisted that since the principle of justice is "an eye for an eye, a tooth for a tooth, a life for a life" (Exod. 21:23-25; Feldman, 1974), one cannot sacrifice one human life for another unless that other is an aggressor or criminal in some way. Consequently, Judaism has resolutely opposed any form of infanticide and has required Jews to accept martyrdom rather than to kill the innocent.

However, in conflict situations where the life of the mother is endangered, the rabbis believed that the child could be considered an "unjust aggressor" or "pursuer" against whom the woman could defend herself. Hence, in such cases, induced abortion was permitted, and the child was not considered to have a full right to life until birth, or "when the head emerges." This reasoning was confirmed by the fact that the Law in Exodus 21:22 does not set capital punishment but only a monetary fine for one who causes an abortion by striking a pregnant woman. Rabbinical casuistry led some to stricter views which drew the line at the stage when the fetus was of human form (as evidenced by the Hellenistic Septuagint translation of Exodus 21:22), while others wished to draw the line thirty days *after* birth if the delivery was premature. There were also wide differences on what degree of danger to the mother justified induced abortion, some even accepting psychological reasons as sufficient justification when they threatened the married life of the couple. However, underlying all these debates is the basic Jewish conviction of the high value of marriage and of children in view of the preservation of the Chosen People.

Jesus did not repudiate the Jewish Scriptures, nor even their rabbinical application, but he gave them his own characteristic interpretation by stressing that God's care extends to every human being no matter how sinful, ignorant, or ritually unclean. Jesus preached the good news of God's love for the "little ones," the outcasts rejected by secular and religious authorities (Gelin, 1964; Dupont, 1973), including powerless little children whom he declared should be given special respect as privileged members in his Father's Kingdom (Mark 9:33-37). Far from being un-Jewish, Jesus' attitude represents the deepest prophetic spirituality of Israel.

The Christian Church, confronted with the widespread Greek and Roman practice of infanticide and abortion, evaluated such customs in the light of this teaching of Jesus on the dignity of children. Luke in his infancy narratives based on Judeo-Christian sources takes up the Old Testament theme of the prophetic vocation and pictures John the Baptist as called to his mission by the Holy Spirit in Elizabeth's womb. In striking parallel to this, Jesus as the new Adam is created by the overshadowing Spirit in the virgin earth of Mary's womb, where he is already Lord, the Holy One, the Son of God (G. Scott, 1974). Thus the Old Testament conviction that God is the creator of human life from the moment it begins to be, so that the human person is defined primarily by this unique I-Thou relation to its Creator, rather than the legal provisions of Exodus, came to be the guiding theme of Christian thinking about the unborn child.

In the practical moral exhortations of the New Testament Epistles abortion is never explicitly mentioned, but in the *Didache*, a manual of Church discipline written in the same period probably in Jewish-Christian circles, it is explicitly forbidden. This opposition to direct abortion has remained what Noonan (1970a) calls "an almost absolute value" throughout the history of the Christian Church.

The consistency of this position has been only partially obscured by the theological controversies which it, like most of the teachings of Christianity, has occasionally engendered. We will only examine them very briefly, while referring readers to the detailed studies of Noonan (1965, 1970a, 1970b), McCormick (1968), Mangan (1970), and G. H. Williams (1970), which recently have been corrected in some details by Connery (1970, 1977).

One difficulty arose from Jewish contact with Greek thought and took the form of the question, When is the human soul infused into the body? Platonists believed that this human animation was at conception, but the Aristotelians, more concerned with biological processes, were of the opinion that it could not be at conception when the embryo is (as they thought) simply unformed menstrual blood, but must be at about forty to sixty days of pregnancy when the fetus has definite organic form. Those influenced by Stoic philosophy even believed it was only at birth that the child breathed in the "vital spirit."

Christian thinkers respected all these views of ancient biology, but the great authority of St. Thomas Aquinas (who was a convinced

Aristotelian) led to the general acceptance of the theory that ensoulment takes place when the fetus has a definitely human form between one and two months of gestation, which (as we saw in 9.1) still has its defenders. For Aquinas abortion was a grave crime because it interrupted the creative work of God in nature, but it was not murder in the technical sense if it took place before ensoulment. Hence Catholic teaching has generally regarded early abortion as a crime equivalent to murder, but not identical with it.

A second difficulty arose from the question of whether the gravity of the crime of abortion was aggravated because it prevents the child from receiving the baptism which Christ required for salvation (John 3:5; G. H. Williams, 1970).

Today the Catholic Church still insists on the importance of infant baptism even in emergency situations such as spontaneous abortion, but theologians generally no longer conclude that this practice implies that unbaptized children cannot be saved (Van Roo, 1954). In chapter 15 we will discuss the reasons for this theological change and also the pastoral administration of baptism in emergency situations.

Other controversies have arisen over the correct way to deal with conflict situations where the life of the mother seems threatened. As we have seen, the Jewish rabbis permitted therapeutic abortion, and as Connery has shown (1977), some Catholic theologians in the past also favored this view, as do Protestant and Eastern Orthodox churches even at present (Grisez, 1970a). Recently, some Catholic theologians are also attempting to revive this opinion. However, since as far back as 1679 the popes have repeatedly repudiated the notion that the killing of one person could ever be a means of therapy for another because such a practice seems utterly inconsistent with the equal dignity of human persons. We must emphasize, nevertheless, that this disagreement on how to deal with conflict cases does not negate the basic agreement among all the Christian Churches (1) that abortion is contrary to the will of God who creates each human person, and (2) that if abortion is ever permissible in a conflict situation (and this is denied by some), it can be justified only by the most serious reasons.

If we ask why the Roman Catholic Church has taken the most strict view on the subject, we will find the most authoritative recent statement on this subject in the *Declaration on Procured Abortion* issued by the Congregation for the Doctrine of the Faith (1974), as well as in important statements by the bishops of the United States (National Conference of Catholic Bishops, 1974). These documents are elaborations of the condemnation of abortion by the Second Vatican Council, which linked it with infanticide (*Church in the Modern World*, 1965c). The *Declaration* argues as follows:

> The first right of the human person is his or her life. A person has other goods and some are more precious, but this one is fundamental — the condition of all the others. Hence it must be protected above

all others. A society nor public authority may not in any form recognize this right for some and not for others: all discrimination is evil whether it be founded on race, sex, color or religion. It is not recognition by another that constitutes this right. This right is antecedent to its recognition; it demands recognition and it is strictly unjust to refuse it. Any discrimination based on the various states of life is no more justified than any other discrimination. The right to life remains complete in an old person, even one greatly weakened. It is not lost by one who is incurably sick. The right to life is not less to be respected in the small infant just born than in the mature person. In reality, respect for human life is called for from the time that the process of generation begins. From the time that the ovum is fertilized, a life is begun which is neither that of the father nor the mother. It is rather the life of a new human being with his or her own growth. It would never be made human if it were not human already. (nn. 11-12).

Note that this authoritative Catholic position does *not* depend upon the view for which we have argued in 9.1 that human personhood begins at conception (cf. Humber, 1975), but rather on the following proposition:

From a moral point of view it is certain that even if a doubt existed whether the fruit of conception is already a human person it is an objectively grave sin to dare to risk murder. "The one who will be a human being is already one." (Tertullian; n.12).

The reason for this is further given in note 19 of the *Declaration*:

This declaration expressly leaves aside the question of the moment when the spiritual soul is infused. There is not a unanimous tradition on this point and authors are as yet in disagreement. For some it dates from the first instance, for others it could at least precede implantation. It is not within the competence of science to decide between these views. It is a philosophical problem from which our moral affirmation remains independent for two reasons: (1) supposing a belated animation, there is still nothing less than a *human* life preparing for and calling for a soul in which the nature received from the parents is completed; (2) on the other hand it suffices that this presence of the soul be probable in order that the taking of life involve accepting the risk of killing a human being, who is not only waiting for, but already in possession of his or her soul. (n. 19)

It would be exaggerated to say that these various church documents, even those of the Second Vatican Council, are definitive and infallible judgments of the pastors of the Church on revealed truth, but the strength and unanimity of the teaching are of very great weight. Furthermore, as Connery's study (1977) shows, the issues involved have been very well debated over a long period, and the advance of medical knowledge far from weakening the Church's position has tended to reinforce and sharpen it.

Why then have controversies arisen among Christians as to the question of therapeutic abortion and other questions arising out of conflict situations (A. Lester, 1971; Rahmeier, 1971)? Some of these disagreements arise from the notion that there is really a strong case for delayed hominization. We have argued in 9.1 that in fact this case is very weak. However, as we have just seen, even the recent *Declaration* seems to grant to this theory at least some probability. Consequently, a few theologians (Wassmer, 1968; Dedek, 1972) have tried to use probabilism (8.1-2) to solve conflict situations. Thus Dedek (1972; cf. 1975 where he omits mention of this reason) argues as follows:

> It seems that the certain rights of the mother prevail over the un-
> certain rights of the conceptus, so that in conflict situations one may
> run the risk of killing a human being because of a reason proportionate
> to the risk. (pp. 80-81)

Dedek is referring to the rule of probabilism that "a doubt as to the fact" (in this case whether the embryo is human in the sense of having human rights) makes it probable that there is no obligation to defer to the rights of another in seeking one's own goals (in this case the mother's life and well-being). Dedek supports his argument by quoting a parallel case from the well-known manual of Prümmer (1960):

> But if the fetus is not certainly but probably dead, many authors
> correctly teach craniotomy is permitted to save the life of the mother,
> since a live mother does not have to give up her life for a fetus which
> is probably already dead. (Vol. 1, n. 136)

However, in the use of probabilism and of probable reasoning in general, it is essential to first determine carefully on which side the presumption lies. In general, the presumption is in favor of freedom from an obligation, but this has to yield in cases where very serious rights such as the right to life are in question, in which cases the *more* probable course must be followed. Then the presumption is in favor of the one who will lose this basic right. Prümmer, therefore, is correct in favoring the rights of the living mother which are certain over those of the child who is probably dead, because in this case the presumption is clearly on the mother's side. The presumption would also favor the mother if it were more probable that a living fetus is not human. However, neither Dedek nor anyone else has established that it is *more* probable that the fetus is not human; rather, as we have shown in 9.1, the arguments for the personhood of the fetus, even from conception, are much the more probable biologically, philosophically, and theologically than the contrary. While it is more certain that an adult woman is a human person than that her unborn child is a human person, nevertheless when it is certain that this woman is pregnant, it is then also certain that a living child already exists who is much more probably human than not and whose basic and very serious rights may not be ignored. Furthermore, these rights require particular advocacy precisely because the child is helpless in its own defense.

Many current Catholic theologians tend to solve such conflict cases not by probabilism in the classical mode, but by the new principle of proportion methodology which we have already discussed and found inadequate (8.1-3). Many Protestant theologians follow much the same type of reasoning, trying to balance the good and evil consequences of abortion in concrete circumstances. However, even if we proceed in this manner, it is not at all clear that abortion can ever be judged the right solution (P. Ramsey, 1973a; McCormick, 1973a).

Woman's Right to Decide

Of course, there are frequently situations in which a pregnant woman may in good faith believe that not to have an abortion will do more harm (not only to herself but to others) than to have one. Magda Denes (1976) has documented this in a very sensitive way from interviews with women in an abortion clinic. Some of the considerations frequently cited in favor of a woman's right to make this decision for herself are as follows:

1. A woman has to bear the risk and burden of pregnancy, delivery, and child care which she will hardly be able to sustain unless to do so is her own choice.

2. Sometimes in the case of very young, inexperienced, or retarded women and in the case of incest or rape, a woman has little or no responsibility for the pregnancy, yet she must bear the consequences.

3. Even when she has shared in the responsibility for the pregnancy, she nevertheless has the right to a normal sex life upon which her marriage and care of other children also depends, yet contraception does not give her complete control over pregnancy. Therefore, she has the right to use abortion as a last resort.

4. For a woman to bear an unwanted child is a disaster for the child as well as for herself, because no matter how she may try, she may not be able to provide the child with the psychological atmosphere it needs, and as a result of her own psychological tensions may be led to child neglect or abuse.

5. A woman who discovers she has a defective child, and especially a genetically defective child who may perpetuate the defect, has an obligation not to bring a child into the world whose life will be one of suffering and a burden to society.

6. Nor can a woman depend upon help from society to care for her unwanted child, nor to provide for its adoption. Such help is often insufficient and given on degrading conditions.

7. Nor should women be forced to obtain an abortion from an illegal and probably dangerous abortionist, perhaps at the risk of death and perhaps of future sterility.

8. Modern women should be free to fulfill their duty of contributing to the solution of the very serious modern problem of population

control by using abortion as a backup when contraception fails or is unavailable.

9. Women should not be inhibited in their use of this right of choice by suffering interference from others who attempt to impose their own religious value systems on others or to arouse neurotic guilt feelings in those who choose abortion.

The advantages for the woman and for society are very tangible and in a concrete situation so many may concur, and the opposite disadvantages of pregnancy seem so overwhelming, especially if the woman is poor, already heavily burdened with children, and physically or psychologically ill, that she may very well believe that there is no other way out. As Rachel Conrad Wahlberg (1973) puts it, "Those who are involved personally with an unwanted pregnancy tend to discuss the philosophical, medical, or moral questions. Those who face nine months of pregnancy and fifteen to twenty years of child raising are more concerned with the immediate crisis" (p. 692).

Faced with a woman in such a dilemma, any compassionate health care professional may also believe that it would be utterly cruel and inhumane to refuse the medical cooperation she requests. Physicians (and also pastoral counselors) dread this situation and find it extremely difficult to refuse the requested help, especially when they are convinced that the woman may very well have the abortion anyway from an illegal abortionist or by self-inflicted methods, or may even commit suicide, so that their refusal will not save the child. Therefore, it is quite contrary to the command of Jesus, "Do not judge, and you will not be judged" (Matt. 7:1) for Christians to condemn as murders such women and the physicians who assist them out of conscientious conviction. Instead of judgment, Christians must seek ways to assist women to escape such anguishing dilemmas, while at the same time show an equal compassion for the helpless child.

The right of the mother to our compassion, however, is based on the same grounds as the child's right to life, so that human sympathy and justice must be given to both. Hence, we must also consider some of the consequences of permitting abortion.

1. By choosing to abort the child, the mother seeks to defend her own rights by destroying another human being, an action which is radically unjust to another and which is contrary to her own moral dignity as a person. It is true that the continued existence of the child places a woman in a unique relation to another person existing within her own body, yet the harm she suffers from this is (except in the most extreme case) only a relative harm for which other remedies may be sought, while the fetus suffers the absolute loss of the right to live for which no remedy is possible.

2. Abortion of children in difficult cases encourages the widespread practice of abortion in much less justifiable cases, because it becomes

the easy way out. Hence, the preponderance of evidence is that the social approval of abortion will imperil many more lives of children than social disapproval, even taking into account the prevalence of illegal abortions. Furthermore, children raised in a society where it is known that abortion is permitted, or that their mothers have had an abortion, lack the important psychological assurance of unqualified parental acceptance if the child once born is found deficient.

3. Women are encouraged and even forced by society to act in a way contradictory to their love and care for their own and others' children. It is risky to suppose that apparent social approval of abortion will do more than cover up the deep conflicts which this introduces in a woman's self-regard or to society's appreciation of the dignity of women as persons. Furthermore, the physical risks of abortion (including sterility) are not negligible, nor is the argument that they are less than the risks of childbirth convincing, since medical science can continue to reduce these latter risks.

4. Abortion policies tend to exclude the father from his proper responsibility for pregnancy for the child and from his role of supporting his wife and sharing her burdens. Hence he, too, is degraded as a person and burdened with deep conflicts.

5. Unmarried women, mentally retarded women, and victims of rape and incest deserve the protection and care of society which is too likely to dispense itself from this obligation simply by providing abortion as a solution. The same is true of poor women whose rights to raise a family are ignored by the encouragement of abortion to keep down welfare expenses.

6. The family institution, which is basic to society, is further weakened when the value of parenthood and of the child as a gift of God is undermined by the spreading practice of abortion. There is little evidence that such practices encourage an attitude of responsible parenthood, but rather that they promote irresponsibility by providing an easy way to escape its consequences. Hence, although very effective in population control, abortion is not a sound long-term solution for a long-term global problem.

7. Easy abortion encourages in society and in individuals an attitude of low regard for the human person as such in favor of a merely functional evaluation of persons in terms of their actual, present contribution to economic productivity and subjective well-being. This goes contrary to the advance of the concept of the dignity of the person and of inalienable rights on which modern democracy is based.

How, then, are we to balance so many positive and negative consequences of abortion one against another so as to apply the principle of proportion without falling into mere utilitarianism? As Richard McCormick (himself a strong proponent of this proportional method) has admitted (1973), it is difficult to see what collection of values favoring putting to death an innocent human being could be proportionate to the one basic value of that person's right to live. How can even the rights of the mother or of society outbalance this, since the mother's rights have the same foundation as those of the child, that is, the human personhood in which mother and child are equal and which it is the prime purpose of society to protect? It should be emphasized that however tangible and certain are the rights of the mother, the evil consequences to the child are still more tangible, certain, and immediate. A woman who threatens to kill herself or who may die in childbirth is still faced only with a possibility of death which may never occur and which it is possible to do something to prevent, but abortion dooms the child irretrievably.

Thus in the abortion question, at least, the principle of proportion brings us right back to the intrinsic and absolute right of the child to life just as does the more traditional position based on the rule that direct killing of the innocent is intrinsically evil and therefore exceptionless. Some defenders of the proportional method (cf. Callahan, 1970b) believe that sometimes the balance of advantages to the mother may outweigh the value of the life of the child, but they never explain how this evaluation can be made. It seems that what really lays back of their position is the view that precisely because the problem is so complex and incapable of an objective solution it must be left to the mother, herself, to decide because she is the one most affected. However, this is to forget the child who is affected even more directly and to abdicate the responsibility of society to protect the child, even against its mother, a responsibility we generally accept without question when it comes to child abuse or infanticide, although infanticide has its current defenders (Freeman and Cooke, 1972; Tooley, 1972). No one, we believe, would argue today that a slave master should be left free to do with his slave what he thinks best because it is *his* property.

Thus authoritative Church documents consistently support the moral rule that direct killing of innocent human beings can never be ethically justifiable. This does not necessarily exclude capital punishment since a criminal is by definition not an innocent. Nor does it exclude killing an aggressor in self-defense or in war, provided that the moral object intended is to stop the aggressive act, rather than the direct killing of the aggressor. However, one obvious exception to the rule has been proposed by some critics of the authoritative Catholic teaching against direct abortion which they believe reduces the position to absurdity, that is, the case where a physician can only save the mother by killing the child, but seems required by this law to let both die.

This criticism can be answered in several ways. Thomas J. O'Donnell (1976) provides a detailed analysis of the so-called medical indications for therapeutic abortion and shows that today the medical profession has solved this dilemma by providing the physician with the means to save both mother and child or at least to deal with the problems of both when both are at risk without attempting to choose the life of the mother against that of the child. Germain Grisez (1970a) answers it by more careful formulation of the Principle of Double Effect which he believes permits the doctor in extreme situations to kill the child *indirectly* in saving the mother. Bernard Häring (1973), in a solution somewhat similar to the probabilistic reasoning of Prummer already quoted, argues that there may be no longer any obligation to respect the rights of a child to life once it is certain that the child cannot live. All these authors agree that the rule against direct killing of the innocent is without exception, and that in practice the physician may not sacrifice the life of the child to that of its mother, but must do whatever he can for both. They do not permit, as would the principle of proportion, that we attempt the impossible task of trying to weigh the many incommensurable advantages and disadvantages involved, instead of facing the clear fact that abortion deprives one human being of its most fundamental right for the sake of another's less fundamental rights.

Finally, it should be noted that some recent authors (e.g., Curran, 1975), after having granted (on the basis of the proportional method) that it is permissible to abort the child to save the mother's life, then go further and argue that since some classical authors not only permitted direct killing an aggressor as a means to defend one's life but extended this to the defense of *equivalent* goods, therefore, it may be permissible to abort a child to save not only the mother's life but also her sanity or to prevent other very grave damage. However, apart from the fact that these "classical" precedences themselves are probably invalid, it is difficult to see how probable injury to the mother can be really equivalent to her death or the certain death of the child.

Conclusions

What practical conclusions for health care professionals can we draw from this discussion? The following norms are drawn from a pastoral document issued by the National Conference of Catholic Bishops (1973) and are helpful in determining what to do in particular situations.

1. Catholic hospitals cannot comply with laws requiring them to provide abortion services, even on the grounds of material cooperation.

2. Catholic physicians, nurses, and health care workers who work in facilities that provide abortion services may not take part in such procedures in good conscience. Their rights of conscience in this regard are recognized by federal law (Reed, 1973).

3. Physicians, nurses, and health care workers should give public witness to their belief in the sanctity of life, the integrity of every person,

and the value of human life at every stage of its existence by their compassion and care for their patients.

4. Physicians and nurses and health care workers who work in hospitals that provide abortion services should notify the hospital in writing of their conscientious refusal to participate in such actions.

5. Abortion is a serious and immoral action. Catholics who perform or obtain an abortion, or persuade others to do so, are doing grave harm to another human being against the Christian commandment of love of neighbor. All who willingly and deliberately assist in abortion procedures share the sinfulness of this destructive act. This is particularly true of the attending surgeon and the health care personnel who administer abortifacient drugs or other abortion procedures.

6. Cooperation in the sinful act of abortion would not ordinarily extend to preparing patients for the procedure or providing aftercare. However, Christian witness may well require Catholic nurses to avoid even those actions which (although not necessarily evil in themselves) may be interpreted as a compromise of Christian values.

7. Under Church law, those who perform or obtain an abortion or deliberately persuade others to do so place themselves in a state of excommunication, and any priest guilty of this is deposed from the priesthood (Canon 2350, no. 1; Huser, 1942; Coriden, 1973). The purpose of these severe penalties is to reinforce the Christian tradition which the Second Vatican Council (1965c) repeated when it declared, "Abortion and infanticide are unspeakable crimes" (*Church in the Modern World*, n. 51). Of course, it must be understood that this excommunication applies only to those who know that they are incurring it, yet freely chose to do so, understanding that they are committing a serious sin. Those who conscientiously dissent from the law do not suffer its spiritual consequences, but they are subject to its canonical consequences. Of course, this excommunication like all others can be removed by sincere repentance and confession, with the purpose of trying to make amends to others for the harm done, insofar as this is possible, but this will not give back life to the child who has been deprived of it. The tragedy of perhaps a million lives a year destroyed in the United States by the medical profession through abortion can only be contemplated with profound sorrow.

9.3   TRIAGE AND THE LIMIT TO EXTENDING CARE

After discussing how to determine who is the human subject of health care, we now need to deal with the question of what health care professionals are to do when they are unable to give full health care to all those who have a right to it. The issue here is not what to do in the long range, because that issue can be settled only by finding ways to provide more health care personnel and more equipment, a problem already treated in chapter 6, but what to do in the short range when resources are fixed.

This is the problem of *triage*, a French word meaning "to pick or sort according to quality." The term came into medical usage as a result of wartime experiences and was first explained by Jean Larrey, chief surgeon of Napoleon in his *Memoirs* (Himes, 1963) as follows:

> . . . those who are dangerously wounded must be tended first, entirely without regard to rank or distinction. Those less severely injured must wait until the gravely wounded have been operated upon and dressed. The slightly wounded may go to the hospital in the first or second line; especially the officers, since they have horses and therefore have transport — and regardless, most of these have but trivial wounds. (p. 9)

In recent discussions triage has come to have a wider significance, applying to any situation where there must be some kind of selection of patients for treatment because not all can be given equal care in a situation of limited resources.

Ethicists generally agree that triage is a just procedure, although as Joseph Fletcher (Lucas, 1975a) points out, the kind of justice involved is not one of strict (commutative) equality, but of distributive equality. In applying triage, we have to ask two questions, Who is in greatest need of treatment? and Who will benefit most from treatment? In the classical cases of wartime or disaster emergencies, these two questions yield a threefold division of victims: (1) the dying, whose need is great, but who will benefit least from treatment and who should be made comfortable and left to die; (2) the wounded who will survive without treatment because their need is little and who can be left to care for themselves; and (3) the wounded who will die unless treated, but who will probably survive if treated. Since these last have both the greatest need and can benefit most, they deserve the chief attention.

Today triage problems arise not only in emergency situations, but also in situations where no real emergency exists. For example, it may be necessary to select which patients are to be given a new vaccine or drug when a sufficient supply for all is not yet available. Again in such supportive health facilities as those which F. D. Powell (1975) has called "coping systems" where patients require almost unlimited attention for chronic, debilitating diseases similar selective problems are common.

In order to apply triage, it may also be necessary to use some random principle of selection not based on need or benefit, such as a lottery (Childress, 1973) or the rule of First come, first served. Such procedures are not unfair if the need and benefit are approximately the same for all, or if there is no way of making a discrimination on a need-and-benefit basis.

The Principle of Subsidiarity (6.1) provides that Charity begins at home, that is, we should first care for those closest to us and whose need is best known to us. Thus, it is not unjust that a family seek the best obtainable care for family members, or that physicians give special attention to their regular patients with whom a special relation of trust has been built up. However, the same principle requires that those who have responsibility for a larger group should attempt to distribute resources in such a way as to protect the basic rights of all, but to give the greatest care to those who have most need and will benefit most.

One of the most difficult problems in applying this kind of justice arises when a choice has to be made between supplying a few patients with expensive and lengthy treatment which may only keep them living for a while in very restricted activity (e.g., kidney dialysis or heart transplantation) and supplying a larger number of persons with simple treatments (e.g., a vaccine or dietary supplement) which may keep them normally active for many years. On the other hand, we can argue that in the second case the benefit for the many is great, while in the first case the benefit for the few is small; but on the other hand, we can argue that for each of the few the need is very great indeed, and the benefit (from their point of view) is very real. Nevertheless, it seems that in the social distribution of health care, priority ought to be given to that kind of preventive medicine or treatment of acute disease which will raise the general standards of health, especially for the young, over elaborate modes of treatment for the aged or seriously handicapped.

The compensation for the individual who is aged or handicapped is to be found not so much in prolongation of life or expensive treatment as in the kind of personal attention which will make what remains of life as meaningful as possible. In this sense, the need of such persons is very great and the benefit they will receive also very great, but what is required is not sophisticated medicine but wise and loving concern on the part of the community. Sometimes such concern is better shown in cultures where medical technology is underdeveloped than it is in our culture.

Even more difficult questions arise when the triage principle is extended to problems of health care distribution on a global scale. We discuss this topic briefly here, although it may exceed the scope of this book, because we believe that American health care professionals must more and more think about health in global terms. This problem of social triage was dramatized by Garrett Hardin (1974) in his proposal of a "lifeboat ethics." According to Hardin, the crisis of the population explosion and world hunger faces us in the developed countries with a hard choice. If we continue to send medical aid and food to such countries, we will only increase their overpopulation, with the result that even more people will starve than if we let them starve now. Consequently, Hardin advocates either we give food only with the condition that these countries institute very stringent (even compulsory) population controls, or we terminate all foreign aid.

Hardin further argues that it would be foolish for us to lower our own standards of living and health for the sake of poorer countries, since we need all we have to raise up healthy, well-educated children who are the only hope of the human race for the future. No matter how much we give to poorer countries, they can never produce such children.

Joseph Fletcher (Lucas, 1975a) points out that Hardin is not advocating mere selfishness, but is using the utilitarian principle, The greatest good for the greatest number, with which Fletcher himself agrees. Fletcher is not sure that the emergency is yet as great as Hardin supposes, but he praises Hardin for his realism. We too believe that ethics should be hardheaded and realistic, but we do not believe that Hardin is so much hardheaded as hardhearted (Faramelli, 1975; Simon, 1975; Shriver, 1976). A realistic effort at distributive justice must take a broader point of view ("Scarce Medical Resources," 1969; Shapiro, 1974).

If Hardin is right in believing that the crisis is so close that only short-range solutions are possible, then it is doubtful that anything at all can be done about the situation since social policy seldom can move so rapidly. Moreover, most experts believe that in the long range, various possibilities are still open by which world population and food resources can be brought into balance. The present situation has come about because the developed countries have introduced modern medical technology into the underdeveloped countries, not merely for humanitarian reasons, but to make possible their policies of political and economic colonialism (Neville and Steinfels, 1972). Unwittingly, the advanced countries by introducing modern medicine also upset the ecological balance and produced a rapid population growth, without at the same time producing the standard of living which in developed countries motivates and facilitates responsible parenthood. Thus, justice demands that the developed countries help restore the balance which they themselves destroyed.

The United States and other wealthy countries need to undertake such a restoration of justice not only for justice's sake, but also for our own self-preservation. It is quite unrealistic to suppose, as Hardin does, that we can sail away in our lifeboat and leave the rest of the world to sink. There is no place to sail to and no ocean to absorb the millions who look enviously to the wealth we hoard. Nor is it true that these countries are without power, since the ultimate weapon may turn out to be not the atom bomb, but sheer numbers.

The popes in their recent social encyclicals (John XXIII, 1961; Paul VI, 1967) have repeatedly declared that the only solution to this crisis of population and resources is distributive justice, with the distribution made not by the superpowers but by international agreement and cooperation. Implicit in the argument of Hardin and other similar positions is the assumption that quality of life and hope for the future depend upon an elite of scientific technologists. Since it is the misapplication of scientific technology which has produced the present crisis, it is not so evident that this elite is really the hope of the future.

Thus in our social triage situation, as Rawls (1971) has argued, the fundamental principle must be equal justice for all members of the world community, even the least privileged. If resources are scarce, then these resources must first be assigned to those members of the community who can use them best and most justly for the good of all. But in making this selection, we must avoid the danger of being judges in our own case. Even according to Hardin's argument, would it not be wiser to attempt to select from *all* countries those citizens on whom the future of the race can most securely depend, rather than waste these resources on so many in our own country who consume much and contribute little?

Health care professionals have a responsibility to employ sound social triage principles in developing health care policies, taking care that all members of the national and the world communities play a role in determining priorities and criteria of selection (P. Ramsey, 1970a; Childress, 1973). When faced with situations in which they find no practical way to achieve this broad justice, health care professionals must do what they can to give the best care to those who most need it and can most benefit from it. In general, these patients are the poor and neglected whose need is greatest and whose opportunities in life will be most enhanced. The privileged have ways to take care of themselves.

9.4   HUMAN EXPERIMENTATION

For Whose Benefit?

After health care professionals have determined who is the subject of medical care endowed with human rights (9.1 and 9.2), they must respect those rights and especially the person's right to health, that is, optimum possible physical and psychological functioning (2.1) insofar as resources are available (9.3).

We have now to consider procedures which are or which appear to be genuinely medical, but where there is real question as to whether the true purpose of the professional is the benefit of the patient, or whether in fact it is the manipulation (Häring, 1975) or use of a human subject not for his or her own benefit but for the benefit of the researcher and perhaps of others who may profit from the researcher's discoveries. We have argued in chapter 1 that the human person is per se an end in himself or herself, so that we can use a person as a means to our own purposes only if that person also somehow truly shares the good we achieve for ourselves as his or her own good, that is, as a common good. To use a person as a means to some goal from which the person is excluded is directly contrary to the Principle of Human Dignity in Community (1.5).

> When science takes man as its subject, tensions arise between two values basic to Western Society: freedom of scientific inquiry and protection of individual inviolability. (p. 1)

These words introduce a major study by Jay Katz and others (1972) concerning the legal and ethical issues of human experimentation. That experimentation on human beings is often useful and often necessary for the common good is without doubt. Many beneficial vaccines and other therapies such as smallpox and poliomyelitis vaccines, open heart surgery, and successful treatment of certain birth defects have required human experimentation, and the whole world attests to its value. At the same time, there is also no doubt that human experimentation has been abused. The world should never forget the horrors of the human experimentation carried out on innocent human beings in the name of scientific progress in the Nazi concentration camps. Aside from such atrocities, other egregious violations of human rights have occurred in the United States, such as the withholding of newly discovered penicillin from patients in the Tuskeegee syphilis study (W. Curran, 1973), the Willowbrook experiments in which retarded children were used as experimental subjects (Diamond, 1973), and the injection of live cancer cells in unknowing subjects in the Jewish Chronic Disease Hospital case (Hersey and Miller, 1976). Psychological experimentation has also given rise to serious debate about behavior control (London, 1969). Such abuses often are not the product of demented or perverted minds; rather they result from lack of care and ethical sensitivity on the part of well-motivated researchers who overlook the rights of human beings in an effort to ensure scientific progress (Barber, 1973).

In his account Katz (1972) states:

> Human experimentation in the practice of medicine is as old as the practice of medicine itself but only during the last hundred years, since the age of Pasteur, has medicine become aware of the need for deliberate and well-planned experimentation. (p. 1)

The heightened concern in regard to human experimentation on the part of ethically serious people is due in part to the growing number of research projects involving human subjects. Since 1947, approximately one-quarter million projects involving human subjects have been carried out, about one-third of which have been supported by the government (Chalkley, 1975). Another source of concern is the fact that the frontiers of science are being rolled back further every day. Hence, human experimentations not only affect the rights of human persons in the future, but may also condition and change the very core of human nature itself.

We can define human experimentation as some deliberate change of condition without foreknowledge of the results but with subsequent observation of them carried out upon living human subjects. Several categories of human subjects may be involved: (1) healthy adults, including the investigator himself, elderly persons, and normal healthy adults; (2) sick adults, usually referred to as "patients," including the acutely and terminally ill; (3) prisoners, soldiers, and students (and even monks) living in highly controlled situations; (4) children, both healthy and ill; (5) mentally incompetent adults and children; and (6) unborn children or still-living aborted fetuses. As we will see, each of these categories present special problems.

Experimentation on these human subjects, or human research as it is often called, may be either *therapeutic* or *nontherapeutic*. Therapeutic experimentation is carried on in order to improve the health of the research subject by prophylactic, diagnostic, or therapeutic methods that depart from standard medical practice but hold out a reasonable expectation of success. The practice of medicine often involves therapeutic research, but practicing medicine should not be identified with therapeutic research. If the effect of medical treatment or other procedures is more or less predictable and standard, then experimentation is not involved. Clearly, what begins as human experimentation may later become standard medical practice.

Nontherapeutic research or experimentation is not designed to improve the health condition of the research subject; rather it seeks to gain knowledge or develop new techniques that will be beneficial for people other than the subject.

The proper manner of conducting these kinds of research on these various categories of human subjects has become one of the most discussed bioethical questions of recent years. Through seminars and studies on the subject, some ethical principles have been developed to serve as a guide for researchers and for those who support research. As a result of such studies by legal, medical, and ethical groups throughout the world, especially in the generation after World War II, these principles have become widely accepted, even though there may be disagreement concerning their application in particular cases. Interestingly, the norms produced by medical and legal experts, such as the Nuremberg and Helsinki statements, are in remarkable harmony with Christian teaching on human dignity formulated by Pope Pius XII.

Principles of Experimentation

We will summarize and discuss these principles, noting first that the ethical issues involved relate chiefly to three ethical principles: the Principle of Totality and Integrity (2.4), which is especially relevant to therapeutic experimentation; the Principle of Human Dignity in

Community (1.5), which relates to the limits of nontherapeutic experimentation; and the Principle of Informed Consent (a corollary of the Principle of Prudent Conscience (3.4; 8.1-1), which relates to the capacity of the various categories of human subjects to participate freely in experimentation.

1. The knowledge sought through research must be important and obtainable by no other means, and the research must be carried on by qualified people.

2. Appropriate experimentation upon animals and cadavers must precede human experimentation.

3. The risk of suffering or injury must be proportionate to the good to be gained.

Because the Principle of Double Effect (8.1-3) is used to justify the possible ill effects of human experimentation, the relation between risk and potential benefit is most important. Of course, predicting the degree of risk with certitude is seldom possible. Moreover, sometimes, as in the case of poliomyelitis research in 1954 when use of some poorly prepared live vaccine resulted in the death of children, some risks are not predictable at all. Hence, absolute certainty in regard to the nature and degree of the risk cannot be required. Pius XII (1952) stated:

> The total exclusion of all danger and risk cannot be demanded. This is beyond all possibilities of human nature, and would paralyze all scientific research and would very often turn out to the detriment of the patient. The appreciation of the element of danger must be left, in these cases, to the judgment of experienced and competent physicians.

Care must be taken, however, to make as accurate a prediction as possible concerning the nature and magnitude of risk eventuating from any particular human experiment, and the bias of enthusiastic researchers in favor of the promise of some new procedure must be subject to cool criticism.

The objectivity of such scientific research depends largely upon the use of controlled experimentation in which a group of experimental subjects is divided into two subgroups, one of which receives the experimental therapy while the other receives the standard therapy or none at all, and especially upon double-blind control in which not only are subjects not informed as to which kind of treatment they have received, but also even those researchers who evaluate the effects of the two treatments are in ignorance as to which subjects have received which. Only the double-blind technique can eliminate the placebo effect, that is, the improvement frequently experienced by patients who expect it and the effect of bias on the part of scientists. However, this raises ethical questions, since it would seem (1) that those patients who do not receive the new therapy are at a therapeutic disadvantage, and (2) that none of the patients in the double-blind experiment could have given informed consent.

We can reply to this difficulty that physicians have an obligation to give patients conservative, standard treatment unless there is a sufficient reason to use a more experimental treatment. This obligation is generally understood and is implicitly contained in the doctor-patient contract. Consequently, in an experiment justice is done to those patients who only receive the standard treatment if nothing more is promised them unless the advantages of the new treatment are very great and the evidence for this already very strong and objectively founded. However, it would be unjust and against the freedom of patients to tell them that they are receiving the new therapy when they are not. Hence, in double-blind experiments the subjects should be informed that if they consent to the experiment some will receive the new treatment and others will not, but that none of the subjects will know. The potential subjects will then be free to consent to these experimental conditions or to refuse to participate. They thus have the chance to choose between the risk that the old treatment might have been safer as well as their chances that they will receive one or the other. Clearly, they should choose to participate only if they see that these risks are fairly equal.

When determining the degree of risk that a person might undergo, one must bear in mind the difference between therapeutic and nontherapeutic research. If experimentation is therapeutic, then persons may undergo greater risk, especially if they might die as a result of the illness or malady that the researcher is trying to cure. The Principle of Totality and Integrity (2.4) is also involved in therapeutic experimentation. As Pius XII (1952) explains, "If the well-being of the whole demands, one may paralyze, destroy, mutilate or separate an organ or member of the body because this is in accord with its natural finality."

The same principle of totality cannot be invoked in the case of nontherapeutic experimentation because one person is not related to another person or to a group of persons (the state) as part of the whole. Although there is a relationship of extrinsic finality between and among different people, there is not a relationship of intrinsic finality or form. Hence, one person does not exist for the other, nor is one person ordered to the other in total finality. Each individual person is an end, or being in himself or herself and cannot be sacrificed for another. This is the basic reason why the public authority has no right to sacrifice individuals for "the interest of the state or for scientific progress" (Pius XII, 1952). Experiments carried out for the good of the state or for scientific progress may provide new knowledge or medical techniques and thus seem to be beneficial, but they do so and are so at the expense of human rights and human dignity and hence are immoral.

Although it is sometimes fitting that researchers themselves participate in experiments, they are bound by the same restrictions as other subjects. The *Nuremberg Code* is rather unclear about this stipulation, implying that researchers may take greater risks than others (n. 5). Pope Pius XII (1952) expresses a more accurate view:

> He (the doctor or researcher) is subject to the same broad moral and juridical principles as govern other men. He has no right, consequently, to permit scientific or practical experiments which entail serious injury or which threaten to impair his health to be performed on his person, and even to a lesser extent is he authorized to attempt an operation of experimental nature which, according to authoritative opinion, could conceivably result in mutilation or even suicide.

4. Subjects should be selected such that risks and benefits will not fall unequally upon one group in society.

Justice demands that the burdens associated with human progress be shared equitably. In recent years, the poor of the world, especially in the United States, have borne an unequal burden insofar as medical research is concerned. The causes of this situation are psychological as well as economic (Ingelfinger, 1975). Research protocols must be designed to offset this imbalance and to assure that when the poor take part in an experiment their human rights are respected and they are given the freedom that their human dignity demands. As one authority points out, given the nature of the situation, it may not be possible to guarantee that the poor will not be numerically dominant in human experimentation, but it is possible to protect their rights. The same consideration holds for those categories of subjects who are chosen because they live in restricted and controlled circumstances where the researcher has easy access to them, for example, prisoners, soldiers, or those confined to rest homes or mental institutions. Such persons are in need of advocacy lest they be too easily persuaded to join in experiments by group pressure or by rewards which their situation makes excessively attractive. Prisoners, offered parole in return for participation in a dangerous experiment, may find this one hope of freedom too compelling to resist.

5. In order to protect the integrity of the human person, free and informed (voluntary) consent must be obtained.

This is perhaps the most important and the most debated of the principles involved in human experimentation and is a form of the Principle of Prudent Conscience (3.4) which is the very basis of all ethical decision. According to one of the more authoritative statements on the subject (Hershey and Miller, 1976), free and informed consent means the following:

> . . . . knowing consent of an individual or his legally authorized representative, so situated as to be able to exercise free power of choice without due inducement or any element of force, fraud, deceit, or duress, or other form of constraint or coercion. The basic elements of information necessary to such consent include: (1) a fair explanation of procedures to be followed and their purposes, including identification of any procedures which are experimental; (2) a description of any attendant discomforts and risks reasonably to be expected; (3) a description of

any benefits reasonably to be expected; (4) a disclosure of any appropriate alternative procedures that might be advantageous for the subject; (5) an offer to answer any inquiries concerning the procedures; and (6) an instruction that the person is free to withdraw his consent and to discontinue participation at any time without prejudice to the subject. (p. 27)

In spite of this rather extensive definition, there are still serious discussions and disputes concerning the concept of informed consent and its application. Many question, for example, whether prisoners can ever give *free* consent because of their situation (Capron, 1973b). Others question whether double-blind procedures, an integral part of some experiments, can ever be employed (Barber, 1976). However, we would hold that both experimentation upon prisoners and double-blind procedures can be utilized if extra care is taken in obtaining consent.

The most puzzling problems, however, are those in situations in which one person gives consent for another for whom the first is morally responsible. This is commonly called *proxy consent*, an unfortunate term since properly speaking a legal proxy is an agent acting on behalf of another by the other's consent, which is precisely what is lacking in the case under consideration. It would be better to call it "vicarious consent" since a vicar fulfills a duty for another irrespective of whether the other has authorized it. It should be distinguished also from *implicit* consent and *presumed* consent. Persons consent implicitly when they actually consent to some general line of action in which is implied more detailed permissions, as when a patient consents to surgery without specifying what anesthetic is to be used. Consent is presumed when it is highly probable that someone who is not able to give consent because absent or unconscious would have given it if present or conscious, as when a surgeon presumes that a patient would expect him to remove a diseased appendix of which the patient was unaware but which the surgeon notes in the course of other abdominal surgery. Proxy or vicarious consent is, according to some, a form of presumed consent, but other explanations are possible. As such, it simply means that one person who represents the interests of another by some legitimate title gives consent for the experiment in place of the subject because that subject is incompetent.

Proxy Consent

Children, the retarded, the infirm, the dying, and recently, unborn children and living aborted fetuses are often suggested as fitting subjects for human research. Sometimes it is argued that this gives them an opportunity which they might not otherwise have of contributing to the common good. Since they are not competent, or at least not fully

competent, to give free and informed consent, the principle can be satisfied in their case only by the proxy or vicarious consent of a parent
or guardian. Decisions of proxy consent must be made in view of the
good of the individual person, not for a higher good or for a class good
which would amount to manipulation of the person as a mere means.
If the experiment is therapeutic, there would be reason for the proxy
to allow risk in proportion to the good that might accrue to the individual in question, since the proxy is acting in that person's best interest.
However, if nontherapeutic experimentation is involved, then the
decision is more difficult.

Some authors (P. Ramsey, 1970a; May, 1976a) maintain that the
person issuing proxy consent has no right to expose a ward to *any* risk.
The justification for this position is that a proxy should make a decision
in accord with the best interests of the subject, but in nontherapeutic
experimentation the interests of the subject are not clearly evident,
and since the subject does not have the capacity to make a free choice
about a free matter, the proxy (guardian) has no right to presume or
say anything on behalf of the ward.

Other authors (McCormick, 1974b, 1976b; O'Donnell, 1976;
Soukup, 1976) would allow exposing children and others who cannot
consent for themselves to "minimal risk." Thus, proxy consent is
interpreted as a form of presumed consent. The justification for their
position is that there are some things a child as a human being *ought*
to do for others, for example, to take part in experiments where there
is hope of "general benefit" and only minimal risk. The United States
Commission for the Protection of Human Subjects, when determining
the norms for fetal experimentation, followed the minimal risk theory
(HEW, August 8, 1975; O'Rourke, 1975).

We would be inclined to follow the more cautious opinion, maintaining that proxy consent is not licit in nontherapeutic experimentation,
even when the risk is minimal. Two considerations convince us of this.

(1) Guardians have responsibility for wards who cannot care for
themselves because of the Principle of Human Dignity in Community
which affirms that no person can achieve fulfillment without sharing
in the common good and contributing to it. Hence, when a guardian
or proxy consents to have a ward subject to experimentation, the proxy
has the right to do so not on the basis of the presumed consent of the
ward which is merely hypothetical, but on the basis of an actuality,
namely, the need of the ward for care. Thus, theories of presumed
consent based on what the ward ought to do if the ward could consent
are weak.

(2) It may be granted that if a guardian in a concrete case is sure
that the ward will suffer only minimal risk and therefore gives proxy
consent, the guardian does not fail in his or her responsibility to care
for the ward, since Little counts for nothing, as the saying of the moralist

goes. However, this cannot be erected into a guideline for general action, since such a rule opens the way for an extensive interpretation under which very serious risks may be taken. In other words, a guardian should be an advocate, jealous of the rights of the ward, not ready to yield these rights for the sake of others who cannot act for themselves, nor for the hypothetical rights of future generations of other children.

The importance of caution in the formulation of guidelines with regard to informed consent by proxy is well illustrated by the recent difficulties of the Department of Health, Education, and Welfare (HEW) over the use of federal funds for research on fetuses alive or dead, in or out of the womb, by either spontaneous or induced abortion. Some researchers had concluded that if the Supreme Court permits abortion, then it is also permissible to use such aborted "material" for experimental purposes, even if the fetus is still alive *ex utero* or at least when it is still alive *in utero* once the mother has decided to have it aborted. While there seems no ethical objections to using dead fetuses produced by spontaneous abortion, provided they are treated with the same respect required in autopsies and the disposal of cadavers (13.4), very serious objections can be raised to the use of dead fetuses if they are obtained by induced abortion because (1) this opens the way to encourage abortion, and (2) it gives to the Supreme Court decision in Roe v. Wade the appearance of moral approval of abortion, which is to go further than the actual force of that decision.

The major objection raised to HEW guidelines was with regard to experimentation on live fetuses, whether *in* or *ex utero*, since this would amount to making the federal government (and hence the citizenry) partners in nontherapeutic experiments on human subjects unable to give free and informed consent, thus setting a precedent which might have extensive and dangerous consequences. The dangers of permitting proxy consent were vividly illustrated in such cases because the guardian in question was none other than the same mother who had doomed her child to abortion and who might even be paid for her cooperation in doing so!

Because of such objections, Congress required a moratorium on such funding until a special commission set up by HEW Secretary Caspar Weinberger could study the matter. On August 8, 1975, Weinberger, as a result of this study, published a new set of guidelines and ended the mortatorium. This effort by the federal government to provide bioethical guidelines of this sort, although open to some criticism in detail, was remarkable and encouraging evidence that wide, even if not perfect, consensus can be achieved by study and dialogue on controversial bioethical questions.

The final guidelines accepted the notion that proxy consent to minimal risk is permissible and also set up a reviewing committee to settle difficulties whose tendency may favor freedom of research rather than protection of the human subject. Consequently, there is still reason to fear that patterns of research will develop in the United States which are dependent upon a constant supply of fetal "material" and that research on fetuses being readied for abortion will become a feature of hospitals and clinics federally funded. The argument for such research is, of course, that it may lead to discoveries highly beneficial for other children who are permitted to live. This supposes that scientific research can proceed only along one line of investigation. Such reasoning, if pressed far enough, leads to the conclusion that all of us should be made subject to experimentation whether we consent or not since this would present researchers with wonderful opportunities to make beneficial discoveries.

6. At any time during the course of research, the subject (or the guardian who has given proxy consent) must be free to terminate the subject's participation in the experiment.

The reason for this guideline is that the consenting subject or proxy may not have been able to correctly anticipate the subjective factors involved, the amount of suffering, or the anxiety or depression until they begin to be actually experienced, or the subject or proxy may even discover that the information given was inadequate or deceptive or imperfectly communicated, or the subject or proxy may have second thoughts about his or her own understanding or freedom when the consent was given. The subject or guardian cannot consent to give away the primary responsibility for defending the subject's own health and integrity since this is an inherent right and obligation. Consequently, if during the course of the experimentation the subject or proxy begins to see that grave risks to the subject's well-being may be involved, the subject or proxy is ethically obliged to stop participation.

Psychological Experimentation

Special problems are involved in psychological experiments (American Psychological Association, 1973; Brody, 1974; Ashley, 1975). In order to discuss these problems more fully, we must defer the topic to chapter 12 after we have explained the nature of psychotherapy and its distinctions from medical therapy more thoroughly. At this point, however, we can state that in such experimentation we must observe all the precautions necessary in medical experiments, especially informed consent, careful calculation of risks and benefits, and precautions against the bias of researchers in favor of their own freedom. We must also add the following special rules.

7. In psychological experimentation, the researcher should experiment with rather than on the human subject. That is, the researcher must gain the cooperation of the subject in the experiment so that the

subject will participate with the purpose of gaining greater insight into himself or herself as a person in order to become free and more realistic in coping with life's problems and also with the purpose of sharing this knowledge and freedom with others.

This guideline is based on the fact that psychological experiments with a human subject are also psychological *experiences* for the subject which can be healthy and psychologically therapeutic or traumatizing reinforcement of bad behavior patterns. In very few cases can such experiences be merely neutral. Even the experience of filling out a questionnaire can be educational or terrifying. Any experience in which the patient is treated as a mere passive object rather than as a person cannot be a beneficial experience. It is questionable whether such treatment can even be experimentally useful since in such a situation the human person is no longer acting humanly, but subhumanly. Thus, human persons should not permit themselves to be treated in this way since those who seek to reduce them to objects are violating their human rights. Psychological experimentation must involve the human, active cooperation of the subject and produce some learning and growth benefits.

8. The researcher must avoid breaking down human trust by lying or manipulation, although subjects can give free and informed consent to experiments in which they have to learn to interpret ambiguous communications or meet puzzling situations.

In many psychological experiments, the experimentalist does not seem to have any qualms about lying to subjects. Not only is lying itself (in our opinion) intrinsically wrong itself and contrary to professional ethics (5.2), it is also psychologically harmful to the subject because it breaks down the social trust on which all human relations is built. Commonsense proof of this is supplied by the fact that those who have been subjected to such manipulation often react indignantly when they discover the deception and feel they have been treated unfairly.

This is especially true when dealing with mentally disturbed patients, since an element of distrust, withdrawal, and paranoia is present in most forms of emotional disturbance which can only be reinforced by deception on the part of professionals who claim to be especially trustworthy and authoritative.

This rule against lying, however, does not prohibit experiments in which previous warning is given that the experiment may involve games in which ambiguous clues are given and embarrassment and defeat possibly experienced. These are risks of the experiment to which the subject must have a chance to give free and informed consent or refusal. Deception in such a case is not what moral theologians define as a "lie," because traditional moral theology has always insisted that it is permissible to use ambiguous clues or language in situations where others are forewarned either explicitly or by the very nature of the situation.

Such games do not usually break down trust if the experimenter sticks to the rules of the game. Moreover, they may be highly educational for the participant since through them the subject gains insight as to how important it is to base one's interpretation of reality on solid evidence, rather than on ambiguous evidence or subjective feelings.

9.   Researchers must not take serious risks of reducing the subjects' ability to perceive reality as it is or to make free choices except as a temporary experience through which the subjects can learn to cope with distortions of truth and attacks on their freedom.

This rule states more exactly the special risks involved in psychological experimentation. It excludes permission for any more than temporary damage to patients' ability to remain or become free in managing their own life. Thus an experiment would be forbidden if it might cause organic brain damage or induce drug addiction, as well as experiments that might make the subject unduly liable to hypnotic control, to compulsive patterns of behavior (as might take place in some forms of behavior modification (cf. Milgram, 1974), or which create recurrent hallucinations. A special case of psychological research which may involve risks to freedom is research in dealing with human sexuality. This issue will be discussed in chapter 12 in connection with therapy of inadequate or perverted sexual behavior.

9.5   LAW, MORALITY, AND PROFESSIONAL LIMITS

Legislating Morality

Since the very nature of a profession involves a certain autonomy, as we have recognized by the Principle of the Common Good, Subsidiarity, and Functionalism (6.1; 8-2), it is understandable that health care professionals are very reluctant to permit laypersons including legislators to prescribe limits to professional activities. Yet the autonomy of a profession is relative to its purpose of serving the health not only of individual patients, but also of the community. Laws have to be made to restrain lawyers, and even the clergy have had to submit to some government regulation of their activities (e.g., the clergy may not perform marriages between parties who do not have a license). The medical profession has generally accepted such regulations as those relating to dispensing narcotic drugs and to issuing of death certificates.

Far more important is the question of the legal definition of the human person which necessarily determines who are the subjects whose rights must be respected in every medical decision. The defining of the human person affects the question of abortion and also concerns many of the problems discussed in chapters 11 and 13. It would seem obvious that our laws should supply such a definition, yet historically it has been assumed the matter is so obvious as to require no definition (St. John-Stevas, 1961, 1971). That this assumption is unfounded is evident from the history of slavery and racial discrimination in the United States where there has been a long struggle to get recognition of the members of racial minorities as full persons having rights equal to those of the majority.

Medieval and British common law regarded abortion as a serious crime, although the courts were not always clear as to whether or at what stage of pregnancy abortion was to be punished as homicide. In 1803, the first statute law in the United States on the subject declared abortion to be a crime punishable by death if the child had "quickened" and by lesser but serious penalties if it had not. Throughout the nineteenth century in England and in the United States, increasingly strict laws were passed against abortion, but with exceptions for therapeutic abortion to save the mother's life. Such legislation was strongly supported by the American medical profession (D. T. Smith, 1967; Callahan, 1970b; Grisez, 1970a), in part because the medical risks for the mother in abortion were still high.

However, a number of factors were at work in the opposite direction. First of all, in Europe and the United States, the value systems of Humanism and Marxism with their emphasis on human technological control over life came more and more to dominate the professions, so that as abortion became medically safer it seemed to many just another effective method of controlling human destiny. Second, the antiabortion laws proved increasingly difficult to enforce equitably since women of means could obtain an abortion on therapeutic pretexts, while poorer women could not. Third, the increasing concern over the population explosion and the growing tax burden for social welfare suggested that abortion was a very effective method of reducing the birth rate, at least as a backup to contraception. Fourth, the feminist movement, which originally opposed abortion, began to favor it as giving women more control over their own lives and greater equality with men. Fifth, the emphasis on the right of privacy in sexual matters increased with the spread of new contraceptive methods.

New York, Colorado, and California adopted very permissive laws with regard to abortion in the 1960s. Finally on January 22, 1973, the United States Supreme Court in Roe v. Wade and Doe v. Bolton came to the decision that it is unconstitutional for any law to infringe on the right of privacy by which a woman has the sole power of decision as to whether to have an abortion, just as couples have the same right to the practice of contraception. While some laws regulating medical procedures, especially after the first trimester of pregnancy and even more restrictively after the second trimester, were not automatically excluded by the Court as having possible constitutional validity, the right of the woman to decide was stated unequivocally, and the Court in later cases reinforced this by declaring that a woman did not need the consent of the father of the child to be aborted, nor did a minor need the consent of her parents. Surprisingly, the Court recently in Maher v. Roe (1977) ruled that this right of the woman to have an abortion does not imply that she has the right to have assistance for such an abortion from state or federal funds, since the government as a matter of public policy can favor childbirth over abortion provided that it does not infringe the woman's freedom. Critics point out that this decision again introduces the inequity which had been one of the strongest arguments for liberalization, namely, that under previous laws poor women could not have an abortion, but the well-to-do could.

The main criticism, however, which can be brought against the present stance of the Court is not that it has moved to protect the rights of the woman, which is entirely in accord with its main historical effort to strengthen and extend human rights (Broderick, 1973), but that it has simply evaded the question of the child's rights on the very flimsy pretext that it is a speculative question on which there is no general agreement. We may well then ask, When has there been general agreement on the issue of rights for racial minorities or for women? It is just because such issues are highly controversial and, if you like, speculative that the Supreme Court has the duty to face them squarely. In fact, it has decided that the unborn child (at least in its first six months of life) is not a human being with human rights, but it has not done so honestly, nor persuasively, as will be evident to anyone who checks the unscholarly history of the controversy with which it documented its decision. As Daniel Callahan (1973b) has said:

> It is often thought that when the State withdraws from resolving "speculative" questions (by definition those which command no consensus?) then freedom is somehow served; that was the gist of all those arguments which would leave abortion decisions up to individual choice and conscience. I have always found that an odd kind of contention, one which, if followed rigorously, would leave all decisions bearing on concepts of "justice," "equality," "the general welfare" and the like up to individual consciences as well. For what notions could be more speculative in their final meaning and implications, to judge from all the disagreement they provoke? (p. 7)

Some who favor the Court's stand have tried to blunt this issue by arguing that the Court has not only considered the mother's rights, but has in effect also protected the right of the unborn child not to be born into a world where it is unwanted and where it may suffer from physical or psychological disabilities (Sprague, 1967). However, as Camenisch (1976) has well argued, if a child does in fact have such a paradoxical right, then it has the right to choose to live or not live, just as the mother has the right to choose to abort or not, and this right of the child to choose to live is denied when the mother exercises her right to abort. Thus, the question of conflict of rights cannot be evaded (Granfield, 1973). Either the rights in question are not truly rights, or some way to balance them must be found. The Court has simply confused this question.

The result of this evasion by the Court of the fundamental issue of whether the child as well as the mother is the subject of human rights has led to a vigorous Pro-Life Movement which favors a constitutional amendment which would permit the states to deal with the question individually. Some urge the adoption of this amendment by the Congress and its ratification by the states; others, a special constitutional convention to debate it. The Catholic bishops have expressed support for some type of amendment, leaving the choice of its exact form to public discussion, and have launched a campaign of education on the "respect life" question. The Pro-Life Movement is also favored by many non-Catholic groups, and public opinion polls seem to show that it has in its favor the opposition of sixty percent of the public to abortion on demand.

However, the Pro-Life Movement is severely criticized by some of the groups in this country who have been the strongest supporters of human rights and social justice. These proponents of civil liberties point out that the Pro-Life members seem to focus all their concern for human rights on the unborn, while showing little concern for the social injustices suffered by those already born. We might ask if there is not equal inconsistency on the part of social justice and civil rights enthusiasts when they hail Roe v. Wade as a triumph for civil liberty (Blanshard and Doerr, 1973) and connect abortion with the cause of women's rights. Both sides need to realize that human rights can only be furthered by a broad and consistent effort to extend legal protection for every human being regardless of race, sex, religion, and age, from conception to death. Moreover, we must not cloud the debate about how best to protect human rights by accusing this or that party to the debate with imposing their religious values on others (cf. Devlin, 1959; Kindregan, 1969; Hart, 1963), when in all such debates every side, religious or secularist, is necessarily advocating a particular value system with which others will differ.

American pluralism demands that minority groups have a right to advocate their own values and to attempt to have these values play an influential role in public decisions. Catholics begin to wonder what will happen to their values if the courts in the name of women's rights begin to require Catholic hospitals and Catholic health care professionals to cooperate in abortion. So far, the law and the courts have been rather careful to protect the consciences of health care professionals in such matters, but this protection may break down as Catholics become more and more integrated into a national comprehensive health care program.

Consequently, in spite of the bishops' advocacy of prolife, some Catholics are hesitant. The congressman priest Father Drinan (1968, 1970a, 1970b; Gaffney, 1974) has strongly arqued that Catholics should work to educate the public to the evils of abortion, but should not favor laws against it, since in a pluralist society this can only be divisive and ineffectual.

Charles E. Curran (1975) in a theological analysis of the problem shows that in the authoritative Church documents, including the *Declaraation on Procured Abortion* of the Congregation for the Doctrine of the Faith (1974), there is some wavering between the older conception of the relations of Church and State and the clearer position adopted by the Second Vatican Council in its *Declaration on Religious Liberty* (1965c). The newer position recognizes that the state, although it has the duty to protect and foster human rights, must also take into consideration that these rights include the freedom of conscience of all groups in the community to make personal decisions about what is right and wrong to the degree that this is compatible with public order and the rights of others. Curran concludes:

> . . . three criteria — as much freedom as possible for the individual, the criterion of public order to justify state intervention by law, and the recognition of pragmatic, prudential and feasible aspects in the law — constitute the framework for the proper understanding of the relationship between law and private morality. Note that in this understanding of law there is what some have called an idealistic function of law insofar as it must support peace, justice, and an order of morality, but there is also the recognition of the rights of freedom of individuals and at the same time the recognition of prudential and pragmatic judgments about the effectiveness and function of law itself. In this way the danger of an idealistic approach, which does not give enough importance to freedom and considerations of feasibility, is avoided as is the danger of a purely pragmatic approach, which sees law as totally distinct from considerations of justice and peace and merely accepting the mores of a particular society at any given time. (p. 134)

Hence, Catholics need not conclude that the only permissible stand for a Catholic in view of the Church's opposition to abortion is to favor a prolife amendment to the Constitution and to outlaw all abortion. Rather, a Catholic must consider all three criteria and favor what course of action will best synthesize all three, a prudential question on which there may well be considerable legitimate difference of opinion (cf. Shinn, 1973). Curran himself favors "a moderately restrictive law such as that proposed by the American Law Institute which would allow abortion in certain particular situations" (p. 136). The main strength of this practical conclusion is that it would be unwise to pass a strict antiabortion law which could not be enforced with a success comparable to that of other criminal laws, since ineffective laws not only do little good, but also do harm to public authority and to their own moral cause.

However, we must also give considerable weight, as Curran himself says in the preceding quotation, to the "idealistic" aspect of law by which it purposes clear standards of right. If this were not the case, then the whole history of the United States with regard to civil rights legislation, which has always proved very difficult to enforce consistently, would be meaningless.

Catholics, therefore, if they are to be true to their belief in the advocacy of the helpless and neglected, need to work for practical legislation which will do as much as possible for the protection of the unborn, while at the same time to work also for the rights of women and other oppressed groups. Curran has wisely urged us to be practical, rather than fanatical, in this campaign for human rights, but political pragmatism does not mean fear to take risks, nor a moral purism which refuses to work with coalitions of people of different motivations and ideologies.

Some fear the Pro-Life Movement because some of its members are too narrow in their social concerns or indulge in distasteful rhetoric. However, to demand in political struggles that all persons working for a particular goal agree on all issues or always have good manners is idealistic indeed. What is rather to be feared is the kind of polarization over an issue which leads people to believe that to favor one set of human rights is to oppose another, as when feminists believe that to support women's rights they must forget the rights of children, or when Pro-Life members believe that to support the rights of children they must oppose the feminist movement. Such polarization has led us in the past into believing that to be against Communism we must favor Fascism, or to favor Israel we must neglect the Palestinians, or to favor peace we must oppose all revolutionaly social movements.

A fair reading of the materials prepared by the American bishops on the respect life issue, however, will show that Church leadership in the United States is making a great effort to propose a consistent program of social justice in accordance with papal teaching, of which the defense of the unborn is only one part (National Conference of Catholic Bishops, 1976b). Our problem is that this consistent peace-and-justice stand is little noticed in the public media, nor well communicated from the pulpit, nor through Catholic religious education.

Undoubtedly the task of Catholics as a community should first and last be educational, rather than merely political. Jesus has taught us to trust more in the power of truth, of love, and of forgiveness than in the power of law or law enforcement. Political action cannot be neglected, but it must be informed by a still deeper educational effort. In this effort to promote respect for life and the rights of the human person, the struggle over abortion is only one element, although a kind of bedrock issue.

The health care professional and Catholic health care institutions have crucial roles to play in this educational effort as regards all medicoethical issues and their social impact. They have the biological and medical information necessary to understand such issues, and they have the professional prestige and influence to be heard. Above all, they deal with the concrete situations in which a respect for life can be most clearly witnessed. In using this legitimate power, they need not feel that they are imposing their religious views on others, provided that they seek to listen to and respect the conscientious convictions of others in the debate, without un-Christian attitudes of judgment and labeling (Tavard, 1973, 1974).

Undoubtedly, the outcome of all the struggles over laws that affect the medical profession will be various forms of compromise which shift and change in each generation. There is nothing wrong with compromise when required by the effort to achieve common action in a society, but it is wrong when the form that this compromise takes is determined by the cowardice of those who should have spoken up for those who cannot speak for themselves.

9.6   SUMMARY

The medical limitations imposed on health care professionals advocated in this chapter can be summarized as follows:

1. Health care professionals have the responsibility to serve the health of every human being from the time that human being comes into existence at conception when it is most probably a person and must be treated as a person with full human rights equal to those of any other person. Consequently, direct abortion is contradictory to the very purpose of the health care profession.

2. Health care professionals must seek to serve all human beings' health needs without discrimination, but when this is impossible because of resource limitations, priorities should be set on the basis of greatest need and greatest benefit from care.

3. Health care professionals should strongly support medical research, but when human subjects are involved, the rights of these persons must be carefully respected. Human subjects should not be used in experimentation unless they give truly free and informed consent to procedures that are for their own therapy or to nontherapeutic experiments in which the risk to themselves is low. The guardians of those who are incompetent to give such consent may consent in their behalf to therapeutic but not to nontherapeutic experiments. Psychological experimentation must fulfill these same conditions and also be a learning and growth experience for the subject.

4. Health care professionals have a public responsibility to help educate others in the value of human life from conception and to play an active role in obtaining the best laws practicable in a given society at a given time to promote and protect the value of this life.

CHAPTER 10 SEXUALITY AND REPRODUCTION

10.1 CONTROVERSY ON CONTRACEPTION

Overview

In 8.3-2 we formulated the Principle of Personalized Sexuality as an expression of ideals developed by the Christian community in its long struggle to understand our present life in relation to resurrected life. In 9.2 we discussed the issue of abortion which is so intimately connected with sexual life. In this chapter, we will deal with optimum functioning of human sexuality as one of the basic aims of the health care profession, reserving, however, the issue of genetic reconstruction of human beings to chapter 11.

Health care professionals are frequently called on to help people make decisions concerning responsible parenthood, yet they themselves often question the realism of the pastors of the Roman Catholic Church who continue to refuse to approve contraception and direct sterilization, although these are generally accepted in modern society as the only practical ways, other than abortion which the Church also rejects, to control reproduction in an overpopulated world.

Our approach to the topic is to accept the painful fact that today the Christian community is profoundly divided over this issue. In many countries there is a deep gap between Church teaching and actual practice, between the way in which this teaching is enforced by some priests and by others, among theologians, and among married couples. Some are convinced that the outcome of this struggle can only be the ultimate defeat of the present official teaching; others, of its ultimate vindication and consistent enforcement. We do not prophesy either outcome, because we believe the process of discernment is still going on within the Christian community. Our aim is to present the different aspects of the question as fairly as we can with special concern to convey correctly just what the official teaching is, since this is essential information for the prudent Christian conscience (3.4; 8.1-1).

Contraception Dilemma

The rise of a new value system in the form of the Humanism of the Enlightment in the eighteenth century and of the immense social changes brought on by the Industrial Revolution in the nineteenth century led to a renewed Christian concern for the family institution. In the twentieth century this concern has been intensified by the rapid rise in the divorce rate and the decline of the birthrate toward zero growth. Humanists generally accept these changes as an inevitable part of technological progress to which social mores must be adjusted by what it often called "the sexual revolution."

Christians have reacted in different ways. Some reassert traditional ideals. Some attempt to rethink these ideals with the purpose of strengthening them through a deeper and more realistic understanding. Some are convinced that Christianity has always taken too negative an attitude toward sexuality and prefer what they regard as the more positive stand of Humanism. The chief point of controversy among Christians, however, has been whether the practice of contraception will further weaken marriage or can be used to strengthen marriage.

Until 1930 the Christian churches generally agreed in regarding contraception as a threat to marriage, but in that year the Anglican Church at its Lambeth Conference declared in favor of some uses of contraception (Spitzer and Saylor, 1969; Shannon, 1970). Catholic theologians had generally opposed this view and Pope Pius XI reacted sharply to this declaration in the encyclical *Casti Connubii* (1930):

> Since, therefore, openly departing from the Christian doctrine handed down uninterruptedly from the very beginning, some have recently decided that another doctrine about this practice should be solemnly proclaimed, the Catholic Church, to whom God Himself has entrusted the teaching and defense of the integrity and purity of morals, standing in the midst of this moral ruin, in order that she may preserve the chastity of the nuptial union from this shameful stain, in token of her Divine ambassadorship, raises her voice on high through our mouth, and promulgates anew: any use of marriage, whatever, in the exercise of which the act is deprived through human industry of its natural power of procreating life, violates the law of God and of nature, and those who commit anything of this kind are marked with the stain of grave sin.

Pius XI's teaching was frequently repeated with greater precision by Pius XII. For example, in 1951 in an "Address to Italian Midwives," Pius XII said:

> Matrimony obliges to a state of life which, while carrying with it certain rights, also imposes the fulfillment of a positive work concerning the state of life itself . . . On partners who make use of matrimony by the specific act of their state, nature and the Creator impose the function of providing for the conservation of the human race. This is the characteristic service from which their state of life derives its peculiar value, the *bonum prolis* (value of children).

By this Pius XII did not imply that every couple has a duty to propagate the race, nor that the use of sex always entails such an obligation, but simply that marriage finds its proper completion in begetting and raising a family (Ford and Kelly, 1964).

On the whole this official teaching was received without much public protest by Catholic married couples, but soon medical discoveries raised new questions. In the same year as *Casti Connubii* was published, 1930, Ogino and Knaus announced their discovery of a scientific way to predict the sterile period of a woman's menstrual cycle, thus making possible the regulation of conception by the exclusive use of this period for sexual intercourse — the rhythm method, or more accurately calendar rhythm since its use depends on the calendar regularity of the cycle.

At first there was considerable hesitation among theologians as to whether this method was simply another form of contraception. However, this controversy was ended by Pius XII in the 1951 address just quoted in which he said that methods of controlling conception basing the restriction of intercourse to the sterile period were licit, even for the whole duration of a marriage, when justified by serious medical, eugenic, economic, or social reasons. Thus, for the first time papal authority was given to the principle of responsible parenthood and to the use of scientific methods to control conception.

Pius XII was convinced that this position was consistent with *Casti Connubii* because the use of the sterile period seems not to involve any positive alteration of the essential meaning of the marital act since this act still retains its natural ordination to procreation. It must be admitted, however, that this ordination is only *remote* and *indirect*, since the act always takes place when conception is impossible.

Many priests hailed and promoted calendar rhythm as a fortunate pastoral solution to the practical dilemmas faced by married couples. Enthusiasm began to wane, however, when it became evident that even normal irregularities in the menstrual cycle can invalidate the prediction of the sterile period, and when many couples reported that the necessary abstention was a source of marital tension.

Soon after this papal approval of calendar rhythm, the first progesterone drug (the Pill) which prevents conception by preventing ovulation became available in 1952. This new method led to a theological debate which, as Shannon (1970) has observed, went through two different phases. In the first of these phases a number of theologians, of whom Louis Janssens of the University of Louvain was the most prominent, argued that the use of progesterones is not contraceptive in the sense condemned by *Casti Connubii*, since it could be regarded simply as an aid to the use of the sterile period since it merely extended this period under effective control (Valsecchi, 1968).

However, the lack of consensus on the validity of this interpretation and especially the discovery that progesterones not only suppress ovulation but also sometimes might be abortifacient by preventing implantation of the fertilized ovum after conception led to a second phase of discussion. Some theologians now began to question the whole interpretation of natural law on which the teaching of *Casti Connubii* seemed grounded and to argue that most contraceptive methods of regulating conception were, from a moral point of view, not essentially different from the use of the sterile period.

In view of the number and authority of the theologians taking this position, many Catholics began to use progesterones or other contraceptive methods and many confessors to tolerate at least this practice. Since many Catholic health care professionals and educated, conscientious Catholic couples who had followed this theological debate with great attention found this new view to support their own experience and reflections, it began to appear that a discernment process was going on in the Church leading to a modification of the previous teaching (Cardegna, 1964; Cavanagh, 1964; Bromley, 1965).

Attempt to Find a Solution

At the same time the broader social problems of world poverty were becoming of great concern to Pope John XXIII as the Second Vatican Council approached, and led him to organize a Pontifical Study Commission on Family Population and Birth Problems to examine the population policies of the United Nations and to recommend a course of action for the pope. This commission met once in 1963 and twice in 1964.

As the Second Vatican Council continued, Pope Paul VI enlarged this commission to fifty-eight members, including three married couples, five laywomen, moral theologians, physicians, psychologists, demographers, sociologists, and pastoral marriage counselors. Its fourth session was held March 25—28, 1965, in Rome. The Council itself concluded with the issuance of the document *The Church in the Modern World* which contained the very important section "Fostering the Nobility of Marriage" (nn. 47-52) in which for the first time (but not without some anticipation in the writings of Pius XII) a new, fully personalistic view of marriage was proposed, along with a renewed condemnation of abortion. The "duty of responsible parenthood" was affirmed and the possible dangers of prolonged sexual abstinence in marriage referred to, but the question of licit and illicit methods of birth regulation was reserved by Paul VI until the completion of the work of the commission.

After the close of the Council, a fifth and final session of the commission, now again enlarged to include sixteen bishops as an executive committee, was held in Rome for two months in the spring of 1966. The discussion centered on two questions: (1) Is contraception intrinsically evil? (2) Can the Church change her teaching?

The result was a sharp division: a majority favored a change in the traditional teaching to permit at least some forms of contraception and a minority opposed this position. The final report sent to the Pope on June 23, 1966, was called "An Outline for a Document on Responsible Parenthood" written by six members of the theological subsection on the commission and approved by nine of the bishops in attendance, opposed by three, and with three abstentions. It was accompanied by a separate document called "Pastoral Approaches," along with a Minority Report and a Rebuttal by those favoring the final Report (Hoyt, 1969; cf. Dummet, 1969).

Paul VI then took almost two years of further study, apparently by private consultation of bishops and theologians, before publishing the encyclical *Humanae Vitae*, July 29, 1968. Because four years of waiting had produced widespread expectation of change, and because practices contrary to the traditional teaching had already been adopted by many, the encyclical provoked still further controversy (Joannes, 1970). The national bishops' conferences of many countries issued pastoral letters attempting to explain the encyclical in terms acceptable to their people and to indicate how it might be pastorally applied.

In the United States, numerous moral theologians have openly dissented from the encyclical and carried on successfully a fight for the right of theological discussion of this and other moral issues (Curran, 1969, 1975; Callahan, 1969a, 1970a). Andrew Greeley has published evidence to show that, while most United States Catholics accepted the changes effected by the Second Vatican Council without great difficulty, *Humanae Vitae* seems to be a major factor in the recent widespread alienation of Catholics in this country from their Church (Allen, 1970; Greeley, 1973, 1976b; Groat, 1975).

The reason this controversy has been so upsetting for United States Catholics is that it seems to many that the strong language of *Casti Connubii* and the milder yet unequivocal language of *Humanae Vitae* involve the infallibility of the pope and the Church. Yet it is clear that these documents do not claim to give a definitive decision about a revealed truth of faith or morals, which is all that the First Vatican Council declared to be an object of infallibility, a declaration confirmed by the Second Vatican Council (1964). That *Humanae Vitae* (and hence *Casti Connubii* itself) does not have infallible authority is evident in several ways, but most clearly from the fact that a number of the national conferences of bishops in their pastoral letters, without ever being corrected by Paul VI, declared to their people that *Humanae Vitae* was not an infallible pronouncement (Russo, 1969; Shannon, 1970). Of course, it is possible that *Humanae Vitae* does contain revealed truths about human sexuality which may later be solemnly defined, but that it does contain such revealed truths can at present only be a matter of theological opinion. Thus its authority is that of an important document of the ordinary teaching of the Church, to which Pope Paul gave great care after attempting to inform himself of all the relevant data through the work of the commission and other consultation. We have already explained in 3.4 the respect due to such teaching, the scope of theological debate which it permits, and the role it should play in forming the personal conscience of Catholics. Further details on this will be developed in 10.6.

This controversy has not only continued, but has also broadened its scope to extend to all the issues of traditional sexual morality, as is evidenced recently by the issuance by the Vatican's Congregation for the Doctrine of the Faith of a document "Concerning Some Questions of Sexual Ethics" and in the United States of a study commissioned by The Catholic Theological Society of America, *Human Sexuality* (Kosnik et al., 1977) very critical of this document. On the other hand, some American Catholic philosophers and theologians (Grisez, 1964; Ford and Kelly, 1964; Kippley, 1970, 1974; R. Connell, 1970; W. May, 1975, 1976b, 1977b) have vigorously supported the traditional position.

In some respects this continuing disagreement within the Catholic community and among the Christian churches has had positive effects. It has made it clear why in the future the discernment process in the Christian community which prepares the way for papal or conciliar teaching needs to engage the whole community in a deeper and more active way (cf. 3.4). Although Paul VI attempted through the work of the commission to inform himself thoroughly before issuing *Humanae Vitae*, as we have shown, the process was inadequate to produce a strong consensus which would have made the implementation of the encyclical effective (Delhaye, 1970). Of course, the problem of securing such a universal participation is enormous, but in today's world it is becoming more and more urgent. At the same time the very fact that public dissent has become possible within the Catholic Church has probably been very advantageous to the ecumenical movement by dispelling the notion that papal authority is absolute and autocratic. At the same time unity of mind and heart within the Christian community and with its shepherds is always an essential ecclesial goal without which the life and witness of the Church is enfeebled. How can we work to achieve greater consensus in this matter? We believe that certain points are becoming clear.

First and most important is the fact that the Second Vatican Council and *Humanae Vitae* clearly situate the problem of sexual ethics in the context of the Christian Church's historical concern for the *family* as an institution but in a more personalistic light. What we have called the Principle of Human Dignity in Community (1.5; 8.2-1) and the Principle of Personalized Sexuality (8.3-2) appear now as first of all to be realized in the family. In this perspective the unifying purpose of sexuality is the faithful *love* of husband and wife which is the source of all its other essential values. At the same time, these other values specify marital love and are inseparable from its essential meaning. This is what *Humanae Vitae*, echoing the Second Vatican Council, means by saying that the *unitive* and *procreative* meanings of marriage may not be separated. This conception of marriage is freed from archaic influences present in some older versions of natural law reasoning, but it is a mistake to think that it rests merely on philosophical theories. At we indicated in 8.3 it is firmly rooted in Scripture and Tradition, although in its present personalized form it is a modern development. Even the theologians who defend the licity of contraception do so with arguments which attempt to show that what they have in mind are only such uses of contraception as they believe will strengthen the family institution and preserve the full meaning of human sexuality in marriage.

Second, it is not helpful for furthering a consensus to connect this specific question too closely to those revisions of moral theology which want to abandon exceptionless moral norms and deny the existence of intrinsically immoral acts. Moreover, it has seemed to some people that the failure of the Final Report of the Commission or the Rebuttal of the Minority Report to deal directly with this issue may have been an important factor in the ultimate decision of Paul VI. In any case, we have argued in 8.1 that a sweeping revision of traditional Catholic moral theology as proposed by the principle of proportion school is highly questionable. If the case for contraception rests on that principle it is a weak case.

Nor is it correct to assert that *Humanae Vitae* builds its case on biologism according to which the morality of a human act is determined merely by its biological structure. Gustave Martelet (1969), reputed to be one of the drafters of the encyclical (Shannon, 1970), has shown that such a criticism neglects the emphasis of the encyclical on the human *meaning* of the sexual act, not simply on its physical structure. We attempted to show in 8.1 that the material and the formal aspects of any human act are so related that while it is always the immediate human intention which gives an act its formally moral character, yet this immediate intention cannot always rectify premoral structures if these by their own intrinsic teleology imply something contradictory to basic human needs. The position of *Humanae Vitae*, right or wrong, is not that a contraceptive act is morally evil simply because of its biological structure, but because the human person who performs the act cannot reasonably intend this kind of a biological act as truly fulfilling human needs, for example, a mature person cannot reasonably perform an act of masturbation as if it really satisfied the true meaning of human sexuality.

Third, if we grant that there are some limits to ethical human intervention in the character of sexual acts (as we have just argued in our second point), and if this limit is set by inseparability of the unitive and procreative meanings of sexuality (as argued in the first point above), then the real point of controversy on which we must focus if we are to promote consensus is the determination of just what these limits are that separate such an admittedly legitimate intervention as the use of the sterile period from an illegitimate one.

The majority-approved Final Report of the Pontifical Commission (1973) asked and answered this question as follows:

> What are the limits of the dominion of man with regard to the rational determination of his fecundity? The *general principle* can be formulated in this manner: It is the duty of man to perfect nature (or to order it to the human good expressed in matrimony) but not to destroy it. Even if the absolute untouchability of the fertile period cannot be maintained, neither can complete domination be affirmed. Besides, when man intervenes in the procreative process, he does this with the intention of regulating and not excluding fertility. Thus he unites the material finality toward fecundity which exists in intercourse with the formal finality of the person and renders the entire process "human."

This is the essential point on which *Humanae Vitae* refused the arguments of the majority of the commission. The commission had argued that contraceptive acts are justified because they can be regarded as "partial acts" whose morality is determined by the couple's sexual life in its *totality*. If this totality is ordered both to love and procreation, then these values are not separated by the contraceptive character of the partial acts. The encyclical, however, insists that these values cannot be separated even in the single marital act, but every act must remain "open to the transmission of life," since if even in the single act these intrinsically related meanings are not objectively present, then it is not an act fitted to express true marital love, and hence is intrinsically contrary to the human meaning of sexuality.

This raises the obvious question: How then are marital acts deliberately confined to the sterile period really an expression of true marital love? The encyclical defends this distinction very briefly and without detailed explanation as follows:

> The Church is consistent with herself and her teaching when she judges that it is licit for married couples to take into account the sterile periods, while at the same time she condemns as always illicit the use of whatever directly interferes with conception, even if such a way of acting is based on arguments which appear serious and decent. In reality, these two cases differ greatly from each other. For in the former case, the married couple use an opportunity given them by nature; but in the other, the couple prevent the order of generation from having its natural processes. (*In priore, coniuges legitime facultate utuntur sibi a natura data; in altera vero, iidem impediunt, quominus generationis ordo suos habeat naturae processus.*) If it is undeniable that in both cases the married couple by mutual and certain agreement for plausible reasons desire to avoid offspring and seek the certainty that offspring will not be born, nevertheless it must also be admitted that in the former case only does it occur that the couple are able to abstain from marital intercourse in the fertile periods, when for just motives the procreation of children is not desired; but that they also use intercourse when the time is not

apt for conception in order to give expression to mutual love and to preserve the mutual fidelity they have promised. By so doing they give proof of a truly and integrally honest love (n. 16). (our translation)

The argument here seems to be that the first condition of the fully human marital act is that it must be freely chosen; that is, it is not a mere instinctual act compelled by a biological drive. Hence, it is possible for a couple without self-contradiction to perform the marital act only in the sterile phase of the natural cycle with the aim of achieving three values: (1) the expression of mutual love through total self-giving (the unitive meaning), (2) rational family planning (the procreative meaning), and (3) freedom from sexual compulsion by the discipline of periodic abstention. On the other hand, when they perform a contraceptive act they positively exclude the procreative meaning and distort the unitive meaning which no longer has the character of total self-giving since it is separated from its essential relation to procreation, and also lose the ascetical growth in freedom (Grisez, 1964).

Some do not find this convincing because the same principle seems to lead to a different conclusion when carefully examined (Dupré, 1964). In what sense is a marital act deliberately placed in the infertile period still "open to the transmission of life"? Certainly this act is not directly and *proximately* ordered to procreation (since it is sterile). Hence the order is only indirect and *remote*. Yet this remote ordination does not seem merely to be through the circumstantial intention of the agents, but to be objective and intrinsic to the moral object, since it consists in the fact that God through nature has provided that human reproduction should normally result not from single acts of intercourse, but from a permanent partnership bound together by frequent sexual acts, only some of which are directly and proximately fertile. The infertile acts, therefore, are naturally ordered to fertility, although only indirectly and remotely. It is in this sense, and only in this sense, that they can be said to be open to the transmission of life.

How then is it true to say that the deliberately infertile contraceptive act is "closed" to the transmission of life? Certainly it is closed if it is employed for merely hedonistic reasons in marriage or if it is used outside marriage by reason of a morally wrong intention which changes the moral object. But when it is employed as an expression of marital love which expresses itself in responsible parenthood, is not such an infertile act still remotely ordered to procreation, just as is the act in the sterile period? Thus it can be argued that the two acts differ only in the mode in which the sterility is effected, and the question again is how this difference in mode differentiates the human meaning of the acts. The difference in mode in one case is said to be "natural" and in the other "artificial," but *natural* here cannot mean "without human intervention," since both modes result from the intervention of human intelligence — in the one case to choose the time of the acts; in the other, to alter in some degree the process of the acts. How are we to determine whether this difference of mode is ethically significant? The answer must be given in terms of the principle, Art perfects nature, which must be judged in terms of the achievement of God-given natural finality. However, it would seem that as regards finality in both modes the marital act is open to the transmission of life only in the sense of an indirect and remote ordination.

Paul VI, however, did not judge this remote ordination to procreation of contraceptive acts to be sufficiently evident or objective to provide for the inseparability of the unitive and procreative meanings of sexuality, because in such acts the relation of these two values seems to depend rather upon a subjective attitude (or circumstantial intention), thus opening the way to other uses of sex which the Christian conscience has always rejected. The encyclical ennumerates these as (1) extramarital sex, (2) exploitation of women as sex objects, (3) governmental intervention in parental rights, and (4) attrition of the Principle of Totality (8.2-3) which sets limits to other medical interventions contrary to human integrity. Thus Paul VI, in spite of the great pressures for him to take a more permissive stand, believed his pastoral duty was to draw the line as regards the methods of responsible parenthood which would clearly protect the essential character of marriage.

That the pope's fears were not wholly imaginary is evidenced by the fact that, since the encyclical, debate on questions of sexual ethics among Catholic theologians has become increasingly radical, so that some now defend as morally justified in certain circumstances the practice of masturbation, homosexuality, and extramarital intercourse (Kosnik, 1977) which the commission majority in 1966 vehemently rejected. Perhaps, however, this is not so much the result of these theologians' stand in favor of contraception as of their adoption of the principle of proportion methodology in its defense. Even if one holds, as we do, that some forms of sexual behavior are *intrinsically* wrong because they violate the separability of the unitive and procreative meanings of sexuality, the question still remains for study: Are the arguments that each contraceptive act is intrinsically wrong more probable than the arguments to the contrary? The authority of the encyclical gives to the affirmative answer a weight greater than that of theological opinions, but the value of the arguments in themselves on their own merits remains open to theological study and discussion.

10.2 RESPONSIBLE PARENTHOOD THROUGH NATURAL FAMILY PLANNING

As we have seen, the Second Vatican Council and *Humanae Vitae* make clear sexuality to be truly human and moral must be the expression of mutual love in freedom and responsibility, which includes also the intelligent planning of parenthood so as to be able to provide for the proper care and education of the children. The primary responsibility for such care belongs to the parents, but they have the right to community assistance in this task, according to the Principle of the Common Good, Subsidiarity, and Functionalism (6.1; 8.2-2) both because the right to marry and have children is a basic human right and because of the fundamental contribution which a family makes to the common good of the community.

Catholics, and especially health care professionals, therefore cannot be indifferent to the population explosion and the ethical problems it raises. Nor can they solve such problems by blind trust in Providence. All recent papal documents dealing with social problems give attention to these issues (Gremillion, 1976), and papal representatives have taken an active part in the work of the United Nations and other international organizations in an effort to plan for the global future. The popes generally have favored a position which, although it is not popular in the United States, is probably the majority opinion in the world at the present time (Berelson, 1975; ITEST, 1973; *Bucharest Report*, 1974; *Population*, 1974).

Briefly, this view can be summed up as follows. (1) In developed countries, including those with a high percentage of Catholics (Janssen, 1975), the growth rate has steadily declined for many years and will soon reach zero. (2) The crisis is a feature of underdevelopment resulting from the ecological imbalance produced when developed countries introduced modern medicine into their colonies or dependencies without at the same time raising the standard of living proportionately. (3) The Malthusian view that population growth must exceed growth in food production has been proved false, and modern technology should be able to supply food for all, provided that the present abnormal population growth can be slowed. (4) The most effective program of responsible parenthood will have two features: (a) it will be supported by strong economic development, and (b) it will promote those methods of birth regulation most acceptable to the value systems of a people, including methods acceptable for Catholics.

Thus, the popes in disproving some methods of birth regulation nevertheless have not neglected to promote a definite social program which includes a reasonable answer to the population problem. Even those who would not agree with that answer should admit that it is more realistic than the two solutions most popular in the United States, namely: (1) the lifeboat ethics we discussed in chapter 9, according to which the United States should maintain its own standard of living and let the rest of the world starve; and (2) the planned parenthood solution which relies on promoting the use of contraceptives by the poor, while ignoring the need for a radical global economic readjustment. Both of these solutions rest on the unrealistic assumption that the United States and the other developed countries can indefinitely continue their present style of life based in large measure on the exploitation of under-developed countries.

If we accept the view that population control has to be achieved by profound social changes, rather than by the use of particular methods of birth regulation, we still have to ask what methods for such regulation are ethically acceptable in view of the Catholic and other value systems which emphasize the intimate relation between sexuality and procreation. How can couples limit the size of their families and still enjoy the sexual expression of their love in a way that will strengthen their permanent commitment to each other, give joy to their life together, and provide a healthy model of sexual love for their maturing children?

The Second Vatican Council (1965c) in *The Church in the Modern World* (n. 51) and *Humanae Vitae* (1968) affirmed the Christian value of abstinence and the acceptability of natural family planning methods, that is, those which make use of naturally sterile periods, but the council also recalled the pastoral advice of St. Paul (I Cor. 7:5) that while it is legitimate for a married couple by mutual consent to abstain from sexual relations for a time, especially for spiritual and ascetic reasons, it can be dangerous to the marriage if prolonged.

As already mentioned, such periodic abstinence first began to be practiced scientifically by the *calendar rhythm* method which depends on the regularity of a woman's menstrual cycle. Because this cycle varies considerably in different women and for some is quite irregular, this method could not be practiced effectively by many couples, sometimes led to insecurity and tension in married life, and gave to the whole theory of birth regulation through natural methods a poor reputation, with the result that many physicians are still not well informed on the whole issue. Today, however, new techniques have been discovered by which it is possible to detect very accurately the time at which ovulation takes place, so that the irregularity of a woman's cycles has become irrelevant (Urrichio, 1973; Kippley and Kippley, 1975).

One technique is based on the fact that the hormonal changes at ovulation cause a distinct rise in a woman's basal temperature. Another, the Billings method, is based on the fact that these changes also result in a thickening of the vaginal mucus and of the position of the cervix which can easily be detected by the woman by a simple self-examination after she has been trained to notice these signs. Both techniques, along with what is called ecological nursing (breast-feeding of the infant, with fondling) form what is now called the symptothermal method, the ovulation method, or simply natural family planning. When properly practiced, it is rated for effectiveness by Tietze (1970) as a Class A method along with use of progesterones and intrauterine devices. At present it is undergoing considerable testing and refinement, and better techniques are being developed to assist women to pinpoint the time of ovulation accurately.

No methods of birth regulation are without some serious disadvantages, and natural methods have been criticized on several grounds. First, while they are highly effective under ideal conditions, they have not been as widely tested in ordinary conditions as have progesterones and intrauterine devices. However, it has been shown that the Billings method can be used with excellent success even by uneducated women (Uricchio, 1973). Second, some (Guerrero, 1973) have theorized that natural family planning may produce genetic defects, since if a pregnancy does occur it is more likely to be at a time when the ovum or sperm are somewhat aged. However, recently Hilgers (1977) has shown that not only is there little evidence for such a theory, but strong reason to think it false. Third, and much more important, is that such methods require a period of continence which if they are to equal progesterones and intrauterine devices in effectiveness may be as long as half the cycle, although with somewhat greater risk this can be reduced to five or six days. Moreover, there is some evidence (Marshall and Rowe, 1973; cf. Bardwick, 1973) that such abstinence produces considerable marital strain and may tempt couples to practice *coitus interruptus.*

In answer to this last and most serious difficulty, proponents of natural family planning point out, first, that as the method is more and more perfected it may become possible not merely to detect the time of ovulation, but to *predict* it, in which case abstinence can be reduced with complete safety to five or six days in a cycle. Next, they emphasize that contraceptive methods also have strong psychological drawbacks, so that fifty percent of couples change their method of contraception in every two-year period because of discontent with it (Bardwick, 1973).

Positively, proponents of natural methods (Ratner, 1968; Max Levin, 1969; Kippley, 1970; Kippley and Kippley, 1975) argue that such methods (1) place responsibility on *both* partners, not merely on the woman as do most methods or on the man as does vasectomy; (2) many women who use such methods have reported an enhanced sense of personal dignity resulting from an awareness of their own body and its rhythms; (3) abstinence from intercourse can help a couple learn to have confidence in the strength of their love for each other and to express it in a variety of ways, without that preoccupation with "total orgasm" which is proving to be a source of tension for many men and women today; and (4) periodic abstinence removes something of the sexual routine and enhances the experience when it is actually decided upon. While it is true that spontaneity is an element of lovemaking (counselors report that fifty percent of college girls who are sexually active refuse to use even contraceptives for this reason [Bardwick, 1973]), a truly mature notion of spontaneity is not just being able to have intercourse at any time, but rather knowing how to give oneself to another at the *appropriate* time, a time which is necessarily determined by the rhythm of some life-style.

Besides these possible subjective psychological advantages, natural family planning has a number of very definite objective merits. (1) When properly practiced, it can be as effective as any method except sterilization and it does not have the obvious disadvantages of a sterilizing operation. (2) Unlike other comparably effective methods, that is, progesterones and intrauterine devices, it has no medical risks. (3) It is never abortifacient as progestrones and intrauterine devices almost certainly are. (4) It is inexpensive and does not require regular medical checkups in order to avoid side effects, but can be effectively taught by simple practical instruction.

Health care professionals need to be well informed on natural family planning and to promote it as a method indubitably in keeping with Christian values, as well as having important medical advantages for couples who can use it consistently and satisfactorily. Catholic hospitals and physicians should provide instruction in this method, but should present it in an honest and objective manner, with correct information about other methods so that couples will not feel themselves being treated as guinea pigs but will have free and informed consent in trying to use the natural method for responsible parenthood. Especially, it is essential that Catholic scientists advance research on natural methods so as to overcome the crisis of conscience among Catholics and to provide others with a method of responsible parenthood and population control that does not tend to separate sexuality from family life as has the spread of contraceptive practices.

10.3 STERILIZATION AND OTHER METHODS OF CONTRACEPTION

Sterilization

Humanae Vitae accepts the ethical concept of responsible parenthood through use of the sterile period, but rejects as unethical other methods widely accepted in our society today:

> Therefore in conformity to these principles of a human and Christian teaching on marriage, we must again declare that the direct interruption of generation already begun as a legitimate way of regulating the number of children, and especially abortion, even for therapeutic motives, are to be altogether rejected. Equally to be excluded, as the teaching authority of the Church has frequently declared, is direct sterilization of a man or a woman, whether this be temporary or permanent. Likewise is every act to be rejected which, either in anticipation of the conjugal act, or in its accomplishment or in its natural consequences, proposes, whether as an end or a means to render procreation impossible.

However, for some the birth-control issue is a purely technical one of calculating the evident advantages and disadvantages of particular methods since they pass over the considerations which have occupied Catholic thinking. For example, a theologian like Joseph Fletcher (1954) concludes that if persons have the right to control parenthood they have the right to use any means that assists to this end unless it has serious medical disadvantages.

From this point of view, the most effective and apparently the least dangerous method of preventing pregnancy (although even it is not one hundred percent effective) is permanent sterilization of the man through vasectomy or of the woman by ligation of the fallopian tubes (Schneiderman et al., 1974). This is termed *direct* sterilization because its direct purpose is contraceptive. Rather than a treatment for pathology, it is intended to render the subject sterile but not impotent.

When sterility results merely as a side effect of a medical treatment directly aimed at specific pathology, it is said to be indirect and can be justified by the Principle of Totality when there is a proportionate gain for health. Thus diseased sex organs can be removed surgically or can be treated by drugs or radiation therapy even if treatment results in sterility (McFadden, 1967, 1976; O'Donnell, 1976).

Because direct sterilization is a form of contraception, it comes under the judgment of *Humanae Vitae* as intrinsically unethical and contrary to the Principle of Totality and Integrity (2.4) since it sacrifices a basic human function without the extreme necessity of preserving life. While it seems medically much safer than oral contraception and intrauterine devices, some physical side effects have been reported such as persistent discomfort from seminal accumulation after vasectomy and tubal pregnancy after ligation. The chief technical drawback is that although surgeons have increasing success in repairing such sterilization for persons who change their minds (O'Donnell, 1976) the risk that it will fail remains high.

As a form of birth regulation, the chief disadvantage of sterilization is that it is a deprivation of the human person of a basic human capacity (May, 1977). Individuals so deprived do not at the time want any more children and commonly report subjective satisfaction with the results. Nevertheless, the ability to reproduce, even when not actually used, relates the individual to the community and its future. The sense of power, of life, and of belonging which this engenders is reflected in the religions and philosophers of all cultures, as the Old Testament testifies by treating sterility in man or woman as a curse (I Sam. 1:5-6; Hos. 9:14). The efforts of Indira Ghandi, politically disastrous to her regime, to enforce a sterilization program on a people of ancient culture illustrates both how tempting this method is to governments seeking a simple and permanent solution to the problem of population control and how deeply it is resented and feared where this sense of the human meaning of complete sexual power is still alive among the otherwise powerless.

Our highly technological culture in the United States is singularly insensitive to deep human needs, which are unconscious or suppressed by cultural pressures. The fact that the majority of the sterilized respond on a questionnaire that they have experienced only a feeling of relief and freedom as a result of their operation is not necessarily a reliable indication of its deeper consequences. Social and psychological research on such effects is still very superficial and the present ecological crisis warns us of the gradual long-term risks of what at first appeared to be harmless and effective technologies. Already some physicians report more and more sterilized patients coming to them to inquire about restoration of their fertility.

The United States Catholic Conference in conformity with papal teachings has insisted on retaining the following statement in its 1971 revision of the *Ethical and Religious Directives for Catholic Health Facilities*:

> Directive 20: Procedures that induce sterility, whether permanent or temporary are permitted when: (a) They are immediately directed to the cure, diminution, or prevention of a serious pathological condition and are not directly contraceptive (that is, contraception is not the purpose); and (b) a simpler treatment is not reasonably available. Hence, for example, oophorectomy or irradiation of the ovaries may be allowed in treating carcinoma of the breast and metastasis therefrom; and orchiectomy is permitted in the treatment of carcinoma of the prostrate.

This directive has been much criticized both by those who dissent from the papal teaching on contraception and by those who believe that the principle of proportion can be applied to difficult cases so that the advantages of sterilization may sometimes outweigh its disadvantages (McCormick, 1971; Kosnick, 1973; Curran, 1973b). Others, leaving aside the contraceptive issue, have attempted to solve it by a different application of the Principle of Totality (cf. Cox, 1972; R. Cooper, 1972), arguing that by this principle some cases of sterilization can be considered *indirect* and therefore licit where medical indications, either physical or psychological or both, have been established. Thus there are many cases in which such indications make it a duty for a woman to avoid another pregnancy, although she is unable (1) to use natural methods because they are insufficiently safe or require a self-control psychologically impossible for her, (2) to abstain because it would disrupt her marriage and interfere with the proper care of the children she already has, or (3) even to use less drastic forms of contraception because of their medical and psychological side effects.

The defenders of the *Directives* reject the application of the Principle of Totality in these cases because in such cases the direct aim is not therapy, but contraception (O'Donnell, 1976). It is true that the purpose in sterilizing is to benefit the woman's health by preventing pregnancy, but the means used is a form of contraceptive sterilization and hence intrinsically wrong. We cannot use an evil means even to achieve a good purpose.

The critics of this directive, however, argue further that in cases admitted as licit by the *Directives* where a healthy sexual function (i.e., secretion of sex hormones) is suppressed because this normal function harms another diseased organ the immediate aim is not therapy, but the suppression of a sexual function. Why is this a licit means? In the abstract it would seem that the suppression of a normal function is intrinsically evil, but in the context of the *whole person* this suppression is judged as not evil because it no longer serves its essential purpose of benefiting the person but has become harmful.

The defenders reply to this that contraceptive sterilization remains intrinsically wrong even in such cases because it is possible for the woman to prevent the pregnancy not by suppressing the function but by abstaining from its use. However, the critics then argue that this answer supposes that the woman is really free to use or not use sex, while she is not free to secrete sexual hormones or not. This distinction may be true in general, but it can be argued that in these cases the woman is *not* free not to abstain. Just as she cannot avoid secreting hormones with a risk of aggravating her cancer, so she cannot avoid continuing sexual activity with a risk of (to her) dangerous of even fatal pregnancy. In both cases, therefore, it seems that the suppression is not intrinsically evil because the normal function in the context of the total person has become harmful, and this harm cannot be prevented in any way except by such suppression.

The difficulty with this extension of the Principle of Totality is that it erodes the distinction between the order of nature in which there is a natural determinism and the order of human culture or social and psychological determinisms which remain under human control in the long run. As we have seen throughout this book this distinction is problematical today (1) because we are achieving more and more technical control over the determinisms of nature and (2) because we are increasingly aware of how imperfect our control is over cultural determinisms. Nevertheless we do not believe this difficulty in precisely distinguishing between nature and culture destroys the significance of the distinction.

In the present case the woman's freedom is certainly greatly reduced, but unless she is actually psychotic it is not wholly eliminated. If she is psychotic, then her husband or guardian becomes responsible to prevent her from becoming pregnant. But as long as she retains some freedom of choice, she must take responsibility for her own decisions about how to control her sexual activities and she must accept the risks involved. Furthermore, in marriage she should seek to share these decisions with her husband in mutual love and responsibility. Whether she can make such decisions or others must make them for her, the problem of whether the *means* by which conception is to be avoided should be sterilization or some alternative cannot be avoided, and this is the problem not of indirect but of direct sterilization. Of course there remains the question of how counselors should act in helping her come to a decision, and we will discuss this later in the chapter.

A second criticism of the *Directives'* treatment of sterilization is that they fail to address the practical problems with regard to this procedure facing Catholic hospitals in our pluralistic country. Certainly Catholic hospitals should not yield to pressures to become sterilization clinics for healthy persons. But what are they to do when staff physicians believe that it is medically wise for them to perform a tubal ligation on a patient at the same time that they perform other abdominal surgery in order to reduce the risks involved in two separate operations, yet it is not clear that this ligation can be permitted under the *Directives*?

Because of such problems a number of Catholic hospitals in the United States and Canada have come to permit tubal ligation in some cases where serious medical indications were established. In Canada the *Medico-Moral Guide* (Canadian Catholic Conference, 1970) seems to leave this possibility open without explicitly authorizing it. In the United States, however, some hospitals, not willing to take the responsibility of interpreting the guidelines in such borderline cases for themselves, requested an official interpretation from the National Conference of Catholic Bishops. As a result, the president of the conference, Archbishop Joseph L. Bernardin, after consulting the Congregation for the Doctrine of the Faith, wrote to United States bishops as follows:

> With the concurrence of the Executive Committee [of the NCCB], I am writing to give assurance that the 1971 guideline [No. 20 of the *Directives* just quoted] stands as written, and that direct sterilization is not to be considered as justified by the common good, the principle of totality, the existence of contrary opinion, or any other argument. This means that Catholic hospitals, as a matter of institutional policy, may not authorize sterilization procedures for reasons other than those contained in the guidelines. If questions of material cooperation arise, the traditional norms of moral theology are to be applied.

The response of the Congregation (1975a) has now been published in which the original of the last sentence summarized in the above letter reads as follows:

> The traditional doctrine regarding material cooperation, with the proper distinctions between necessary and free, proximate and remote, remains valid, to be applied with the utmost prudence, if the case warrants . . . In the application of the principle of material cooperation, if the case warrants, great care must be taken against scandal and the danger of any misunderstanding by an appropriate explanation of what is really being done.

When this is compared with the similar instruction of the United States Catholic Conference on the question of cooperation in abortion a very significant difference is obvious. Hospitals were strictly forbidden to cooperate with abortion in any way, even *materially*, but they were left to decide conscientiously for themselves (under the authority of the local bishop) when it was ethical for them to cooperate *materially* in procedures involving direct sterilization.   The difference does not means that the Congregation or the United States Catholic Conference has approved direct sterilization.   On the contrary, they have repeated the condemnation of direct sterilization as intrinsically wrong and have rejected the various arguments which have attempted to justify it or to extend the concept of indirect sterilization to cover the sort of cases which the *Directives* reject.   But they have conceded that in some cases Catholic hospitals may *tolerate* some degree of material cooperation with such illicit acts (O'Rourke, 1976).

What kind of situation might warrant such material cooperation? We have explained previously (8.1-4) what the traditional norms of moral theology in regard to cooperation are.   Formal cooperation with ethically wrong actions is never permissible, but material cooperation in many wrong actions is not only permitted but ethically required in a world where without such cooperation many good actions would be frustrated.   If Catholic hospitals are to carry out their ministry, they cannot avoid sometimes engaging in activities with such double effects, some of which involve working with persons who choose to do things which we would not feel ethically justified in doing ourselves, but which we must tolerate for the sake of the mainly good results of the cooperation.   We may believe that those with whom we cooperate in such cases are themselves acting in good faith (so that no actual sin is involved), although their actions are objectively wrong.   Even if they are not in good faith, yet we do not approve what is wrong in their actions (and would prevent it if we could), but only support what is objectively good in their activities.

Thus all Catholic doctors who pay dues to a county medical association are giving some support and approval to the activities of fellow members although they know that some of the members engage in overcharging, fee splitting, excessive surgery, negligence, sterilization, and abortion which they consider unethical yet which they cannot prevent simply by resigning from the association, while their failure to cooperate materially by belonging to the association would endanger their own ability to pursue their profession and would also weaken the work of the association to uphold medical and ethical standards.   This is also true of all United States tax-payers who know that some of their tax money will be used to promote unethical medical activities, for example, Medicare abuses.

In the case of direct sterilization, however, a Catholic hospital (unless it chooses to dissent from the *Directives* and thus come into conflict with the local bishop) cannot approve such procedures since that would be *formal* cooperation.   A Catholic hospital is, indeed, obliged to express its disapproval of sterilization explicitly and officially as a matter of hospital policy and do whatever it can to avoid or minimize even material cooperation with it.   Consequently it is not proper for a hospital to propose in its ethical code a list of "medical indications for which sterilization is permitted" since this amounts to an approval of elective sterilization.

Nor would this be permissible if the cooperation of the hospital is material but *immediate* (8.1-4), nor if cooperation would give rise to serious scandal because others would believe that the hospital condones or promotes an illicit operation. Recently, William B. Smith (1977) has argued that such material cooperation by a Catholic hospital would never be sufficiently remote to be justifiable unless perhaps under the coercion of a court order. However, it seems to the authors of this book that it is best to leave questions of proximity of cooperation to prudential judgment since they can be very complex. On the other hand, we would be inclined to the view that a hospital faced with a court order should *not* cooperate because of the scandal that such a submission of freedom of conscience to public power might entail. The instruction of the Congregation for the Doctrine of the Faith makes clear that in making this decision Catholics must use "the utmost prudence," especially as regards the danger of scandal. The administrators of a hospital which would find such cooperation necessary would be required to explain its dealing with exceptional cases very carefully to the staff (as well as to the public if this becomes necessary) and must take care that its toleration remains *restrictive*, not merely routine. It is desirable that a hospital have a *medicomorals committee* with adequate theological consultation to deal with such exceptions.

What is the role of the bishop of the diocese in such matters? He has the responsibility of overseeing the medical institutions of his diocese which identify themselves as "Catholic," to keep informed of controversial matters, and to intervene to prevent grave ethical abuses. However, the primary obligation to apply the *Directives* rests first on the hospital itself. Hence it appears more prudent for the bishop not to interfere with a hospital's decisions on cooperation since these decisions involve a detailed knowledge of the exceptional cases and the local siutation unless it seriously abuses its discretion. Through his own diocesan agencies, therefore, the bishop may require annual reports from the hospital on how it has dealt with such cases.

The basic issue remains. Catholic hospitals either must decide to hold the line by adhering to a strict interpretation of the *Directives* in order to give an unambiguous witness to a distinctly Catholic position, which has the risk of forcing such hospitals to gradually withdraw from serving the general public because of lack of financial and professional support and earns for them the reputation of sectarian unreasonableness. Or they must allow a much broader interpretation of the *Directives* that permits material cooperation. If a hospital chooses the second option, it is in danger of gradual secularization — increasingly the fate of Catholic universities and colleges — in which true Catholic witness becomes less and less possible. Perhaps the only way open in some more difficult situations is a middle course in which material cooperation is kept strictly limited and under vigilant control. This approach, however, also has its difficulties. All in all, the authors feel the stricter policy should be maintained if at all possible.

The declining birthrate in the United States has recently led to a strong movement for hospitals in a city to consolidate obstetrical departments so that a single center located in one of the hospitals can afford the highest quality care. However, such a center will probably be guided ethically by a Humanist value system, which many suppose to be simply neutral. Catholic hospitals entering into this form of cooperation are in effect handing over all patients to a center where sterilization and perhaps even abortion will be treated as normal options or even encouraged. If they do not cooperate, they will be accused of wasting health resources and frustrating an effort to provide women with quality care. We believe that Catholic hospitals should not abdicate their mission to provide women and children with the best care possible in accordance with a Christian value system. Consequently, they should insist on cooperative arrangements which fully protect these values and their constitutional rights in a pluralistic society, or they should retain their own department.

Other Contraceptive Methods

Sterilization is the most drastic form of contraception because it is permanent, but other methods also raise special questions. The only method classified by Tietze's study (1970) as belonging to Class A of most effective methods, other than natural family planning and sterilization, is oral contraception in its various forms (with the exception of a reduced-dosage regimen, the so-called mini-pill). As we have already seen, some theologians have considered it as approximating natural methods because (1) it is not permanent, (2) it operates by artificially extending the natural period of sterility by suppressing ovulation, (3) it does not alter the sexual act psychologically or esthetically, and (4) it seems simple to use in a pill-consuming culture.

Most theologians consider it permissible to use various contraceptive drugs if the purpose is to treat menstrual disorders. Many believe this also includes use to regularize the menstrural cycle so as to permit more effective natural family planning, including the maintenance of the normal sterility of the lactation period (provided that the mother supports this by actually nursing the child). It would include also uses of such drugs to promote fertility. Finally some argue that these drugs can be used to determine the exact time of ovulation provided that the cycle of fertility is not suppressed. However, all these uses of contraceptive drugs have been questioned from a medical point of view (Mintz, 1970). The ethical questions to be asked are these: Is there true pathology? Is the use of progestational drugs aimed to correct this pathology so that the resultant sterility is not the direct aim of the medication?

As a method of contraception, however, progesterones have two very grave medical drawbacks. More and more evidence shows many undesirable side effects; at least sixty have been reported. (cf. *Index Medicus, passim*, "Contraception: Adverse Effects.") Some are dangerous or even fatal to those suffering from circulatory disease, especially older women. In spite of apparent simplicity in use, therefore, contraceptive drugs have to be taken under medical supervision not always accessible to the poor. This disadvantage is offset in the opinion of some doctors by the statistical evidence that these risks are considerably less than the risks of the pregnancies which the method prevents. However, a statistical comparison between the risks of pregnancy for all women (including, for example, minority women who in the United States do not receive adequate maternity care) does not tell us much about the comparative risks for a woman given high-quality care. In any case, to risk death to bring a child into the world and to risk death to avoid one are not easily compared.

The second and much graver drawback of a contraceptive drug, ethically speaking, is that it not only operates as a contraceptive by suppressing ovulation, but sometimes (perhaps as high as fifty percent of the time) it also so alters the uterine lining and vaginal secretions of the woman that she discharges an ovum which has already been fertilized. Thus we are dealing not with contraception, but with abortion, or a high risk of abortion. It can still be argued that the woman who takes such a drug intends the contraceptive effect, and that the abortion, therefore, is indirect. However, even in this case a proportionate reason for the contraceptive use of the drug must exist, equal or greater than this serious risk of destroying the unborn child, a condition not easy to verify.

In Tietze's Class B of effectiveness are a number of devices (intrauterine diaphragm with cream or contraceptive jelly, condom, and reduced-dosage hormonal drugs). The reduced-dosage drugs have less risk than full-strength progesterones, but are otherwise essentially the same. Intrauterine devices share the same disadvantages as progesterones: medical risk and sometimes abortifacient action. In fact, it is probable that the effectiveness of these devices is due *mainly* to their abortifacient action (Hilgers, 1974).

The diaphragm with jelly and the condom are probably medically safe and are contraceptives in the strict sense, that is, they prevent conception rather than destroy the conceptus. However, against them it can be objected not only that they are esthetically displeasing, but also that as the sterilizing methods suppress the generative significance of the sexual act these methods diminish its unitive significance. They resemble, to a degree, *coitus interruptus*, which all would admit cannot express total self-giving.

The methods which Tietze lists in his Class C (vaginal foams and jellies, the old calendar rhythm method, and coitus interruptus) and Class D (post coital douche and prolonged breast-feeding) are not in themselves effective enough to be widely recommended, although breast-feeding can be a useful element in natural family planning programs.

The pastoral principles for dealing with persons involved in conflict situations with regard to these various methods of birth regulation will be discussed in 10.6.

10.4 ARTIFICIAL INSEMINATION AND IN VITRO FERTILIZATION

We have just argued that persons have a real need to have children not only because of the continuation of the human race, but also because human sexuality finds its complete expression of love not simply in orgasm but ultimately in family life. Evidence for this is found in the demands by infertile parents to adopt children and also in the increasing practice of artificial insemination (Gilbert, 1976).

Artificial insemination is any process by which fecundation of an ovum takes place not as a result of the act of sexual intercourse, but as the result of sperm being introduced into the vagina by means of an artificial process. The sperm which is used in artificial insemination may be from the husband of the woman who wishes to conceive; if so, the process is referred to as homologous insemination, or artificial insemination by the husband (AIH). If the semen is from another than the husband, it is known as heterologous insemination, or artificial insemination by a donor (AID).

Though the feasibility of artificial human insemination was known in the last century, it was not practiced to any significant extent until the 1930s. Today it is not an unusual occurrence. However, people who have children in this way usually do not care to reveal the fact, and hence it is difficult to collect accurate statistics. Judging from the number of scientific and popular articles written on the subject in the last few years in the United States and elsewhere, many thousands of children are conceived and born as a result of artificial insemination (Ciba, 1973).

People who request artificial insemination are usually married, childless for a number of years, and unwilling or unable to adopt children. Sometimes fear of hereditary deficiencies rather than infertility leads them to seek this service. Physicians who perform this procedure often refer to it as "therapy," although it can hardly be called a healing process. Most refuse to inseminate single women, nor will they inseminate a married woman if the purpose of having a child is to hold the marriage together. Moreover, some require a series of psychological tests and inquiries to determine whether the couple will be able to handle the strains and tensions that may result in married life as a result of this procedure. Even these minimal standards, however, are not observed by all physicians who practice artificial insemination (Haman, 1973).

The process is comparatively simple (Strickler et al., 1975). Semen is collected, usually by masturbation, into a sterilized container. Sometimes the semen might be frozen and used at a later date, but frequently it is used within a few hours. If the semen of a donor is used, usually some attempt is made to screen him in order to avoid transmitting a debilitating hereditary disease. Results of screening, however, are at best uncertain. The semen is introduced into the vagina as close as possible to the day of ovulation by means of syringe or plastic cap which is placed at the cervix. Recent studies show that conception results in about sixty percent of the cases, a higher percentage resulting if insemination is repeated over a number of cycles (Strickler, 1975). The process is so simple that one theologian (McFadden, 1967) remarks:

> Traditionally, the practice of medicine has been associated with the treatment of disease . . . there is surely no knowledge or skill proper to the medical profession which is involved in the procedure. Members of dozen walks of life — such as veterinarians, biochemists, biologists — would be equally capable of executing the action. (p. 58)

The human results of artificial insemination insofar as the family unit is concerned are difficult to ascertain empirically. One study of AID parents has been made and the results would seem to indicate that slight harm results (Strickler et al., 1975). However, in this study the process of evaluating the impact was entirely subjective. Moreover, the study did not allow sufficient time to elapse to study the impact upon the child or upon the husband or wife in later years. It would seem that there comes a time in the development of a child when the child feels that its very existence depends upon the secure love of the parents for each other and their identification with the child. While undoubtedly it is better for a child to be adopted by a loving family than to be raised in an institution, the adopted child may suffer some disadvantage compared to the natural child. This is evidenced by the frequently reported cases where adopted children feel a great need to discover their biological parents. Such needs cannot be reduced to purely conscious factors, but arise from unconscious sources not under voluntary control.

As one physician who has practiced artifical insemination (Horne, 1975) states:

> The success or failure of "treatment" should not be solely measured by whether or not a pregnancy occurred, and was delivered successfully, but also by the long-run sociological and psychological effect on both the unfertile couple and the child as revealed a generation later . . . I believe without reservation that the future of the "potential child" be of first consideration and the wishes of its proposed parents second. (p. 873)

From a legal point of view, artificial insemination is in an ambiguous position (Hoffer, 1975). In some countries, there are laws which treat heterologous insemination (AID) as adultery. In the United States no laws have been enacted regarding it, but several bills, some favorable and some unfavorable, have been introduced in state legislatures. Some of the favorable bills would legitimize children born of AID and bestow the usual rights of inheritance upon the child so conceived. These rights are subject to challenge, especially in the case of AID children. Though there is no established jurisprudence in the courts of the United States in regard to artificial insemination, the courts tend to approve AIH, but to consider AID contrary to public policy and good morals.

In judging the morality of artificial insemination, we are implicitly judging the morality of several other actions similar to it which will become more controversial in the future. For example, if artificial insemination for childless couples is licit, why would it not also be licit to inseminate women in order to modify or improve the human species? Why could not single women be inseminated if they thought having a child would lead to greater fulfillment? Moreover, if conception outside of intercourse is fitting for human beings, why not approve conception in a test tube (*in vitro* fertilization) when both egg and sperm become subject to human manipulation? In the latter case, the fertilized ovum might be placed for gestation in the womb of the woman whose egg is used, in the womb of another woman, or in an artificial placenta (Francoeur, 1970).

In this matter, as in the discussion of contraception, we need to go back to the basic principle of the inseparability of the unitive and generative meanings of sexuality. The objection to contraception is that it deprives the act of sexual love of its relation to procreation, and attempts by Catholic theologians to defend it depends upon arguments attempting to show that this relation is not completely removed. Similarly, but conversely, the issue regarding artificial insemination is whether the procreative process is in this way separated from its relation to the expression of sexual love. As Pius XII (1951) said:

> To consider unworthily the cohabitation of husband and wife, and the marital act as a simple organic function for the transmission of seed, would be the same as to convert the domestic hearth, which is the family sanctuary, into a mere biological laboratory . . . . The marital act, in its natural setting, is a personal action. It is the simultaneous and direct cooperation of husband and wife which, by the very nature of the agents and the property of the act, is the expression of the mutual giving which, in the words of Scripture, results in the union "in one flesh." (n. 295)

Most Catholic theologians reject donor semination (AID) as a method of solving the problem of childless couples (McCormick, 1969). As George Lobo (1974) writes:

> The bond of mutual and exclusive human sexual love between the parents is violated if the sperm of another man is introduced into the woman's

vagina. If conception occurs, the child has no relation to the love that binds man and wife together. (p. 150)

This is in accord with the teaching of Pius XII (1949) who said:

> Artificial insemination in marriage, with the use of an active element from a third person, is equally immoral and as such is to be rejected summarily. Only marriage partners have mutual rights over their bodies for the procreation of new life, and these rights are exclusive, nontransferable and inalienable . . . Between marriage partners, however, and a child that is the fruit of the active element furnished by a third person — even though the husband consents — there is no bond of origin, no moral or juridicial bond of conjugal procreation. (n. 176)

A woman has a true need to bear children, but it is obviously not an absolute need, and it does not justify the risk that her husband will be unable (even if he originally consents) to accept the child which he knows to be another man's without unconscious hostility, nor the risk that the child will suffer from this disruption of the basic order of the family which is so deeply ecological and a work of God's providence. Furthermore, she does an injustice to the donor, since although he is willing he is being sexually exploited much as a prostitute is. He is the true father of the child and responsible for it, and yet he is induced (usually by payment) to surrender his responsibility in a dehumanizing way. Thus AID is intrinsically wrong because it is contrary to the basic significance of sexuality.

However, when it is possible to use the husband's semen (AIH), the case is less clear, and some Catholic theologians believe it can be permitted, either because they dissent from Pius XII's teaching or because they believe his condemnation falls only on the use of masturbation to obtain the semen (Häring, 1973; cf. Van Allen, 1970). They would argue that as some justify contraception by saying that the act remains *remotely* ordered to procreation, so in AIH the artificial procreative process remains remotely ordered to the unitive act of love. The partners express their love regularly by intercourse which they would render fertile if they could, but since they cannot, they use an artificial process to achieve this legitimate purpose.

It is undoubtedly legitimate to use medical art to find remedies for sterility and even to intervene in the marital act itself to promote its fertility, for example, by techniques such as the use of a syringe or cervical spoon, or methods of concentrating the sperm density of the semen emitted in intercourse (O'Donnell, 1976). Thus Pius XII (1956b) stated:

> One does not necessarily proscribe the use of certain artificial methods intended simply either to facilitate the natural act or enable the natural act, effected in a normal manner, to attain its end. (n. 659)

In all these cases the child is begotten as the fruit of an actual expression of unitive love. It is difficult, however, to establish convincingly that this essential significance of parenthood is retained when there is a complete physical separation of the insemination from the act of unitive love. Papal teaching considers this as contrary to the essential finality of sex and as an opening to the unlimited manipulation of the sexual powers which will damage the institution of the family, as the widespread practice of contraception already seems to have done.

Thus, the objection to AIH does not rest on the method used to secure the semen. All theologians who have written on the question of licit methods of obtaining such a sample for diagnostic purposes admit the licity of prostatic massage or aspiration from the epididymis or testicles, but generally they have rejected the much simpler and medically more useful procedure of induced ejaculation on the grounds that it was masturbation, which we have already argued is depersonalized use of the sex act which is intrinsically wrong and cannot be justified by a good intention. However, it could be argued that there is an essential moral difference between masturbation as an act whose moral object is sexual satisfaction and the same physical act whose moral object is the obtaining of a sample of a body fluid for an examination, with the accompanying pleasure as a foreseen but not intended double effect. In which case the man obtaining the sample in this manner would not be masturbating provided that he did not consent to the second effect.

Although artificial fecundation is illicit, it would seem that artificial gestation might be licit provided that there would be sufficient reason for so extraordinary a procedure. If a couple conceive a child in the natural way, and if for one reason or another the woman would not be able certainly to carry the child to viable term, it would assist the natural process, rather than subvert it, to transfer the child to an artificial womb and thus protect its life.

Would it also be licit to transplant an embryo naturally conceived from the uterus of its mother to a foster mother for the good of the child or because of serious danger to the mother? Would the foster mother be justified in thus lending her womb to carry the fetus of another? Though one study group has rejected this form of artificial gestation, some say that it does not seem beyond the realm of ethical intervention. Certainly, it would not be mutilation of the woman's sexual organs, nor would it destroy her personal bodily integrity. It would be similar to the age-old custom of the wet nurse, which in cases of real necessity seems entirely justified.

10.5 TREATMENT OF RAPE VICTIMS

Rape is one of the more common social crimes in our society. Because many rape victims hesitate to expose themselves to shame and notoriety, and because false charges of rape are often filed, it is difficult to ascertain with any degree of accuracy the number of rapes committed in the United States each year. However, when crimes of violence are tabulated the percentage of rapes increases each year. There is evidence that rape is motivated by hostile impulses, a desire to assert the aggressive power of the rapist and to humiliate the victim, just as much as by a desire for sexual pleasure (Brownmiller, 1975). Strange to say, some people would actually defend rape in some cases and justify it within marriage on the ground that it meets masculine needs. However, without or within marriage, it is contrary to the meaning of sexuality as an expression of mutual love for the sexual act to be performed against the will of the partner.

A victim of rape should be given the most sensitive and charitable care possible. Such victims often complain justifiably that they are treated by the police and medical personnel alike as though they were responsible for provoking the attack, thus compounding the grave injustice from which the woman has suffered. Many cities now have formed rape treatment task forces, not only to help educate police and medical personnel concerning humane treatment for rape victims, but also to prevent the crime by alerting the public to the signs of impending attack and to the measures that might prevent or ward it off. Hospital procedures developed by such task forces are designed to accomplish four things:

1. To offer the psychological support and counseling which the woman needs to work through the trauma of the attack and its aftermath. Often this will require follow-up treatment with a counselor or psychologist.

2. To provide medical care for injuries or abrasions that might have occurred.

3. To gather evidence to be used if the rapist is apprehended and prosecuted. This usually consists of a rather extensive examination of the vagina, pelvic area, and clothing.

4. To provide treatment to prevent possible veneral disease and pregnancy.

The last point just mentioned raises special ethical problems. Although the chances of conception after rape are in fact very low statistically (Wilke and Wilke, 1975) (as is evident from the fact that married couples desirous of children achieve a pregnancy on the average only once in one hundred acts of intercourse), it is a very serious concern to the victim and she deserves every help that medical professionals can give her, provided that help is ethically licit. Since the victim is in no way responsible for the possible pregnancy, she has both the right and the serious duty to avoid it. She has the duty to avoid it because it will put a burden on her very difficult for her to deal with, and also because a child who may be conceived in these circumstances cannot easily be provided the proper setting for personal development.

It follows from the discussion of abortion in 9.2 that once the woman has conceived she cannot take any action or request others to do so, nor may they cooperate with her in doing so, which would abort or destroy the fertilized ovum. While she has the right to protect herself from the effects of the aggression, she does not have the right to do so at the expense of the life of an innocent child. Nor is there any proportion between the child's right to life, itself, and her right to be free of the injury done her, grave as this is.

She does, however, have the right to prevent conception taking place. A woman who has consented to intercourse takes responsibility as a free person to use the sexual act in keeping with its intrinsic significance of love and procreation. On this responsibility the arguments of *Humanae Vitae* against contraception are based. The rape victim, however, has no such responsibility because she has never consented to use the sexual act. Nevertheless, some thologians, taking the position that the only human dominion over the sexual process is to use it or abstain from it, would not permit any human interference with the sexual process once begun. Hence they would deny the woman the right to remove or destroy the semen once deposited. We have already argued that *Humanae Vitae* does not reject all human intervention in the sexual process, but only that which separates the unitive and generative meanings of the act. The rape victim has assumed no responsibility to give this proper meaning to the sexual act which has been unjustly forced upon her.

Therefore most Catholic moralists today admit that a woman who is in real danger of rape may, prior to the attack, if the danger is real take a contraceptive drug or even insert a diaphragm (Curran, 1974). After the rape she may through her own action or that of a medical person do what is possible to render the sperm inoperative, to prevent it from joining the ovum, or to delay the production of a fertilizable ovum.

Problems arise, however, when it is proposed by physicians to use methods which do not prevent conception only, but which may be or actually are abortifacient. As we have already said, such methods are illicit because the woman is protecting her rights at the expense of the rights of a child already in existence. This is true even in the period before the implantation of the fertilized ovum in the uterus because, as we argued in 9.2, it is probable that the zygote is truly human even before implantation and that this probability benefits the rights of the fetus. On the other hand, however, as to the *doubt* as to whether conception has in fact taken place, the probability should benefit the rights of the woman. This means, therefore, that as long as it is truly doubtful that the woman has conceived she can take means to prevent conception, even if these means might in some cases actually be abortifacient if conception has taken place without her knowing it. But once it becomes certain or highly probable that conception has occurred, she must then give the benefit of the doubt to the rights of the fetus to life and avoid any serious risk of abortion.

For years, Catholic moralists when discussing licit methods of attacking the sperm before conception recommended (with some limitations as to time) curettage (D and C), vaginal douche, or intrauterine douche (O'Donnell, 1957). Today from both the medical and moral points of view, none of these methods are an acceptable approach to the problem.

The vaginal douche may be used for cleansing and sanitizing purposes, but is unlikely to prevent conception. Conception takes place ordinarily in the fallopian tubes, not in the vagina or uterus, and recent studies show the sperm enters the tubes in five to thirty minutes after intercourse (Settlage et al., 1973). Hence, the vaginal spermicidal douche might attack some of the sperm remaining in the vagina, but would be ineffective for most of them. The intrauterine douche is considered too dangerous because the fluid it introduces could flow through the fallopian tubes into the peritoneal cavity and perhaps cause serious infection. Competent gynecologists do not employ this procedure today.

The theologians who formerly allowed dilation and curettage realized that the scraping of the womb made it impossible for an already implanted zygote to survive or for a fertilized ovum to be implanted. But they argued that the principle purpose of this action was to eliminate the sperm, and if this were done soon enough after the attack, the Principle of Double Effect could be used (Healy, 1956). Given the new evidence of the motility of the sperm, it no longer seems reasonable to say that curettage is a specific remedy to remove the sperm when the significant sperm is probably already out of the uterus.

The usual medical procedure recommended in most rape protocols today is an injection of antifertility steroids or oral medication with these drugs over a period of a few days. One of the more common synthetic antifertility steroids prescribed is diethylstilbestrol (DES). One effect of DES is to prevent ovulation. Thus if the woman who has been raped is at a point in her cycle when ovulation is imminent and the risk of conception high, DES will act as an antiovulatory agent and render fertilization impossible because the sperm will have died by the time a fertilizable ovum is available. (Rudel and Kincl, 1966; Middleton, 1965).

Some moralists, apparently unaware of the antiovulatory effect of DES, condemn outright its use in the treatment of rape victims (O'Donnell, 1976). These moralists are correct in being concerned about the possible abortifacient effects of DES, since these steroids also render the endometrium of the uterus hostile to implantation. For some time it was thought that this was its only effect (Morris, 1966). However, the antiovulation effect must also be considered in the ethical evaluation. Granted that the act of administering DES has two possible effects, one licit (antiovulatory) and the other illict (abortifacient), can we apply the Principle of Double Effect to justify its use for the sake of a licit result? Since the women's intention in using DES is not abortion but the prevention of pregnancy (which for her is legitimate), and since the evil effect is not a means to the good effect, the only real question is whether there is a proportionate cause. We have already stated that the woman may not risk an abortion if she knows herself to be certainly or very probably pregnant, but if this is in doubt, the doubt favors her rights of self-defense. Thus the problem resolves itself into the factual question about whether the chances are high that she is already pregnant when the drug is taken so that the risk of abortion is notable. In a recent article Donald McCarthy (1977) has attempted to calculate this probability and concludes:

> The use of DES or hormone injections should not be simply described as an abortifacient procedure. It might accomplish this unwelcome effect in 2.5 percent of the situations, but does not do so in 97.5 percent of the situations.

Thus we can conclude that the use of DES in rape cases is probably licit as long as there is serious doubt that pregnancy has occurred. Some would support this conclusion by pointing out that the doubts about when animation or hominization takes place are strongest for the first week after conception. While this doubt in our opinion is not well-grounded according to current knowledge (9.2), it is still conceded as plausible in the *Declaration on Procured Abortion* of the Congregation for the Doctrine of the Faith (1974), although it cannot be used to justify direct abortion. However, in this case abortion is not intended even as a means, but is only an accidental effect, and the benefit of the doubt favors the rights of the woman who has suffered unjust aggression.

We can conclude that Catholic health care facilities have the following responsibilities to rape victims.

1. They should prepare and carefully observe a protocol for the treatment of rape victims in which the first concern is respect for the dignity of the woman, regardless of her character or socioeconomic condition. This should include both medical and counseling help to reduce the harm she has unjustly suffered and should shield her as much as possible from embarrassment.

2. The protocol should include medical effort to prevent pregnancy, but not by the use of abortifacients as such. However in the present state of our knowledge it is licit to use DES or antiovulant drugs with the intention of suppressing ovulation, even if there is some accidental risk of abortion, provided that there is still serious doubt that pregnancy has already resulted. Since, however, such treatment is controversial, if the woman, herself, or the medical staff object on grounds of a conscientious desire not to risk cooperation in abortion, their consciences should be respected.

3. The protocol should also provide for the collecting of adequate and accurate information for the police so that the aggressor can be brought to trial and conviction.

A warning might be added that a hospital, depending upon state laws, may be liable to legal suit if it fails to provide the women with the opportunity to avoid pregnancy. Consequently if a Catholic hospital believes in conscience that it is unable to provide treatment which can be established as adequate in the local courts, it should make sure that victims can be promptly referred to their own physicians for whatever antipregnancy treatment they themselves choose.

10.6 PASTORAL APPROACH TO MEDICAL SEXUAL PROBLEMS

Pastoral Implications of Humanae Vitae

Difficulties of conscience experienced by Catholics in sexual ethics in relation to health are usually referred by health care professionals to a priest, often the chaplain in a health care facility. In chapter 14 we will discuss the chaplain's role in ethical counseling. However, it is also important that all Catholic health care professionals understand the changes in pastoral practice which are under way in the Catholic Church since the Second Vatican Council, some of the most controversial of which relate to sexual ethics. Consequently in the last section of this chapter we will deal at some length with the way in which the teaching of *Humanae Vitae* is being pastorally applied and the implications this has for the instruction of Catholics in sexual ethics, a task in which members of the health care profession often play an important role.

Many of the criticisms which have been raised against *Humanae Vitae* and also against the subsequent *Declaration on Certain Questions Concerning Sexual Ethics* issued by the Congregation for the Doctrine of the Faith (1975) have complained that the pastors of the Church seem content to pronounce moral judgments but do not provide much pastoral help for dealing with problems Christians experience in everyday life. However, when we read *Humanae Vitae*, as well as Paul VI's (1968b) explanation of his personal intentions in issuing this encyclical and also the pastoral letters of the various national episcopal conferences explaining it (Delhaye, 1970; Shannon, 1970), we are struck not only by the intransigent way in which the pope maintains Christian ideals as traditionally understood, but also by the fact that Paul (whose whole pontificate shows him to be a pastor of great forbearance and mercy) sought for a more compassionate approach to sexual problems.

Previous popes have denounced contraception in very strong language as a "shameful stain on marriage," "moral ruin," and "a grave sin." For a time confessors were required to question every married couple if there was any suspicion they might be practicing contraception (Creusen, 1932). Although this pastoral severity was later somewhat moderated, the ordinary practice up to the controversy over oral contraceptive drugs was to refuse absolution and communion to those who would not promise to abandon this practice. At that time the Church's discipline was aimed at halting the spread of contraception. In the United States this policy was surprisingly successful, as proved by the fact that the Catholic birthrate for a long time remained significantly above the national average.

However, this battle eventually was lost. We have already mentioned in 10.1 that in the United States *Humanae Vitae* produced a catastrophic negative reaction among Catholics which largely offset their positive reaction to the reforms of the Second Vatican Council. Church attendance fell markedly, and it seems the great majority of younger married Catholics ignore its conclusions in practice. Of course such statistics cannot determine whether Paul VI was doctrinally mistaken. Experience with the effects of a contraceptive society could ultimately vindicate his position. Further ethical debate may reveal that in this matter liberal opinion was inconsistent with authentic Christian humanism, so that the price of maintaining doctrinal truth, however heavy pragmatically, had to be paid (Von Hildebrand, 1969).

Perhaps it would be fairer to say that the catastrophe was due, in part at least, to the fact that the pope took what appeared to many to be an *ambiguous* stand: too hesitant, then too intransigent; too firm on principles, too vague on how they could be pastorally applied. Yet it must be admitted that any change in moral discipline is likely to meet such difficulties. What is this change in pastoral practice? It consists in the fact that Paul VI no longer insisted on explicitly labeling contraception as a "grave" or "mortal" sin, nor did he insist that those continuing to practice it should be refused absolution or denied communion (Godden, 1968; Martelet, 1969; Delhaye et al., 1969; Gallon, 1968). Thus *Humanae Vitae* gives the following instruction to married couples:

> We do not at all intend to hide the sometimes serious difficulties inherent in the life of Christian married persons; for them, as for everyone else, "the gate is narrow and the way is hard, that leads to life." . . . Let married couples, then, face up to the efforts needed, supported by the faith and hope which "do not disappoint . . . because God's love has been poured into our hearts through the Holy Spirit, who has been given to us"; let them implore divine assistance by persevering prayer; above all, let them draw from the source of grace and charity in the Eucharist. And if sin should still keep its hold over them, let them not to be discouraged, but rather have recourse with humble perseverance to the mercy of God, which is poured forth in the sacrament of penance. In this way they will be enabled to achieve the fullness of conjugal life . . . (n. 25)

And to priests:

> Your first task — especially in the case of those who teach moral theology — is to expound the Church's teaching on marriage without

ambiguity. Be the first to give, in the exercise of your ministry, the example of loyal internal and external obedience to the teaching authority of the Church. That obedience, as you know well, obliges not only because of the reasons adduced, but rather because of the light of the Holy Spirit, which is given in a particular way to the pastors of the Church in order that they may illustrate the truth [Vatican II, *On the Church*, n. 25]. You know, too, that it is of the utmost importance, for peace of consciences and for the unity of the Christian people, that in the field of morals as well as that of dogma, all should attend to the *Magisterium* of the Church, and all should speak the same language . . . To diminish in no way the saving teaching of Christ constitutes an eminent form of charity for souls. But this must ever be accompanied by patience and goodness, such as the Lord himself gave example of in dealing with men. Having come not to condemn but to save, he was indeed intransigent with evil, but merciful towards individuals. In their difficulties, many married couples always find, in the words and in the heart of a priest, the echo of the voice and the love of the Redeemer. (nn. 28-29)

Also to doctors and medical personnel:

We hold those physicians and medical personnel in the highest esteem who, in the exercise of their profession, value above every human interest the superior demands of their Christian vocation. Let them persevere, therefore, in promoting on every occasion the discovery of solutions inspired by faith and right reason, let them strive to arouse this conviction and respect in their associates. Let them also consider as their proper professional duty the task of acquiring all the knowledge needed in this delicate sector, so as to be able to give to those married persons who consult them wise counsel and healthy direction, such as they have a right to expect. (n. 24)

And to medical researchers:

It is particularly desirable that, according to the wish already expressed by Pope Pius XII, medical science succeed in providing a sufficiently secure basis for a regulation of birth, founded on the observance of natural rhythms. In this way scientists and especially Catholic scientists will contribute to demonstrate in actual fact that, as the Church teaches, "a true contradiction cannot exist between the divine laws pertaining to the transmission of life and those pertaining to the fostering of authentic conjugal love" [Vatican II, *Church in Modern World*, n. 30]. (n. 24)

Some national episcopal conferences (McCormick, 1969; Shannon, 1970; Delhaye, 1970; Horgan, 1972) simply urged their people to obey the encyclical. This was the position of many Third World bishops (India, Ceylon, Phillippines, Mexico) as well as those of Spain, Scotland, and Ireland. Others (Italian, Swiss, German, England, Japan, and United States) urged confessors to deal with those practicing contraception in a very compassionate way and to avoid anything that might make these couples give up the regular use of the sacraments. Finally, the French, Belgian, Dutch, Austrian, Scandinavian, and Canadian bishops openly raised the question as to what the confessor's attitude was to be to those who believed that it would be morally wrong for them to give up the practice of contraception in their present circumstances and concluded that it was not always necessary for the confessor to refuse absolution. The Austrian bishops pointed out that the pope had refrained from speaking of contraception as a "grave sin" and advised:

> If someone should err against the teaching of the encyclical, he must not feel cut off from God's love in every case, and may receive Holy Communion without first going to confession. (*New York Times*, October 4, 1968)

Since Paul VI has tolerated these more liberal interpretations of the pastoral application of the principles which he enunciated in *Humanae Vitae*, we may conclude that they are not evidently inconsistent with his own pastoral purposes in issuing the encyclical (Zalba, 1970; McCormick, 1973c; but cf. Lynch, 1977). But how can they be understood theologically? The most radical interpretation would seem to be that of the Austrian bishops, namely, that although individual contraceptive acts are *objectively* "disordered," this moral evil may be only venial, unless aggravated by hedonism, irresponsibility, and so forth (Shannon, 1970).

There are three obvious objections to this view about the gravity of the moral evil of contraception.

1. Pius XI and Pius XII, whose condemnation of contraception Paul VI reaffirmed, clearly considered it an objectively grave or mortal sin (10.1). However, as Valsecchi (1970) and others have emphasized, these popes were considering the hedonistic use of contraception. Paul VI, however, had before him the commission report of theologians who attempted to make a case for the use of contraception not for egoistic motives, but precisely to promote marriage and family. It would seem, therefore, that his omission of any attempt to characterize the gravity of contraception in such cases is significant.

2. If contraception is not a mortal sin, then why didn't the pope say so and quiet the whole controversy? It seems to trivialize the encyclical to say that it is dealing only with venial evils. However, this objection overlooks the fact that the pope is not merely interested in the issue of gravity, but in proposing a Christian view of sex in the face of an increasing erosion of Christian values (Schall, 1968; O'Callaghan, 1970; MacDonald, 1975). Even if in such cases contraception is only a venial sin, the principle of chastity which it violates is of very grave importance. Moreover, the pope undoubtedly believed that once the principle is violated, even in small matters, the way is open to hedonistic uses of contraception and then to still graver evils. Finally, it may very well be that the pope believed that contraception is per se mortal, but did not wish to bind the faithful to this opinion because he saw it as less clear and certain than his principal message and hence prudently refrained from committing himself on this point.

3. Much more serious is the objection that there is no reason to believe that the pope intended in the encyclical to abandon the traditional teaching of moral theology that any deliberate sin against the right moral

order in sexual matters is per se a grave or mortal sin, because it violates the God-given order in a matter of great importance not only for the individual but for the race. This is the well-known axiom, In regards to the Sixth Commandment there can be no light matter. It would seem, therefore, that Paul VI supposed that this axiom would make it clear to priests that if contraception is per se wrong it is a mortal sin against the Sixth Commandment.

However, today this axiom is disputed by some moral theologians, and Meier (1966) and Kleber (1971) have shown that historically it has had a checkered career. We have already argued (3.4; 8.1-2) that a sin is mortal because it is an act by which we turn away from friendship with God either *directly* or *indirectly* by turning away from friendship with our neighbor, since to hate our neighbor is contradictory to our loving God who loves us both alike. But we destroy our friendship with our neighbor only by wishing him or doing him a *serious* harm. Thus contraception is not a mortal sin unless it is of the nature to cause serious harm to ourself or another.

Theologians have never considered sexual sins as direct acts against God. They are not (ordinarily) sins of malice, but of weakness, since they are done for pleasure, not to harm others, with the exception of rape, sadistic acts, or those performed to humiliate or out of revenge. Undoubtedly they become mortal when aggravated by such malicious purposes, but this is exceptional.

How, then, can most sexual acts be mortal? What serious harm do they do? Humanists generally argue that they are harmless. Christian theologians, however, have generally believed that as sexual acts can do great good they can also do great harm. Classical moral theology argued that adultery is mortal because of the injustice it does one's spouse to whom fidelity was promised. Fornication was said to be mortal because of the danger of harm to the illegitimate children who might be born. In general, it was argued that they violated the divine order in a very serious matter, namely, the good not of the individual (as sins of gluttony and drunkedness) but of the race. It is hard to see, however, that every inordinate sexual act really threatens the survival of the race! So it was finally argued that if exceptions are allowed, then the whole order of sexual morality will be endangered because sexual pleasure is so great that if indulged it will move beyond all limits (Connery, 1977).

Thus the ultimate reason given by classical moral theology for rating as mortal *every* sexual sin was a slippery-slope argument based on the tendency of human beings to regress to an egoistic level. Yet this argument is firmly rooted in sad experience of the ambiguity of human sexuality. Sexual need can become an addictive egoism that is destructive to self and others, or it can become the opening out of the person to genuine love and creativity. The adolescent, once initiated to sexual pleasure by masturbation or fornication, lacking the social discipline and support of marriage, will probably have great difficulty in keeping under control the addictive drive to repeat such experiences. It is the acquisition of this addictive egoistic hedonism which is the harm done by illicit sexual acts. Such sexual addiction, of course, does not do the physiological harm that drug addiction causes, but in another sense it may be more harmful because it distorts what is most intimately personal in the human being, the capacity for self-giving in love.

However, it is not so clear that sexual acts performed within marriage which are less than ideal cause this kind of serious harm. Classical theologians held that when married couples perform the normal sexual act, not as an expression of love but in a merely selfish way, they sin, but only venially, because such acts still take place in the context of committed love (Noonan, 1965). Could not the same reasoning be applied to the contraceptive act when it is used to express love and in an effort to fulfill the duties of responsible parenthood? It is disordered because of its departure from the natural process with its objective order to generation on which *Humanae Vitae* insists, and hence in some measure it opens the way to hedonism and the other possible consequences mentioned in the encyclical, but is this danger so great as to be qualified as mortal sin?

Whatever may be thought of such an argument, the issue can perhaps be more securely and practically treated in terms of *subjective* or *developmental* morality, to which we turn next.

A Developmental Approach

When it is healthy, human life, is a process of growth and development. The Christian view of human life emphasizes this developmental thrust and understands it also as a process of liberation from the bondage of sin and retrogression. Yet we have often considered ethical life in purely static, legalistic terms of laws observed or broken. Thus, formerly it was assumed that if the pastors of the Church had condemned something as sinful then no one who had been informed of this condemnation could be subjectively justified in acting against it. Today, it seems extreme to draw such a conclusion.

First of all, there is the possibility of honest dissent from teaching that is admittedly not infallible and which has been so embroiled in controversy (Fitch, 1969). Thus, the Belgian bishops in their pastoral (Delhaye, 1970) assert that it is possible for Catholics to be in good faith when they say they cannot in conscience follow the practical conclusion of the encyclical when it forbids them to use contraception in fulfilling their obligations of responsible parenthood.

Second, persons who do not dissent from papal teaching, as the French bishops noted in their pastoral letter, may yet find themselves practically perplexed in conscience (Delcaration of CLER, 1968; O'Callaghan, 1970). As Sahuc (1970) has explained, such couples find themselves faced with the duty of simultaneously (1) preserving their marriage by sexual expression of love, (2) being responsible parents, and (3) refraining from the practice of contraception which for them is the only practical way of meeting the first two obligations. In the hierarchy of values, the first two are clearly of greater weight than the third. Consequently, they rightly choose to seek the greater good at the expense of the lesser evil. The French bishops in their pastoral adopt this lesser-evil solution in cases of conflict of duties (to which several other of the pastorals also refer) and assert, "Contraception can never be good. It is always a disorder, but this disorder is not always culpable."

Some commentators on the French pastoral have pointed out that this seems in flat contradition to a passage in *Humanae Vitae*:

> To justify conjugal acts made intentionally infecund, one cannot invoke as valid reasons the lesser evil, or the fact that such acts would constitute a whole together with the fecund acts already performed or to follow later, and hence would share in one and the same moral goodness. In truth, if it is sometimes licit to tolerate a lesser evil in order to avoid a greater evil or to promote a greater good, it is not licit, even for the gravest reasons, to do evil so that good may follow therefrom; that is, to make into the object of a positive act of the will something which is intrinsically disordered, and hence unworthy of the human person, even when the intention is to safeguard or promote individual, family, or social well-being. Consequently, it is an error to think that a conjugal act which is deliberately made infecund and so is intrinsically dishonest could be made honest and right by the ensemble of a fecund conjugal life. (n. 14)

However, the French bishops were certainly aware of this passage. They are not denying that contraception is intrinsically wrong and always disordered, but agree to this. In the abstract or essential order, of which the pope is speaking, there cannot be an irresolvable conflict of duties. However, in the concrete or existential order we may not be able to discover what that solution is, and it is in such perplexity that we are bound to choose the greater good at the expense of the lesser evil. A counselor dealing pastorally with persons in such perplexity can ordinarily help them to a correct solution, but when persons in good faith remain perplexed, then the confessor without approving the doing of evil for the sake of good should not reject their decision to do what seems to them best. We should add that when a counselor deals with someone who is *not* wholly in good faith, but who is debating between two evils acts, the counselor (without approving either act) may assure him it is better to choose the lesser evil. Thus, he might point out that contraception is certainly better than abortion if he sees that the person is likely to choose the latter.

Third, since the evil in question is at worst a sin of weakness, we must admit that many people are caught in addictive life patterns and lack perfect freedom of decision. Much of this bondage is the result of moral education and social support in a society where Christian ideals are little understood and often contradicted by social insitutions. We have only to think of the prostitute who seems to have no other way of making a living, the man in a bad marriage, the lonely celibate who is caught in a habit of masturbation, the homosexual who cannot marry. It is true that all such persons can live chaste lives if they are open to God's grace, but here and now such persons, while sincerely desiring to live as Christians and striving not to harm others or to go deeper into depersonalization, lack the strength to pull out of their situation all at once. Can we say that every new act of impurity is mortal sin? The older theologians would have said that in such cases culpability is reduced, perhaps to the point of venial sin. The important thing is whether such persons can be helped to begin to free themselves to the point that a way of life conformed to the Christian ideal of sexuality can be freely chosen.

Thus from a pastoral point of view, a counselor has to decide how to help such persons move closer to the ideal, without further burdening or discouraging them (Mulligan, 1969; Kelly, 1972; Shehan, 1973; Lobo, 1974; Delhaye, 1975). The practice of confessors formerly was to insist (1) that such persons promise to give up the sin here and now, (2) that they not commit the sin again before going to communion, and (3) that they come again to confession and renew their promise before going to communion if they had backslid. The rationale was to keep the objective ideal clearly before the sinners' mind and to get them to renew regularly their sincere promise of amendment, with no risk of receiving communion insincerely.

Today, with a more nuanced understanding of the psychology of sin, many confessors would consider this method to be sometimes counterproductive in helping the penitent move forward. It would seem that such persons can have true contrition if they are sincerely trying to eliminate from their life the worst and most harmful elements of what they are doing which lie at the limits of their actual freedom. Thus the prostitute will start looking for another way to support herself, the masturbator will begin to seek a less introverted life-style, the homosexual will cease promiscuity. It can then be judged that the continued immoral acts are subjectively venial and need not keep these persons from communion, provided that they keep trying and continue to come regularly to confession, trying to be freed from bondage step by step. Above all, the confessor needs to communicate to these persons that God has not rejected them, nor has the Christian community of the Church, but that the confessor wants to help them in every way possible, and does not demand a heroic moral transformation all at once. This attitude is not essentially contrary to that of good confessors in the past, but the pastoral strategy is somewhat different.

The pastoral directives of *Humanae Vitae* seem to leave the way open to some such pastoral procedure in dealing with those who practice contraception not for egoistic reasons but in an effort to fulfill their marriage obligations. Paul VI clearly wants confessors to keep couples receiving the sacraments while educating them to seek a more natural method of regulating family life. The bishops seem to have understood this as evidenced either by their explicit pastoral instructions or at least by their toleration of the widespread employment of such an approach by their priests. Unfortunately, in the United States too many Catholics, educated in a somewhat mechanical morality, have become alienated from the Church because they believe they cannot without hypocrisy continue to go to the sacraments unless they promise to cease contraceptive practices absolutely, while those who continue to go are alienated from the pope because they believe they are defying him.

Good pastoral care will work to heal these wounds and divisions by creating an atmosphere in which the conscience of individuals, accepted at a particular stage of their lives and their spiritual and moral development, is truly respected. At the same time such care must encourage individuals to open themselves to the guidance and support available in the community of the Church and of society.

Education for a Sexual Future

The sexual revolution projects a future in which the Christian vision of human sexuality will appear ridiculous and unrealizable. Yet for Christians human sexuality is governed by norms of *hope*, a hope on which a truly human future must be built. Perhaps, as George F. Gilder (1975) has argued, the sexual revolution is really sexual suicide.

To build a healthier future it is essential to help Christians develop a fully human understanding of their sexuality. Catholic health care professionals and health care facilities can play an important role in this developmental task. We suggest three contributions for which there is urgent need.

1. The first responsibility of Christian health care professionals and facilities in the area of sexuality is to promote and cooperate with sound programs of sex education. Sound sex education is primarily spiritual and ethical, not medical, but health care professionals have an essential role to play in it because of its close connection with bodily life. While many sex education programs today provide excellent biological and psychological information, they also promote the value system of Humanism which Christians find quite inadequate. We can hardly criticize such programs, however, unless we provide superior ones. A Christian program should begin with helping parents succeed in their natural role as the principal sex educators. Today, many

parents suffer from (a) the predominant influence of Humanist values and (b) from incorrect, distorted views of Christian values which stress negative, repressive aspects of sexual morality based on fear, rather than a positive, but realistic view based on a true understanding of God's gifts and their stewardship.

A sound program of Christian sex education should provide the following kinds of instruction:

(1) Understanding of the unitive-procreative meaning of sexuality in sacramental marriage

(2) Knowledge of mental hygiene and essential biological knowledge about sexual differences and equality, lovemaking, intercourse, pregnancy, and birth

(3) Information on why people have a need for children and on the problems of sterility, adoption, and limits on the right to have children

(4) Information on the problems of responsible parenthood in present-day society, natural family planning methods and alternative methods, and ethical evaluation of all birth regulation methods

(5) Explanation of the rights of the unborn child

(6) Discussion of the problems of genetic defects and the Christian attitude toward defective persons

(7) Consideration of the problem of homosexuality and similar difficulties in psychosocial development

Such programs can be considered preventive medicine since they might go a long way to reduce the frequency or severity of many of the problems described in this chapter, but they will not have a widespread effect unless they are also joined to social programs aimed at improving the climate of our society.

2. Sound sex education must be based on continuing research and open discussion. When sexual issues are involved, such objectivity is difficult to achieve. It has taken a real struggle on the part of some physicians and nurses to get a hearing for natural methods of delivery and breast-feeding, because such an approach seemed like a conservative attack on medical progress. Similarly, in ethical questions dealing with sexual matters our culture has a strong bias toward voices announcing the coming of new "freedoms" and a suspicion of those who are concerned to retain and strengthen traditional values of modesty and chastity and the disciplined restraint they require. To arrive at an atmosphere in which both sides can be fairly heard when discussing sexual issues is extremely difficult. A Christian identity committee of a Catholic health care facility should be developed as the proper forum where such discussions can take place in a truth-seeking atmosphere.

3. Catholic health care professionals who play a role in public and social agencies that deal with sexual problems should take care that these agencies do not content themselves merely with promoting birth control. Granted that responsible parenthood must be an important objective of any such agency, this objective should not be conceived in merely negative terms. Rather the principal goal of all such work should be to strengthen and promote the family as the basic institution of society. Only in an atmosphere of good family life based on faithful love can the next generation develop toward a mature fully human sexuality.

CHAPTER 11 RECONSTRUCTING HUMAN BEINGS

11.1 PRESENT AND FUTURE CAPABILITIES

In recent years medical technology has moved from the mere capability of repair of the human body to new capabilities of remodeling the body by surgical reconstruction and even by genetic reconstruction which will alter not only an individual, but also all his or her descendants. Some of these new capabilities are already practical, others still futuristic. In this chapter we will deal in some detail with certain present problems associated with modifying the human person but will only touch on the futuristic ones for purposes of illustration.

A basic axiom of medicine has always been the Greek dictum, Art perfects nature, which implies that a human person can be healed (or patched up) and developed to maturity, but cannot be essentially remade. Today, however, we must face the questions, Is it right for us to become our own creators? Can we and should we remake human nature? (Packard, 1977). Can we hasten the processes of evolution by eliminating our troublesome wisdom teeth or our appendix by genetic engineering, or least by some type of surgery at a very early age, before trouble arises? Might we in the future greatly reduce the complexities of the digestive system which so often becomes diseased and feed human beings in some simpler way, perhaps by a more effective intravenous method? Might we sterilize all human beings and reproduce artificially? Robert Francoeur (1972b) has answered that because "we can, we must," and calls this the "technological imperative."

In this chapter we will first discuss organ transplants which are already a partially successful means of patching up the body including the special case of transsexual surgery and then in the latter part of he chapter will discuss more briefly the issues that radical reconstruction by surgery or genetic engineering may raise in the future.

We here enter into issues which are largely futuristic, but which by no means can we now ignore, since the first steps are already being taken into this forbidding if not forbidden territory. Three levels of physical remaking are possible. (1) We can use surgical procedures which would replace existing organs with transplants, biological constructs, or artificial organs which are not mere substitutes for natural organs but which expand old or introduce new functions into the body. We have given the examples of replacing the digestive system with a new way of nourishing the body and of eliminating much of the reproductive system and producing children in a test tube and incubating them in an artificial womb. We might also mention possibilities of expanding the human senses so as to make it possible for us to see or hear beyond the present or upper range of sight and vision. (2) We might influence embryological development by drugs so as to mold the development of the phenotype (the actual body) while not changing the genotype (inherited characteristics). Thus conceivably the phenotypic sex of a child could be determined at will in spite of the genotype by altering the course of development very early in embryonic life. (3) Ultimately we may be able to employ genetic engineering to actually produce any gene combination in the fertilized ovum that we desire, thus creating human beings by "recipe." Related to this is the production of clones from the somatic cells of a parent or artificial reproduction of multiple individuals all having the same genetic composition.

The basic ethical issue, here, is seen by some theologians to be the question of the extent of man's dominion over nature. This is a classical way of posing the issue, but it is perhaps too much influenced by the Greek image of God as a jealous monarch who becomes angry when Prometheus infringes on his prerogatives. Others would see such attempts to improve on man as an insult to the work of the Creator whose masterpiece is man or at least as a fatal temptation to pride (Ellul, 1965).

Today, however, in considering radical human development, we need to stress two theological points. (1) God is a generous Creator, who in creating us also called us (by gift of intelligence) to share in his creative power. Consequently, God does not want us to leave fallow the talents He has given us, but encourages us to improve on the universe He has made. (2) Such improvement is possible because theology can accept the idea that God has made an evolutionary universe in which man has been created through an evolutionary process that is not yet complete. Thus God has called man to join with God in bringing the universe to its completion and in doing this He has not made man merely a workman to execute God's orders, or to add trifling original touches on his own, but has made him a genuine co-worker and encourages him to exercise real originality.

Granted this view, however, it is not so clear that the remaking of man's body on new lines is really the appropriate place for man's creativity. We have enough to do remolding our environment and creating human culture. No doubt with greater knowledge we may be able to tidy up some of the business of evolution by removing such vestiges as our wisdom teeth or appendix if, indeed (which is not really known for sure), this would be a real improvement. Some day we may also be able to eliminate genetic disease and even advance human health eugenically. However, we must remember that our human creativity depends upon our human brain. Any alteration of man that would injure the brain and hence his very creativity would indeed be a disastrous mutilation, especially if this were to be transmitted genetically, thus further polluting the gene pool with defects which might be hidden and incalculable.

It is generally admitted that our knowledge of this wonderful brain is still in its beginnings (Rose, 1973; ITEST, 1975). The complexity of the brain is beyond any other system which we can imagine, and this complexity is reduced to a relatively very small organ capable of self-development from the embryo and of self-maintenance, but not of self-restoration. Our brain may be near the limit of complexity and integration possible in an organic, living system. In this case any radical improvement may be illusory, while even slight alterations may be very damaging. Thus, to say the least, radical attempts to alter the structure of the human brain must be viewed with the utmost caution, since the risk is very high that we will only produce persons of lowered intelligence.

This is certainly not so true of other organ systems, and it is possible to imagine that someday in other environments it might become necessary, for example, to replace the human lungs with other ways of obtaining oxygen. In principle it would seem that such changes would be ethical (1) if they gave support to human intelligence by helping the life of the brain and (2) if they did not suppress any of the fundamental human functions that integrate the human personality. Thus alterations that would make it impossible for a human being to directly sense the external world at least as effectively as we now do with our "five senses" would be contrary to the Principle of Totality and Integrity (2.4). So would alterations which would make it impossible for human beings to experience the basic emotions since emotional life is closely related to human intelligence and creativity. Again, alterations which would make human beings sexless and incapable of parenthood would also be antihuman.

We can draw the following conclusions:

1. Genetic engineering and less radical transformations of the present normal human body would be permissible if they improve rather than mutilate the basic human functions, especially as they relate to supporting human intelligence and creativity. Transformation would be forbidden, however, (a) if human intelligence and creativity are endangered and (b) if the fundamental functions which constitute human integrity are suppressed.

2. Experimental efforts of this radical type must be undertaken with great caution and only on the basis of existing knowledge, not with high risks to the subjects or to the gene pool.

11.2 ORGAN TRANSPLANTATION

Any surgical procedure involves some reconstruction of the human body, but there is a striking difference between procedures such as setting a broken bone or sewing up a wound or removing a tumor, which assist a natural healing process or remove a diseased part, and a procedure by which an organ orginally belonging to another is transplanted into the human body in place of one of its own parts which becomes dysfunctional. The latter procedure involves the rights not of one person but of two and hence raises a new moral question.

Two types of organ transplants are possible, one involving an organ or tissue taken from a dead person and given to a living person and the other involving an organ taken from one living person and given to another living person. When an organ or tissue is taken from the body of a dead person and given to a living person, there is no ethical problem by reason of the transplant. With few exceptions, religious groups as well as Humanistic ethicians have recognized the worth and ethical validity of such transplants (Pius XII, 1956a; Daube, 1964; Simmons, 1973). If some serious question arises concerning this type of transplant, it stems from factors other than the transplant itself. For example, concern has been expressed about the worth of heart transplants, most of it arising either from the great expense of money and personnel involved in a medical procedure that brings very little substantive value to the human society (Fadali, 1973; P. Ramsey, 1970a) or from fear that in some cases the organ donor had not actually expired (P. Williams, 1973). But these concerns are not focused on the transplant as such. Pope Pius XII (1956a) summed up Catholic teaching on transplants involving an organ from a dead person thus:

> A person may will to dispose of his body and to destine it to ends that are useful, morally irreproachable and even noble, among them the desire to aid the sick and suffering. One may make a decision of this nature with respect to his own body with full realization of the reverence which is due it . . . this decision should not be condemned but positively justified." (n. 646)

However, there are far more difficulties and less consensus concerning an organ transplant between living persons. Although transplants of other organs such as the heart, liver, and pancreas have been attempted, only kidney transplants have become numerous, and "nonrenal human solid organ grafting must still be considered experimental rather than truly therapeutic" (Amos, 1973). The first successful kidney transplant was done in 1954 and by 1977 a total of 24,193 such transplants have been performed involving 19,631 patients (Rapaport, 1977). Those alive today with kidney transplants number some 13,000 persons. Prior to 1950, the morality of transplanting an organ from one living person to another was discussed by Catholic theologians from a theoretical point of view (Cunningham, 1944). Although an interesting question, it was an impractical question because transplants between living persons were contemplated but not yet possible. Most theologians who considered the subject did not approve of it. These theologians argued that the Principle of Totality would justify mutilation or injury to one part of the body provided it was done in order to preserve the person's own health or human life. However, the principle would not justify transplants between living people because one person is not related to another person as means to end or as part to whole. Thus, one person's bodily integrity could not be sacrificed for another. Although they could not use the Principle of Totality, other theologians sought other ways to justify transplantation (Kelly, 1956).

Whatever the theoretical discussions, organ transplants from living donors were performed in the early 1950s. Although many of these early transplants were not successful because the transplanted organ was rejected by the immunization reactions of the recipient's system, it was clear that organ transplants were a reality. Scientists began to argue that unless there is freedom to undertake such daring experiments medical progress will be hampered (Fox and Zwazey, 1970). Hence, ethicians and moralists gave the problem closer scrutiny.

Gerald Kelly (1956), a leader in this development, wrote, "It may come as a surprise to physicians that theologians should have any difficulty about mutilations and other procedures which are performed with the consent of the subject but which have as their purpose the helping of others. By a sort of instinctive judgment we consider that the giving of a part of one's body to help a sick man is not only morally justifiable, but, in some instances, actually heroic" (p. 246). In developing the rationale for a more liberal opinion, Kelly maintained, "It is clear from reason and papal teaching that the principle of totality cannot be used to justify the donating of a part of one's body to another person." Moreover, he acknowledged, "It is also clear from reason and papal teaching that, since man is only the administrator of his life and bodily members and functions, his power to dispose of these things is limited." But he sought to delineate as clearly as possible the limits of this dominion, especially insofar as organ transplants are concerned.

Hence, Kelly asked, is there any other way in which this seemingly worthwhile and Christian action could be justified? He suggested that the principle of fraternal love, or charity (cf. our Principle of Common Good, Subsidiarity, and Functionalism [6.1], would justify the transplant provided that there was only limited harm to the donor. Although it was not unanimously accepted, some theologians agreed with this opinion and expounded upon it. Distinguishing between anatomical integrity and functional integrity, they stated that the latter, not the former, was necessary in order to ensure human or bodily integrity (McFadden, 1977). Anatomical integrity refers to the material or physical integrity of the human body. Functional integrity refers to the systematic efficiency of the human body. For example, if one kidney were missing from a person's body, there would be a lack of anatomical integrity, but if one healthy kidney were present and working, there would be functional integrity because one healthy kidney is more than able to provide systemic efficiency. If a cornea were to be taken from the eye of one living person and given to another, however, the case would be different. Not only would anatomical integrity be destroyed, but functional integrity would be destroyed as well. The loss of sight in one eye severely damages vision, especially insofar as depth perception is concerned. Hence, in this case more than anatomical integrity is involved.

This distinction between anatomical and functional integrity which we have incorporated in our formulation of the Principle of Totality and Integrity (2.4) explains why the Church has approved blood transfusions and skin grafts and why theologians have approved elective appendectomy if the abdominal cavity is open for another legitimate reason. In these situations, loss of anatomical integrity may occur through loss of blood, skin tissue, or an internal organ, but no loss of functional integrity occurs.

Thus the concept of functional integrity is the key factor in addressing the morality of transplants between living persons. Certainly, a risk is involved if a donor surrenders an organ to another person, even if the donor has two of them. Aside from the risk involved in the surgical procedure, such donors take the risk of serious illness themselves if the one remaining organ becomes damaged or diseased. But the risk, although serious, is thought to be justified by the fact that donors share in the common good of the community to which they contribute by helping another, that is, by love (cf. P. Ramsey, 1970b).

Clearly, organ donation is not an obligation (Daube, 1969); rather it is something chosen in the freedom of charity (P. Ramsey, 1970b; Rappaport, 1973). Motivated by the same charity, one could decide not to offer an organ. Such a decision would not be unethical. For this reason, it is imperative that a donor's free and informed consent be obtained (3.4). Given the fact that the more successful transplants are between members of the same family, familial or social pressure to offer oneself as a donor may at times be severe (Bernstein and Simmons, 1975; Greenberg et al., 1973). Physicians who perform transplants sometimes assure greater freedom to family members by declaring them physiologically unacceptable if they are reluctant to offer their organs (Haney, 1973).

About half the kidney transplants in the United States are derived from cadavers; the other half are derived from living donors, usually members of the same family. Transplants from living donors are far more successful. Whether this is because the living donor is usually a relative, and thus has a similar genetic disposition, or for some other reason is not clear. The technique of using cadaver kidneys should be concentrated on and perfected. In this way, the very difficult question of ensuring free and informed consent will be eliminated and the risks that are incumbent upon donors will be lessened. One aid to increasing the supply of renal transplants from cadavers is the donation of organs in accord with the Uniform Anatomical Gift Act (Sadler, 1968). Enacted in all fifty states, this legislation allows persons to will their organs to others after death by signing a statement to that effect. Naturally, this practice is acceptable and even laudable from a moral point of view.

We agree with Kelly and others that organ transplants between two living persons are licit if functional integrity is maintained in the donor, but we would caution that when assessing the risk-benefit ratio clear thought to be given to the risk and to the potential benefit. Consent should not be given unless the prognosis is good. Many recipients of kidney transplants, for example, die within a short time even if the transplant is "successful" (Rappaport, 1977). Therefore, it is necessary to weigh the value of such a brief prolongation of life against the life-long risk to the donor.

In addition to the rationale put forward by Kelly and others to justify transplants between living persons, some Catholic theologians go a step farther and seek to justify these procedures either by expanding the Principle of Totality or by treating the whole process as a curative action, even though two people are involved and one will be injured (Nolan, 1968). In so doing, they destroy the limits so carefully delineated by Kelly and others to protect human integrity. The human unity predicated on body and soul is destroyed according to these theories, and the body becomes something used by the person, some of which is at the disposal or "over against" the person and thus may be sacrificed by the person for any higher good. Falling heir to Cartesian dualism that makes appreciation of the body-soul unity of human nature impossible, one author even concludes that both eyes may be given to the disposal of, or "over against," the person and thus may be sacrificed why we believe such views do not do justice to the Christian view of the integrity of the human person (cf. P. Ramsey, 1970b).

The development in the last thirty years of the moral teaching of theologians concerning organ transplants between the living is of more than antiquarian interest. First of all, it shows clearly that the opinion of theologians can develop. Second, it shows that by refining accepted principles, and not by denying them, a way can be found to prove new positions. Third, it demonstrates that most ethical problems are solved by starting with intuitive judgments and then examining the principles in light of the solution proposed in the intuitive judgment.

Finally, it should be noted that the arguments for the gift of human body parts lose their force when it is a question of sale, even the sale of blood (Titmus, 1973; "Sale of Human Body," 1974). Such a sale is ethically objectionable for two reasons: (1) it is contrary to the dignity of the human body and depersonalizing, and (2) those who need such a gift should receive it, rather than only those who can pay.

In summary, the transplanting of organs or tissues from a dead person to a living person does not offer any intrinsic ethical problem. Transplanting organs from one living person to another is also ethically acceptable provided that the following criteria are met:

1. There is a serious need on the part of the recipient that cannot be fulfilled in any other way.

2. The functional integrity of the human person will not be impaired, even though anatomical integrity may suffer.

3. The risk taken by the donor as an act of charity is proportionate to the good resulting for the recipient.

4. The donor's consent is free and informed.

11.3 SEXUAL REASSIGNMENT

A special type of reconstructive surgery which has been recently introduced is transsexual surgery. Such surgery, along with hormonal treatment and psychotherapy, is part of the procedure of sexual reassignment which has been developed as a way of dealing with the puzzling and painful condition called transsexualism or more accurately gender dysphoria syndrome. Such procedures raise the ethical question of whether it is within the scope of medical care to attempt to change a person's biological sex for the sake of the good of the whole person.

Transsexualism is used as a diagnosis in medicine even though it has no definite meaning. In general, transsexualism is "a condition in which there is apparent psychological and social identification with attributes of the opposite sex" (Meyer, 1974). But there are no definite medical symptoms, nor is there a known dynamic that gives rise to symptoms, nor is there a known etiology for the diagnosis (Fisk, 1973). In spite of the ambiguity concerning this "disease," people are said to be transsexual, and the transsexual surgery performed is supposed to alleviate or cure this condition (Feinbloom, 1976).

Transsexual surgery, or sexual reassignment, has become more common in the past ten years. Although the procedure is performed at some fifteen different centers in the United States (Leff, 1977), the pioneer and renowned center for treatment and surgery for transsexualism is the Gender Identity Clinic at Johns Hopkins University School of Medicine, founded in 1966. About nine out of ten people who are patients at this clinic are males who wish to have the physical characteristics of a female. In either case, the patient's sexual organs are restructured to resemble the sexual organs of the other gender (Markland, 1975). However, a complete change in physical gender is not achieved. The male transsexual can neither ovulate nor conceive a child, and the female transsexual cannot generate sperm. The simulation of external sexual organs from male to female is much easier than vice versa, and both are accomplished through surgery and continuous use of synthetic hormones. The surgery may entail considerable risks of failure or complications requiring more than one operation, and the hormonal treatment runs the risk of breast cancer (Markland, 1975).

Each applicant at the clinic receives physiological and psychological testing, and only those who have lived for a time as transsexuals and who have no apparent signs of psychosis are accepted as candidates for sex alteration (Meyer, 1974). Precautions are taken to ensure free and informed consent. Often the chief motivating factor on the part of the patient requesting the procedure is a desire to perform sexual acts in a manner congruent to the opposite sex. The desire to dress or live as a member of the opposite sex, which characterizes some transsexuals, can sometimes be satisfied without surgery.

Someone suffering from this syndrome sometimes conceives of himself as a "woman in a male body." Such a dualistic notion which seems to identify personhood with a soul emprisoned in the body is philosophically false. Nor can we agree with some authors (Dedek, 1975) who seem to accept without question the possibility that a person can have the true psychological identity of one sex and the physical identity of the other. Even the present director of the Gender Identity Clinic, J. K. Meyer (1974), states, "I have seen any number of men who would like to live as female and vice versa; I have never seen one with a reversal of core gender identity" (p. 278).

Undoubtedly sexual identity is not only a physical fact, but an aspect of self-identity, that is, a person's consciousness of who he or she is in relation to other persons (Sapp, 1977). However, we ordinarily judge the psychological normality of human perceptions and feelings by their congruence with physical reality, so that we identify ourselves first of all by our bodily identity, and when our feelings and fantasies are incongruent with physical reality, we judge that we suffer from some degree of mental disturbance and illusion. Few psychotherapists would treat their patients by trying to make reality congruent with the patient's illusions, rather than vice versa. It seems, therefore, that however sympathetic we may be with persons who report they *really* are of another sex than their body we do them no favor by helping them live out this illusion. If Meyer is correct, then it is *prima facie* unlikely that persons who experience psychic anguish because of this feeling of incongruence can ever achieve permanent relief by an effort to realize their fantasies.

The causes of transsexualism are not known. Research indicates that transsexuals as a group have not been shown to differ genetically, hormonely, or anatomically from normal persons (Money, 1971). In general, psychological gender identity arises from many factors: genetic complement, familial experience, anatomy, sex assignment, and influence of being reared as a boy or a girl. Often childhood trauma or parental influence disposes one toward a transsexual personality (R. Green, 1974).

Transsexualism or gender dysphoria is a grave and painful malady and people with this condition should be treated with great compassion. Moreover, the increase of people with this condition demonstrates the need to develop a well-balanced sense of personal identity in young people. Through psychiatric or psychological care, readjustment of this condition can be successful, especially if the person being treated is still young. According to one study, treatment for young people should follow this pattern: (1) selection of a therapist of the same sex as the disordered child, (2) involvement of the parents in the treatment program, (3) consistent disapproval of the cross-gender behavior and consistent approval of sex-appropriate behavior, and (4) continuous effort toward shoring up the family role of the same sex parent and his relationship with the dysfunctional child (Green, 1974).

Some phychiatrists regard the person with a transsexual personality as severely disturbed and emotionally immature. They interpret the patient's request for removal of the sexual organs to be self-mutilating, masochistic, and suicidal (Meerlo, 1967). Psychiatrists who share this view urge surgeons not to join in the patient's delusions by performing sex-reassignment surgery.

On the other hand, when psychological or psychiatric treatment does not seem effective, other psychiatrists recommend the surgical procedure just referred to. One physician (R. Green, 1970) has stated, "The critical question is no longer whether sex reassignment for adults should be permitted but rather for whom." Those who hold this position argue that some help is given to transsexuals through this procedure in that they suffer less from internal conflict and are able to adjust better to society. Proving that better adjustment takes place is rather difficult, however, and as one expert (Meyer, 1974) states, "Transsexual surgery, even in the most difficult case of gender dysphoria, must be recognized as palliative, rather than curative."

Those Catholic theologians who follow the principle of proportion or a theology of compromise solve cases of this sort by evaluating the proportion between the good and bad consequences of this procedure. At this level, it is very difficult to make a judgment because we are dealing with a relatively new and experimental mode of treatment. Those engaged in the experiment have invested a good deal of concern and reputation in its results and are perhaps somewhat biased in their claim for good results, as is so often the case with new therapies.

In many cases, even with data which seem to show that sexual re-assignment is successful, the ethician has to ask questions about the criteria of evaluating the success. Can we really say that a former male transsexual who could only find sexual satisfaction in promiscuous sexual contacts and who now feels happier with the same pattern of promiscuity is better off as a person because he is now psychologically more comfortable? For such data to have much ethical meaning, it would be necessary to decide not merely whether after the treatment these persons are more comfortable, but also whether they are less compulsive and more in control of their actions and more morally responsible about them. Sound psychological therapy is not aimed merely at comfort or adjustment, but at helping the patient face the world with realism and an enhanced freedom of choice. Today, the published data do not permit us to come to conclusions about these questions. What we do know is that the best centers engaging in sexual reassignment reject almost eighty percent of those applying and do not report a very great success with the twenty percent selected. Does this not suggest that even after this selection the risks are so high that there is no proportion justifying the taking of such risks, which are not only psychological but medical (Markland, 1975)?

From the viewpoint taken in this book, however, there are other considerations than a balancing of success and failure defined in such terms. If we hold that homosexual acts are objectively speaking intrinsically wrong, then we must ask whether in fact such surgery is merely a kind of facilitation of such acts.

Of course there is no ethical objection to operations performed on persons whose biological sex is ambiguous when the purpose is to improve sexual identity in favor of what seems to be the predominant sex of the person, a matter which is not always easy to decide because of the numerous types of genetic hormonal defects in sexual development which have been discovered (Leff, 1977). If this predominance cannot be determined, then either sexual role can be selected, although today sex determined genetically would seem to give the most definite answer.

However, when the person is biologically of one sex, but claims to be psychologically of the other sex, it would seem that the following conclusions can be made. (1) The treatment is not properly psychotherapeutic, since it yields to the neurotic illusions of the patient rather than attempts to ameliorate them. (2) As one author (McFadden, 1967) says, "To destroy wholly healthy organs in the body and to supplant them with imitation 'organs' . . . is a gross and grotesque form of mutilation" (p. 283). (3) The result does not cure the psychological abnormality of gender dysphoria. (4) The newly created "male" is not given the sexual potency necessary for a valid marriage and the newly created "female" is not capable of children, not merely because of sterility, but because of a radical incapacity which would also invalidate marriage. The surgery is correctly considered a mutilation in the strict sense because it destroys the bodily integrity of individuals with regard to a basic function, rendering them permanently sterile.

Thus it seems this type of surgery is intrinsically outside the limits of ethical medicine since its purpose is not genuine treatment of a psychological illness, but an illusory adjustment involving a destructive loss of bodily integrity.

Undoubtedly those who have undertaken this type of work have done so out of compassion for the very genuine suffering of the psychologically disturbed patient tormented by compulsion and sometimes threatening suicide. On a theory of compromise (Curran, 1977a), it may be said that at least a percentage of sufferers may be relieved of incapacitating anxieties and adjusted better to life. However, to follow such procedures cooperates with illusion and magical thinking which we should not encourage in any sufferer and certainly not in society. The fact that even those who advocate such surgery find it prudent to reject eighty percent of the applicants seems to indicate how quick troubled people are to place their hope in medical miracles which are at best of doubtful efficacy.

11.4 GENETIC SCREENING AND COUNSELING

Screening

The medical speciality of diagnosing inherited or genetic defects and their treatment, as well as the task of screening populations for these defects, and of counseling couples who are or may become parents of defective children is developing rapidly, and special institutes dedicated to it are being founded throughout the United States (Powledge, 1973; Epstein, 1975).

Three basic discoveries have made it possible to predict the sex and inherited traits of a child from the moment of conception (Reisman, 1969; Bergsma, 1972, 1973). These discoveries are as follows: (1) Gregor Mendel's theory of the laws of the combinations of units of inheritance, (2) the fact that these units or *genes* are located in the chromosomes of the nucleus of every cell, and (3) the fact that the genetic code consists in variations in a fundamental substance, deoxyribonucleic acid (DNA), out of which the genes are composed. Techniques of diagnosing these defects at early stages of child development are being perfected, such as *amniocentesis* by which the genetic condition of the unborn child can be determined in some respects by examining the amniotic fluid in which the fetus floats in the womb. Also techniques to counteract some of the deleterious consequences of genetic defects are being worked out, and there is even prospect of methods for correcting the defective genes themselves.

Why such advances are medically important is evident from the following statistics (Osmundsen, 1973):

> . . . there are now almost 2,000 verified or suspected single-gene defects, and each of us carries between five and eight mutant lethal equivalents (genes), which we are all able to transmit to subsequent generations.

Thus, we are all mutants, in the strictest sense, although only about 5 percent to 8 percent of us actually manifest some form of genetic mutation. An estimated 0.4 percent of all live births are attended by chromosomal imbalances such as trisomies and chromosome maldistributions . . . Three-quarters of these, or 0.29 percent, are deleterious defects. (Also, an estimated 9 percent of all early embryos are chromosomally abnormal, most of them lethally so.) Major single-gene mutations — homozygous and heterozygous — such as the autosomal dominants and recessives and the x-linked disorders occur in 1.8 percent of the general population. The polygenic conditions such as diabetes mellitus, gout, and some allergies occur in 1.7 percent to 2.6 percent of all live births. (These figures appear to remain fairly constant throughout the globe.) Add the figures, and we have the 4.8 percent to 5 percent incidence of genetic disease in all live births. (p. 27)

In view of these facts some scientists in the name of preventive medicine advocate *genetic screening* of the whole population for four purposes: (1) for scientific research, since such research is necessary if we are to achieve full understanding and control over human inheritance; (2) to assist responsible parenthood so that carriers of genetic defects may not pass them on; (3) to make possible early therapy before the malfunctioning of defective genes has caused extensive damage; and (4) to give the parents the option of aborting the child when the defect is serious and no therapy is yet known (cf. Gaylin, 1973a; Lappé, et. al. 1974a; Singer, 1974).

We have already given reasons why this last purpose is ethically unacceptable, but the first three are certainly legitimate. However, they raise serious questions (Emery, 1973, 1974, 1975). First of all, the research purposes of genetic screening must be regulated in the same way as any other kind of experimentation on human subjects (cf. 9.4). Thus it would seem that since amniocentesis involves significant risk (at least in one percent of the cases) it cannot be used for research purposes unless there are also proportionate benefits for the fetus. However, most screening techniques used postnatally only involve the withdrawal of an insignificant amount of body fluid or tissue and are harmless. Nevertheless, informed consent is required in all such cases, and it is highly questionable that it is legitimate to enact laws which require compulsory screening for research purposes alone. Even when consent is given, care must be taken about how the information is used. If the results are made known to subjects, there is danger that they may misunderstand or exaggerate the seriousness and possible consequences of their condition or the condition of their children. If the results are known to others, there is danger of stigmatization, that is, that victims will be regarded by others as humanly inferior or dangerous. For example, it is unfair to label blacks who are carriers of the sickle-cell trait diseased or defective or carriers.

Second, the use of screening to promote responsible parenthood is in general a laudable purpose, since there can be no doubt that couples should not bring into the world children for whom (with the reasonable assistance of society) they cannot adequately care, and the care of defective children presents special burdens. Consequently, prospective parents have the duty to seek the scientific information useful to such decisions, and society has the duty to assist them in obtaining such information (Kushnick, 1976). We have already noted (10.2) that the right of married couples to beget children is conditioned by their capability to provide for them.

Nevertheless, caution is necessary in the face of programs of *negative* eugenics advocated by certain enthusiasts (Osmundsen, 1973; Glass, 1975) who argue that modern medicine has upset the ecological balance by saving the lives of more and more defective persons who would formerly have died before they could reproduce. Thus the genetic load of defective genes in the gene pool is increasing, and we may soon be faced with a much higher level of genetic disease in the population. However, as Marc Lappé (1972a) has written:

> The consensus of the best medical and genetic opinion is that whatever genetic deterioration is occurring as a result of decreased natural selection is so slow as to be insignificant when contrasted to "environmental" changes, including those produced by medical innovation. (p. 421)

If we prevent only those persons who themselves suffer from a particular genetic disease from reproducing, this still does not eliminate heterozygous carriers who will continue to transmit defects dependent on recessive genes. At present we are far from being able to detect all these carriers. Even if we had this ability, not only would such elimination extend to a great number of people, but would probably also mean the elimination from the gene pool of many desirable traits since the same persons carry both good and bad traits which sometimes are genetically linked in ways still very obscure to us. Thus programs of negative eugenics based on present knowledge would achieve their goals only very slowly, over many generations, and might have side effects worse than the evils they remedy. Moreover, as defective genes are eliminated from the gene pool, they are constantly being replaced by mutations caused by environmental factors.

It seems, therefore, that such information cannot be used to compel persons to refrain from reproduction, but it may be supplied to them to enable them to make responsible personal decisions (Annas, 1975; Frankel, 1974). Even here, however, there needs to be some public caution (Murray, 1972). Some states have adopted compulsory screening of newborn infants to detect those afflicted with phenylketonuria (PKU), a genetically based metabolic disease which results in mental retardation and which can be treated by diet. After these programs were instituted, it was discovered that some persons who test positively do not develop mental retardation, and that the dietary treatment to which they were subjected may even have been harmful (W. J. Curran, 1974a; Lappé et al., 1974). Thus such programs have to be carefully designed. A task force of the Institute of Society, Ethics and the Life Sciences (1972) has suggested guidelines which can be summarized as follows:

1. The attainability of the aims of the program should be pretested by pilot projects and other studies and the program should be constantly evaluated and updated.

2. Community participation in planning and executing the program should be secured to educate the public as to the true significance and legitimate use of the information obtained.

3. The information obtained should be made available according to clearly stated policies known to those participating before they consent, and their privacy should be carefully protected.

4. Screening programs should be voluntary. The rights of parents to make their own decisions about the use of the information in family planning should be protected and care taken to avoid stigmatizing them or their offspring.

5. Information about screening should be open and available to all, with priorities given to well-defined populations suffering from frequent defects.

6. Programs should not be instituted unless the tests used are able to give relatively unambiguous information and this should be precisely recorded.

7. The general principles with regard to experimentation with human subjects, such as informed consent, protection from risks, and so forth, should be observed.

8. Persons to be screened or have their children screened should be informed before they consent as to the nature and cost of therapy and its risks or that no therapy is available.

9. Counseling to help the subjects understand and deal with the information should be provided.

We would also add that it is important to consider whether the cost in money and personnel in administering such programs give them high priority in view of the rarity of most of these conditions. However, it must be recognized that in some cases (PKU, for example) the testing per subject is quite inexpensive, while the cost of caring for even a few mentally retarded children in institutions may be very high.

Counseling

If such screening programs are to be voluntary, then the question becomes chiefly that of counseling parents as they attempt to decide how to use this information in planning their families (Motulsky, 1974).

A family comes to a genetic counselor because of fears about possible defects in children already in existence or about their responsibilities for future pregnancies (Lebel, 1977; Fraser, 1974; M. G. Wilson, 1975). These fears may have arisen because of positive test results in mass screening, or because of a record of genetic disease in parents, previous children, or near relatives (Gordon, 1971; G. Smith et al., 1971).

Some argue that if serious reasons exist to believe a fetus is gravely defective, the parents should be persuaded to agree to abort the child if this suspicion is confirmed by amniocentesis (John Fletcher, 1972). Otherwise it is hard to justify the risks (perhaps one percent chance of death) of the amniocentesis procedure. Granted that abortion is ethically unacceptable, the counselor should not recommend amniocentesis unless it is justified by the possibility of intrauterine therapy of some type proportionate to the risks — a possibility which at present is still largely theoretical. Nor is this risk justified by the hope of saving the parents anxiety, a hope which may not be realized.

Again, some counselors would suggest that even when amniocentesis cannot determine genetic defect with certainty, the parents should be left to decide whether they wish to take the risks or to abort (cf. Lappé, 1971, 1973; Lappé and Brody, 1977). This means that if they decide to abort they are also risking the destruction of a normal child since such tests are not infallible, nor do they perfectly predict the degree of phenotypic impairment. We believe that counselors not only should not recommend abortion as a solution, but also that they should compassionately persuade the parents to find another solution. If the parents declare a firm intention to abort, the counselor should not cooperate in any way with them. The reason is that the rights of the fetus to life should be protected by counselors, exactly as they would protect the rights of a child already born against the infringement of these rights by the parents, however well intentioned they may be. However, a counselor in doing whatever possible to avoid abortion should exercise great prudence, avoiding threats, pressures, and recriminations because they will only aggravate the situation. The counselor should respect the conscience of the parents while doing everything possible to protect the child.

We may agree with Margery W. Shaw (1974), Director of the Medical Genetics Center, University of Texas, when she writes:

> Professionals in general, and physicians in particular, tend to adopt a paternalistic attitude in dealing with patients or experimental subjects or relatives. But only those who desire "parenting" will blindly follow another's advice. The rest will be influenced to a greater or less degree by the prescriptions of the counselor who is directive rather than permissive. Those who would argue that the counselee needs protection from directive counseling are themselves being paternalistic. (p. 251)

However, Shaw is overly optimistic when she also writes:

> I am not afraid that genetic screening will lead to genocide, nor that

> abortion will lead to infanticide, as many have warned. If we need checks
> on our behavior the law will provide them. (p. 251)

The law once prevented abortion as a form of infanticide and genocide.
Today the law has been reinterpreted by the Supreme Court in the
opposite sense. The law is only as firm in its protection of human rights
as are the convictions of the public about who and who not is the subject
of such rights, and the attitudes promoted by health care professionals
are influential in changing these convictions (cf. 9.5).

Is it permissible for a counselor to give information to parents whom
the counselor only suspects may resort to abortion? In the present
ethical climate this suspicion always exists, and it has deterred Catholic
health care facilities from instituting genetic counseling centers. However, parents have a right to such information which has good as well
as bad uses, and the counselor who supplies it cooperates only materially
and remotely if the parents use it for a purpose which the counselor
considers unethical. In our opinion Catholic health care facilities have
a duty to provide such counseling in accordance with Christian moral
standards, since otherwise parents will be forced to obtain information
from centers where abortion will be an accepted and even encouraged
solution. For reasons already given in 9.2 we reject such arguments
as that of Bentley Glass (1972) who writes:

> Is it not equally a right of every person to be born physically and
> mentally sound, capable of developing fully into a mature individual?
> Has society, which must support at great cost the burden of genetic
> misfortune resulting from mutation, chromosomal accident, and prenatal
> harm inflicted by trauma or virus no right at all to protect itself from
> the increasing misfortune? Should not the abortion of a seriously de-
> fective fetus be obligatory? Should not the loss of a defective child be
> recompensed by the opportunity to have another, a sound child by
> prenatal or postnatal adoption? (p. 252)

It certainly is a right for a child to be free of every defect which we
have the power to prevent or correct. But it is paradoxical to believe
that this right is protected by destroying the child whom we have not
been able to save from defect. Glass is really talking about the concern
of the parents and society to save themselves from the burden of defective
children. Parents may have the responsibility not to produce such
children, but having produced them they also have the duty to care
for them, and they cannot lighten their burden by destroying the unborn
child any more than an infant or adolescent. Underlying such arguments
is the basic conviction that it is better never to be than to be a defective.
This is an assumption of some Humanists, but it is not consistent with
a Christian view of the value of a person.

However, it remains true that couples have the duty of responsible
parenthood, and society has a legitimate concern to support and encourage this responsibility. The genetic counselor, therefore, has the
function of helping prospective parents prepare themselves for the
possibility that a fetus will be defective and to plan ways to provide

for this eventuality. The counselor also has the task of helping them decide whether they will run the risk of future pregnancies or of helping single persons to decide whether or whom they will or will not marry.

In the past some would have argued that a person or a couple at risk of begetting a defective child or children or of transmitting defective genes to future generations should fatalistically marry and beget children, and "leave it to God." This fatalism, as we have already pointed out, has not been as damaging to society as some eugentic enthusiasts have thought, since it does not upset the ecological balance established by evolutionary selection. Even today when medical advances have upset this balance by counteracting this selective process such fatalism can only very slowly increase the social burden about which Bently Glass is so concerned. Nevertheless, Christian teaching does not favor fatalistic attitudes, but advocates parental responsibility.

Prospective parents, therefore, have to consider these factors: (1) their own need to have children as the completion of their mutual love, (2) their own capacity to care for these children, and (3) the risks that each particular child may suffer from grave handicaps which require special care, including the possibility that this child will be faced in its turn with the question as to whether he or she should pass on defective genes to the next generation. Some significant risks of defect exist for *every* child and could not be eliminated even by the most radical use of abortion. Thus in all cases of parenthood it is a question of the relative balance of risk of defect in proportion to parental capacity to care, as Lappé (1972a) has stressed. Furthermore, it is the duty of the counselor and of society to assist the parents in accepting and meeting reasonable risks. For counselors or society at large to encourage in parents the attitude that they should not have children unless the children are perfect and require the least care possible is as reprehensible as to encourage parents to reproduce fatalistically.

Certainly, the correct professional attitude for genetic counselors is to give the parents reliable, objective information as to the probabilities of defect and its consequences and the type of therapy and care which will be required. Counselors should also help them (directly or by referral to others professionally competent) to deal with personal, economic, and social factors which determine the parents' capacity to meet the demands of care if a child has a particular defect and the social resources which may be available to help. On the basis of this objective information and counseling support the individual or couple must make their own decision about whether their need for children justifies taking the risks involved (Pearn, 1973). Such decisions must be made not merely by some persons, but by everyone, since begetting new life is essentially a risky business. The reason that genetic counselors are needed today is that now we have available more information about the risks involved in reproduction and need more help in dealing with the complexities this information discloses (Veatch, 1972c).

We have already argued in 10.4 that the need and right of a couple to have children is not absolute. Hence if the risks are high, for example, twenty-five percent, of begetting a child so defective as to require care that the parents, even with reasonable and available social assistance, cannot supply, then they have the responsibility not to beget such a child and are required to use methods of birth regulation which are licit to prevent this. Counselors, therefore, should do what they can, while respecting the consciences and psychological freedom of their clients, to dissuade persons at this high risk from reproducing and should see they are properly informed about the various available methods of birth regulation, especially natural family planning and the ethical evaluation of these methods (10.3).

Problems also arise with regard to adults who have a genetic defect which will eventually become a serious handicap or lead to early death, for example, Huntington's chorea which in middle life results in progressive neurological degeneration. On the one hand is the responsibility of the person not to pass this defect on to children and on the other, the personal difficulty of living under a sense of doom. Undoubtedly as people become more aware of the existence of genetic defects, it will become impossible to keep such knowledge from individuals. It would seem that all individuals should have the freedom to decide whether they wish a diagnosis. Nevertheless, we would argue that individuals who seriously suspect they have such serious defects would be wise to have the matter settled by a reliable test and to adjust their life plans accordingly (Lynch, 1972; Hemphill, 1973; Bok and Lappé, 1974).

At the same time the right of persons to make decisions about reproducing genetic defects should be respected both by the Church and by society, and they should not be stigmatized because of their decision. The reasons are these. (1) The balance of factors cannot be reduced to objective certitude, especially because involved is weighing of personal needs and capacities. (2) The great value of personal responsibility in the use of sex and the living of family life greatly outweigh the damage done society by the increased genetic load which cannot be significantly lightened in the short run, and which we do not yet know how to significantly lighten in the long run. (3) If the parents prove mistaken in their decision, society can and should assume the responsibility for adequate care of the children, a burden which is not great compared to many other health problems. Clearly, if society promotes adequate education about genetic hazards, in our society where the birth rate is low and falling it is probable that negative voluntary eugenics will become a part of our general social pattern. Genetic counseling will promote this, and Catholic genetic counseling will also promote it without encouraging abortion or neglecting the freedom of decision of the parents, while actively promoting a more optimistic and life-affirming attitude toward the inevitable risks of parenthood.

11.5 GENETIC RECONSTRUCTION

Gift or Order

This issue of the parents' need and right to have children or even to *order* the sort of child they want is also at the base of the host of new problems which now loom on the horizon concerning genetic engineering or to use an expression which has less pejorative connotations genetic reconstruction, that is, the effort to repair genetic defects at their genotypic source in the genes and chromosomes rather than in their phenotypic effects and, further, to control and produce at will new combinations of genetic traits in offspring (Etzioni, 1973; "Genetic Engineering," 1974; English, 1974).

The first and probably simplest form of such engineering would be to determine at will the sex of the fetus by selecting sperm which do or do not have the Y chromosome that determines maleness and then using selected sperm for artificial insemination or *in vitro* fertilization and implantation (Lappé and Steinfels, 1974). In 10.4 we have discussed the ethical issues involved in such methods. Even if a technique could be invented which would promote or suppress the production of one or the other type of sperm in the male parent without interfering with the normal process of sexual intercourse, the social and ecological consequences of such intervention could be counterproductive.

Biologists are convinced that evolutionary selection has developed the process of sexual differentiation by a genetic mechanism of the sort we find in the human species because this ensures an approximate fifty-fifty distribution of the sexes. Some additional mechanism not fully understood even produces a slightly higher number of male zygotes to offset the higher mortality of males. Studies made in the United States (Westhoff and Rindfuss, 1974) show that most young couples now want two children, preferring a boy first, but once the boy is assured, then want a girl. These studies predict that if sex selection was widely adopted there would first be a marked rise in male births, but then a levelling to a fifty-fifty distribution. It seems, therefore, that the promotion of sexual selection might not be seriously deleterious to society, although it certainly would have risks and would have few if any social advantages over leaving it to nature. Its only advantage would be that parents would have freedom of choice, provided that overall they use this choice to have equal numbers of boys and girls.

We should ask, however, whether ethically speaking this free choice of a boy or a girl is an advantage to the *child*? After all, parents should not let their subjective preferences operate at the expense of their children in this matter, just as it is unethical for them to insist that the child be a doctor or a lawyer if this is not truly for the best interests of the child. It might be argued that it is some advantage for a boy to have a sister and vice versa, rather than a sibling of his or her own sex, but it would be hard to prove that such an advantage, if it exists, is of major significance. On the other hand, as we argued in 10.2 Christian teaching shows us that it is a major significance to children that they be accepted by their parents as a divine gift to be loved for what they uniquely are and not merely because they conform to the parents' hopes or expectations. At the present time we are becoming more aware of the immense injustice and harm done to women by the fact that our culture has built up patterns and structures which constantly say to a girl, "You should have been a boy." Sex selection by the parents will either reinforce this male preference pattern, or if parents can be reeducated to equal preference, it will still say to the individual child, "You are loved because you conform to your parents' preferences." This seems an injustice to the child and further reinforces the cultural message that children exist primarily to fulfill the needs of the parents rather than for their own sake. This implication is already built into many of our cultural structures, and there is an ethical responsibility to fight against it. The health care profession should discourage such attitudes, not promote techniques to further them.

The same consideration applies to more complex forms of genetic reconstruction. While some progress has already been made in genetic recombination at the level of simple organisms, the possibility of using such methods to correct genetic defects or to create new genetic structures in human zygotes or embryos is still remote (Shinsheimer, 1973; Freidmann and Roblin, 1972; Davis, 1970; Eckhart, 1971; Danielli, 1972).

If the purpose of such techniques is therapy of an individual fetus, the only ethical issue is the proportion of probable benefit to risk. However, the issues already discussed concerning *in vitro* fertilization and artificial insemination and implantation arise if these techniques can be used to produce a healthy embryo only at the expense of creating a number of embryos from which one will be selected and the others allowed to perish (cf. 10.4; Edwards and Fowler, 1970).

What if the purpose is not therapy of an existing fetus, but the production of superior human beings? Two methods have been proposed. One is to replicate many genetically identical individuals by cloning. In such a process nuclei from the somatic cells of a "superior" individual would be transplanted into denucleated ovum which would then develop into an identical twin of the nuclear donor. This would require *in vitro* fertilization and implantation into a foster mother's womb (Watson, 1971; Stinson, 1972). Another method is to recombine genes in the nucleus of a zygote, probably by using viruses which have the capability of incorporating a section of a chromosome derived from one nucleus and fixing it in a chromosome of another (transduction) (Davis, 1970; Eckhart, 1971). Theoretically it may become possible to synthesize chemically new genes which have never existed in the gene pool or to produce them by artificial, controlled mutation. Thus it might be possible to produce a human being according to recipe, with just the height, complexion, physiological traits, and mental abilities which we desire. While this is still very remote (Chakrabarty, 1976; Cohen, 1975), we would not rule it out ethically merely on the grounds that it would be usurpation of God's creative power, since we believe that God wishes to share this creative power with us insofar as we are capable of using it well (Principle of Stewardship and Creativity, 8.3-3).

However, grave ethical difficulties do arise when we ask whether we have either the knowledge or the virtue to take the responsibility for creating these superior members of our race (Gustafson, 1973a, 1973b). Attempts to define *superior* (Shinsheimer, 1973) eugenically are so amgibuous as to be arbitrary. Because humans are evolutionary and historical beings, *superior* does not mean a being with what seems to be superior to one age and culture, but rather a being with capabilities of meeting the challenges of new and unpredicted situations. Genetic variation assists this flexibility, while the production of many identical human beings or of favoring certain supposedly superior types amounts to a restriction on this genetic variability. At the most, a eugenic policy would have to be content with introducing into the gene pool some new, apparently valuable traits or increasing somewhat the percentage of their presence. Furthermore, all the difficulties already raised about the way in which such techniques tend to separate the child from its relations to parents and family arise once more.

The following conclusions can be drawn:

1. It is more feasible, technically and ethically, to improve the human condition by improving the environment and development of the individual, that is, the *phenotype*, than by modifying genetic endowment, that is, the *genotype* and priority in research and investment of medical resources should be given to the former effort. Genetic research is extremely important, however, if we are to understand the interactions of genotype and phenotype (Szebenyi, 1972).

2. Presently proposed methods of genetic reconstruction of human beings involve *in vitro* fertilization and other procedures which are ethically objectionable because they separate reproduction from its parental context and involve the production of human beings some of whom will be defective because of experimental failure and who will probably be destroyed. This contravenes the basic principles of ethical experimentation with human subjects (cf. 9.4; cf. Lappé, 1972b; P. Ramsey, 1970a, 1972; but see also Joseph Fletcher, 1954, 1971a).

3. Proposals to improve the human race by sex selection, cloning, or genetic reconstruction are ethically unacceptable in the present state of our knowledge. Unless limited to very modest interventions, they would restrict the genetic variability important to human survival, and they would separate reproduction from its parental context.

4. If the foregoing problems can be overcome, it will be ethically

desirable to develop and use genetic methods for therapy of genetic defects in existing embryos, keeping in view the risk-benefit proportion (Fackre, 1971).

Apart from efforts to reconstruct human genes, much discussion has been given recently to the possible effects on the ecological balance of experimentation with recombinant deoxyribonucleic acid to produce new forms of life which might have many technological applications: for example, to produce food plants which could directly utilize atmospheric nitrogen and thus eliminate the use of fertilizers. The risk of producing dangerous forms of life against which no natural defenses exist seems real enough. The same basic ethical principles that govern any form of experimentation apply here (9.4) including legal restraints (H. Green, 1973), but at the same time such research should be positively encouraged (Walters, 1972; Lederberg, 1975; Powledge, 1974, 1976; Lappé et al., 1975-1976; Berg et al., 1975).

11.6 SUMMARY

The Principle of Stewardship and Creativity throws light on many of the problems of human reconstruction. We should not conceive of natural law as a fixed pattern of human life to which we are forever confined. Rather, the Creator has made us human beings free and intelligent, and it is precisely this intelligent freedom which *is* our human nature and the foundation of natural moral law. Our human intelligence, however, is not disembodied, but is dependent upon a brain and a body which have a specific structure. In caring for our total health as persons, we not only have the right but the obligation to understand ourselves in our psychological and biological structure and to improve ourselves even in ways that may seem novel to past generations. Such improvement is good stewardship of the share in divine creativity with which God has endowed us.

At the same time, we must use this creativity with profound respect for God's existing creation and especially for our own psychological and biological mode of existence, lest by tampering with our brain or the rest of our personality we should undermine the freedom and intelligence upon which this creativity depends. Consequently, the use of surgery and genetic manipulation to improve our bodies is ethically good, provided that we take full account of such risks and are not carried away by a false ambition to work technical miracles without regard to their real meaning for human living. In particular, Christians should be concerned that such innovations do not weaken the fundamental relations within the family or the sense of the child as a unique gift of God.

CHAPTER 12   PSYCHOTHERAPY AND BEHAVIOR MODIFICATION

12.1   THE CONCEPT OF MENTAL SICKNESS

In dealing with ethical problems in psychiatric medicine a very special problem arises: What is the difference between mental illness and ordinary physical illness? In chapter 2 we have already tried to clarify this point by presenting a four-dimensional model of human personality. In this model the *psychological* dimension is closely interrelated with the *physical* dimension but also clearly distinct from it, as well as from the ethical and spiritual dimensions. The failure in the history of medicine to make these distinctions has been a source of vast confusion, and this remains a source of current controversy (Schwartz, 1974).

Thus a group of antipsychiatry psychiatrists has made a strong, if exaggerated, case against the whole concept of mental illness (Sedgwick, 1973) and the medical model of psychiatry. The most eloquent is Thomas Szasz (cf. also Torrey, 1972; Laing, 1976). In books like *The Myth of Mental Illness* (1961) and *Ethics of Psychoanalysis* (1968) Szasz has argued that the concept of mental illness is completely invalid and that the greater number of psychiatric illnesses are really social maladjustments between the behavior of a nonconformist individual and the demands of a social system. The cause of these maladjustments is to be located in our modern social system, which is unable to deal with individual differences. Szasz (1970) has even compared modern psychiatry and mental hospitals to the medieval religious Inquisition, that is, institutions whose purpose is to enforce conformity on the part of more highly individualized personalities to a rigid and oppressive social system through a cruel process of interrogation and torture. One group of psychiatrists call themselves "radicals" and see the whole mental health establishment as an instrument of oppression (cf. Talbot, 1974).

That these accusations are not without serious foundation is also evidenced by such books as that of Roy Medvedev (1971) who has shown that in the USSR the government has repeatedly incarcerated social reformists in mental institutions under the pretext that anyone who criticized the regime must be insane. The same issue was raised in the United States after World War II by the treatment given to leading literary figure Ezra Pound whose prison term for treason was commuted to incarceration in a mental hospital for several years.

The novel of Ken Kesey (and even more the movie based on it) *One Flew Over the Cuckoo's Nest* in 1962 dramatized the way in which patients, even those self-committed to a mental institution, can be reduced to robotlike conformity by the "system." The tragedy of this story was that the "monster" Nurse Ratchett was in fact a dedicated, well-meaning, and highly professional person who quite unconsciously had become a manipulator of people. Clearly in such cases it is not the individuals who are sick, but a system which makes both patients and health care professionals into a mutually destructive gestalt.

This accusation is also further strengthened by recent discussion of the effect of the total institution on human beings (Goffman, 1962; Rothman, 1971), which indicates the dangers of a closed social system in which people so live within a rigid set of man-made ideas and behaviors that they are cut off from contact with a reality that is beyond and different from their limited perception. This often leads to a distorted, *paranoic* way of perceiving and interpreting the world. The only difficulty with this analysis of Goffman is that we are beginning to see that not only an asylum, a prison, or a hospital can become a total institution, but also in fact modern society with its technological organization, its mass media of brainwashing and its all-seeing surveillance can itself act as a total institution, so that there is no escape unless (as in Kesey's novel) we can sail out to sea in a boat.

This problem comes to a climax in the great current problem of penology (Wilkins, 1975). In former times, punishment was sharply distinguished from treatment. The assumption of the legal system was that a crime, unless committed by persons so mentally disturbed that they did not know they were committing a wrong (i.e., a breach of law), was the responsibility of the agent. The proper way to deal with crime was by death, corporal punishment, or imprisonment. These were considered as *deterrents* to future crime by the criminal or others because the fear of punishment would be an element in the rational calculus of anyone tempted to commit a crime.

However, in recent years another theory has more and more obtained acceptance according to which many or even most crimes should not be considered punishable acts for one of two reasons (Menninger, 1968):

1. The person is suffering from some psychological maladjustment whose roots are unconscious and uncontrollable.

2. The person has been led by social injustices and by acculturation in a subculture to follow a set of standards in judging what is right and wrong different from the laws of the dominant culture.

In such cases the person has not in fact committed any *ethical* wrong, and the proper means of social control is not punishment, but in the first case treatment and in the second, reeducation.

Consequently, in our present society the line between punishment and treatment has become obscure (Van den Haag, 1975). Criminals are incarcerated not to make them fear future incarceration if they commit crimes again, but to cure them of mental illnesses and to educate them to conformity with accepted social standards of behavior, sometimes with little protection of their basic human rights (Rudkovsky, 1973). On the other hand, the patients in mental institutions, even those who at first voluntarily accept confinement, come to feel that their condition is no different from that of prisoners, since they are subjected to treatment which they do not understand and concerning which they can make no real choice.

From this vein, Richard M. Restak has argued in *Pre-Meditated Man* (1975) that most of the problems of bioethics are not really ethical in the ordinary sense, but *politcal*, that is, questions of power as to whose will concerning human behavior is to prevail. The line between normal behavior and abnormal behavior thus turns out to be only a question of who is deciding what *they* want *us* to do.

Granted that this obliteration of distinctions is a social reality today and a very dangerous one, we should take the warning, but we should not let the outcries against the system confuse the problem of medical care still more.

First of all, it is necessary to hold firmly to the fact that there is such a thing as human behavior which is dysfunctional and which is caused by organic and physiological defects (Snyder, 1973; Rose, 1973). There can be no doubt that not only lesions of the central nervous system, but also a wide variety of physiological disorders can make it difficult or impossible for human beings to sense and perceive the world correctly, to live in a state of emotional balance and sensitivity, to think clearly, and to make decisions free from uncontrollable impulses (Siegler, Osmond and Mann, 1972; Siegler and Osmond, 1974; Osmond, 1972). Moreover, there is increasing evidence that there may be a genetic basis for some mental illnesses, particularly for schizophrenia (Rosenthal, 1971; McClearn and DeFries, 1973).

The problem here, of course, is not that these physical disabilities (except in the most severe cases) automatically lead to highly abnormal behavior. Rather, it is a matter of tension between the innate capacities of the individual and the demands of the environment. For example, a patient with a respiratory disorder may be relatively comfortable under some atmospheric conditions and intensely uncomfortable under others that would not greatly distress a normal person. This disparity may also prevail among people with an inadequate or impaired capacity to adjust to certain environmental and social stresses. Clearly this suggests that the mental health of a society is to be achieved not only by treatment of the individual, but also by political and social readjustment of the environment to more adaptive life-styles. It would seem that modern society has the means of social control which should make it possible to be highly tolerant of varied human capacities.

A recognition of this fact has led recently to the policy (made possible by the use of psychotherapeutic drugs and under the pressure of economic considerations) of sending as many patients as possible back into the community, supported by outpatient treatment. The difficulty with this trend is that it frequently leads simply to hiding the problem, to neglect, and thus to further social disorder.

The general conclusion, therefore, is that there are indeed a large number of people in our society who require psychiatric care that is impossible without hospitalization, but that there must be great caution within practical limits (Treffert, 1975; Perrucci, 1974) to protect the human rights of the patient (Ennis, 1972; Ennis and Siegel, 1973; "Conflict over Patients' Rights," 1975), especially as regards both voluntary (Olin and Olin, 1975) and involuntary commitments ("Developments in the Law," 1974) and retention (Rosenham, 1973), the right of treatment during the patient's stay (Birnbaum, 1960; Bazelon, 1969; Robitscher, 1972a, 1972b; Torrey, 1974; Stone, 1974, 1975), and even the right to refuse some forms of treatment (Himmelstein and Michels, 1973; Murphy, 1975).

This psychiatric care must include an educational component by which patients are taught to cope with the social situation in which they must live after leaving the hospital and which they ordinarily cannot much alter. The patient's family must share in this education so as to assist in the patient's reentry into normal living or a halfway house should be available to facilitate this difficult transition. It is essential, moreover, that Christians recognize and respond to the need of a profound social transformation of our culture so that it will be able to meet the needs of so-called deviants who are precisely the "little ones" to whom Jesus went out (Douglas, 1970; Kittrie, 1971; Horton, 1971; Gaylin, 1973a).

Even antipsychiatrists have to admit the truth of these conclusions when a demonstrable physical or physiological basis of mental problems is in question. Such critics, however, tend to minimize this class of problems and to emphasize that in most cases so-called mental illness seems to be purely functional or largely functional. The strength of this position is that at present we cannot demonstrate such a strong organic basis for most mental illnesses. Clearly, medical research must continue to seek possible causes, especially in those disorders such as schizophrenia which are extremely resistant to psychotherapy.

As for those mental disorders in which there seems to be no organic defect or it is only secondary, we are dealing with what might more accurately be called a mental illness or emotional disturbance. Here it does seem misleading to continue to use a medical model if by that we mean the same model as is used for organic diseases (Veatch, 1973b). Psychotherapy as such is a different kind of therapy than that used for physical disease. To treat patients by talking with them or guiding them in recalling and reenacting past experiences is a very different process than to treat them with drugs.

Mental illness, therefore, in the strict and proper sense refers to mental disorders as they result from faulty development and use of our human cognitive and affective capacities ("Mental Illness," 1974). Physical and physiological impairments may contribute to this faulty development and function because they inhibit the adaptive capacity of the person.

Thus psychotherapy is sometimes more like education or re-education than it is like the medical model of treatment (London, 1964). It is based on the assumption that the mentally disturbed person has at least some capacities for normal mental life, but that these capacities have not been properly developed, are malfunctioning, or are being poorly used. In other words, the mentally sick person has adaptive capacities to cope with life situations in a satisfactory manner, but has not learned how to use coping mechanisms in an effective way, or is inhibited from such use by abnormal fears and faulty perceptions of reality.

12.2 PSYCHOTHERAPEUTIC METHODS AND GOALS

Methods

There is, however, a very important difference between psychotherapeutic or mental health education and other types of education. *Education* in the ordinary sense of the word as it is a function of an academic institution is the development of human capacities at the rational or conscious level (the ethical level in terms of 1.4 and 2.3), while psychotherapy deals with psychic processes less conscious and free than the level of rational thought, just as education at the spiritual level deals with psychic processes which transcend the level of discursive rational thought. Physical education as such deals with the training of processes that are physiological rather than psychic.

At present there is a plethora of psychotherapeutic methods (Harper, 1959), but two very different conceptions of human psychological development are reflected in the two main current schools of psychotherapy. Perry London in *Behavior Control* (1969; cf. also London, 1964) calls these "insight therapy" and "action therapy" (cf. Kanoti, 1971). In practice these therapies overlap, but they have different theoretical and clinical sources. The insight therapies derive largely from Sigmund Freud and the psychoanalytical school, although they have now moved on to include a great variety of therapeutic methods other than psychoanalysis, and especially to take into consideration the social group aspect of behavioral disorders (Small, 1971). What characterizes these therapies is that they aim at helping individuals *understand*("have insight into," "get in touch with") their own behavior and its affective sources and thus to learn how to deal with life situations in an effective way. It is assumed that mental disorder means simply that patients lack this insight or the skill to deal with their emotions and interpersonal relations because during the course of their psycho-social development they have been traumatized or wrongly guided. Thus psychotherapy of this type especially deals with lack of coordination between the rational level (and in the case of the therapy of Jung, perhaps also with the spiritual level [V. White, 1952; Moreno, 1970]) and the psychological level of the personality. Normal persons have this co-ordination between rational and subrational processes, while neurotic or psychotic persons do not.

On the other hand, action therapy (Wolpe, 1966, 1973) is the out-come of the behaviorist school of psychology which rejects or bypasses the whole notion of the subconscious because it does not even find the notion of consciousness of any great help in psychological theory. Even those who do not go to these theoretical extremes understand human be-havior in terms of "operant conditioning." Human beings behave as they do because they live in a physical and social environment which has edu-cated them to behave in a certain way by a kind of education which consists in an ordered series of rewards and punishments (positive and negative reinforcements) which favor some forms of behavior and eliminate others.

In such a view, mental illness is behavior which is unacceptable to society and which may be also internally so self-inconsistent as to cause painful conflict in the organism. Action therapy, therefore, is a process of reconditioning the person to a more self-consistent and socially acceptable type of behavior. Its methods do not depend upon a growth in insight on the part of subjects, who need not know how their mal-conditioning has arisen or even how the therapy works, but are aimed simply at distinguishing undesirable behavior patterns and developing new ones.

However, it should be noted that action therapies include not only reeducation by means of external rewards and punishments (e.g., by administering painful electric shocks), but also extend to reeducation of the person's fantasy life by desensitization, as when a patient over-comes a phobia by imagining painful situations and gradually comes to feel less anxious about them. Thus methods that rely on suggestion are considered action therapy, although they may look very much like what goes on in insight therapy.

The controversy between these two points of view still continues and is often obscured by bitter polemics, but it probably reflects two aspects of human psychology which are not necessarily contradictory. Action therapy reflects the fact that human behavior which at first may be conscious and deliberate quickly takes on a patterning and becomes automatic and subconscious. Thus when I am learning to drive a car or play the piano, each motion is conscious and deliberate, but once I have acquired the habit, I can perform these actions without conscious attention. This applies also to motivation, because in general we find it easier and more pleasant to perform in a habitual manner and more difficult and even painful to go against a habit or routine response. The advantage of such automatization of behavior is obvious: it frees my attention from the details of routine behavior and permits me to concentrate on decisions about new or unusual situations, problems to be solved, and new skills to be acquired. Without this capacity to form habits, our energies would be wasted on the routine acts rather than concentrated on the adaptive and creative ones.

Furthermore, in psychosocial development the formation of such habits in the child precedes the time when the human person is mature enough to have full self-consciousness and control. No wonder then that children who have been badly trained by their social environment arrive at the stage of self-control with many faulty, and perhaps disastrously restricted or inconsistent and conflictual, patterns of behavior whose origin and even existence they do not understand. These may even lie in the unconscious part of the psyche. Thus children may have developed irrational fears by associating fear reactions with harmless stimuli, but they no longer understand why they are afraid.

The action therapies, based on a highly developed theory of learning through conditioning, seek to reeducate the patient by extinguishing undesirable patterns of behavior and establishing or strengthening desirable ones. Included are not only external behavior, but also emotional reactions which are undesirable, especially the hampering and disorganizing kind of fear that we call neurotic anxiety.

The insight therapies agree that the human being has many automatisms, and that aberrant adult behavior is basically due to faulty conditioning in early childhood when the organism is highly impressionable and the power of the ego to resist environmental influences is low. However, the emphasis of insight theories is on the emergence of the ego or self as controlling behavior in an adaptive manner in the face of the natural and social environments. Consequently, simply for the therapist to correct faulty habits in the client is only a treatment of symptoms. The real problem is to help patients develop a strong ego and to understand how they came to have faulty habits so they will be able under their own choice to form better ones. Hence, it requires at least some measure of exploration of the past and a growing insight into one's own personality structure.

It would seem, therefore, that the two therapies can complement each other. Clients who have acquired insight into their own behavior and unconscious motivation may still need to be taught how to recondition themselves and to be aided by others in so doing. Freud and the psychoanalytic school too quickly assumed that a person who understands why he acts irrationally will then spontaneously be free to act rationally. This failed to take into account that reeducation in the form of breaking old habits and forming new ones is a complex task. Here learning theory is extremely important. On the other hand, the goals of action therapy seem too limited because they are based on a narrow, behavioristic conception of human life. Most such learning theories have been developed from animal experimentation and have proved themselves most practical in dealing with subnormal intelligences, just as insight therapies are most successful with highly intelligent, verbal, and creative personalities. Learning good habits is not all there is to having an integrated personality. It is also necessary to develop an autonomous ego.

Thus, insofar as it is distinct from medical therapy, psychotherapy is not so much a process of healing a defective organic structure, but of reeducation, not at the level of fully rational behavior, but rather at the level of automatic, conditioned, or subconscious behavior. Its purpose is to free the individual from undesirable patterns of behavior, especially those which are inconsistent, so that rational free life becomes more possible.

Goals

This definition, however, raises the very serious question of what is *normal* (Horton, 1971; Gaylin, 1973a). The action therapist Joseph Wolpe (1966) quotes R. P. Knight (1966) with approval, saying that the criteria of successful psychotherapy of any type can be summarized as follows:

1. Relief of undesirable symptoms (e.g., excessive anxiety)
2. Increased productivity in the person's work
3. Adjustment and satisfaction in sexual relations
4. Better interpersonal relations
5. Increased ability to endure the stresses of life

Another author, Robert A. Harper (1959), after surveying the bewildering array of therapies now current, sums up by saying that most therapies today have to settle for the following results to consider themselves successful:

1. The weak ego of the patient is supported by the stronger ego of the therapist.

2. The lack of realism of the patient is corrected by the more realistic attitude of the therapist.

3. The patient comes to see that many things he fears are not so terrible.

4. The patient learns to be more patient in solving problems, less impulsive and panicky.

5. The patient acquires a greater or new faith or "life-myth" from the example of the therapist who represents a hope for health.

6. The patient gets a more objective perspective on his problems from discussing them with the therapist or with his therapy group.

7. The patient focuses his floating anxieties on the outcome of the therapy process, so that he feels less isolated and helpless.

At the present time, psychotherapeutic methods do not have a clear record of efficiency. Psychoanalytical methods are extremely time-consuming and expensive. The action therapists have argued that the insight therapists have very little objective proof that their methods succeed better than natural processes; furthermore, it seems that the success they have is largely independent of the mode of therapy and mainly dependent upon the personal relation with a therapist who is a sensitive, realistic, and caring person.

The action therapists claim to have a better and more demonstratable record of success, but on examination it appears that this success is mainly in rather restricted areas of neuroses, and its permanence is often questioned (Birk, 1974). Furthermore, it does not seem to go very far in achieving the ultimate aim of developing a strong autonomy in the patient. At the present it must be concluded that this type of problem is very complex and our knowledge and ability to cure still very limited. Nevertheless, there is no doubt that therapy is sometimes successful. Perhaps this is not so different from many other areas of medical care, let alone of ethical and spiritual guidance.

Clearly, the goals listed by Wolpe and Harper are rather modest. Other therapists speak in terms of "the mature personality." However, this is ambiguous. If by *mature personality* we mean that therapy extends to total development of the human person, that is, to the development of what used to be called "the virtuous man," who is morally excellent and also spiritually profound and creative, it is clear that we have passed beyond the level of the psychological and encroached on that of the ethical and spiritual. It is true that some therapists, particularly those of the Jungian and existentialist schools (Rollo May, 1969, for example) have come to be not only therapists in the ordinary sense, but also something much more like a guru or spiritual guide. Their work is more like that of a philospher, educator, or spiritual director than of a health care professional. While not denying the great value of the work of some of these persons, it seems that we must put some limit to the task of psychotherapy. Its work is complete when the person becomes psychologically normal (i.e., in a state of normal adult health). After this kind of normality is attained, there still remains much growth for the individual throughout the whole of a human life, but guidance of this growth seems to exceed the work of psychotherapy and to demand ethical and spiritual counselors.

How then can we draw this line? If we look at the insight therapies, the answer is rather clear. Psychoanalysis, for example, is terminated at that point when patients are sufficiently *free* to manage their own life in a realistic manner, independent of the therapist, and no longer hampered by unconscious motivations or self-deluding excuses which would prevent patients from perceiving the world as it is, making free choices and carrying them out effectively (Menninger, 1958). In short, the patient now has a self-determining ego, which realistically recognizes its own emotional complexity, its innate needs, and its limitations and also realistically recognizes the practical and human situations of life to which it must accommodate itself in achieving a sufficient satisfaction of its needs. This does not mean that all terminated clients will live their lives well in an ethical sense. A psychologically healthy person can, theoretically at least, also be an ethically bad person and a spiritually undeveloped person, but this is due to his own free choices, not from compulsions imposed by his background or social situation (Menninger, 1973). At the point when the client can live by free choice, she no longer needs the therapist or therapy. Of course, a client may later regress under new stresses and have to return to treatment.

This notion of autonomy or freedom as defining the term of therapy is not so acceptable to action therapists. Under behavioristic influences they often reject the notion of freedom altogether. Thus B. F. Skinner and his followers carry on systematic war against the whole notion of human free will (Skinner, 1953, 1964, 1971, 1974). However, as many critics (Machan, 1974; Neville, 1971) have pointed out, Skinner and other behaviorists unconsciously contradict themselves. They assert that the therapist can assist the client to behave more realistically, that is, as the therapist himself behaves. This makes sense if the therapist is *free* to choose between alternative modes of behavior for himself and for the client, while the client, although still *not* yet free, wants to become free. But it makes no sense if both are equally unfree and merely conditioned by their environment (as Skinner's theory asserts).

Therefore, even extreme behavioristic therapy really aims at freeing the patient (cf. Jones, 1964). It does not merely substitute one determinism for another, but substitutes a type of determinism which is instrumentally consistent with self-determination at a higher level for a type of determinism (neurosis) which is incompatible with such self-determination. Thus skill in typing is a conditioning consistent with the freedom of the writer to create an original composition and is preferable to a neurotic compulsion to repeat a fixed pattern of words, which would be incompatible with creative writing.

Therefore, mental health is psychological freedom based on a realistic perception and understanding of the world, and it involves self-understanding, self-consistency, and self-control. By *self-control*, however, we mean a realistic self-control, that is, one based on a realistic recognition and practical provision for one's intrinsic needs as a human being. *Mental health is prior to the ethical questions of moral right and wrong, since only when a person is free can there be a question of moral choice and moral responsibility.*

It is important, however, in view of the multidimensional and integral character of human personality to emphasize that no human being is *totally* free. Human freedom is limited (1) by innate biological structure, determined genetically and by various accidents of development, with its innate needs or drives, (2) by unconscious conditioning of the sort already described with which therapy deals, and (3) by limitations of our knowledge of the world and ourself, set largely by the culture in which we live and the scope of our experiences and education. Psychotherapy deals principally, but not exclusively, with limitations on human freedom that arise from the level of unconscious conditioning.

It is best to conceive this limited human freedom in terms of the *area* in which a given individual is free. Thus recent studies on members of extremist groups like the John Birch Society began with the assumption that racists are people of authoritarian personality type. To the surprise of the researchers it turned out that these people who appear to be imprisoned by political views that approach a paranoic view of reality were on the average perfectly normal from a psychological perspective. Perhaps determinism here was more at the level of socialization rather than of unconscious conditioning and can be corrected only by ethical education, not by psychotherapy.

At the psychological level, the area of freedom is very limited in the psychotic who is out of touch with reality. But even here it is probable that most psychotics have some areas of freedom, at least at sometimes, and this is why they can be reached by psychotherapy or chemotherapy as the case may be, which aims to gradually extend this area. Neurotics are decidedly more free, but have some areas of unfreedom which do not occur in normal persons. The normal person also has a limited area of freedom, but its limits lie near the level of the necessary determinisms of automatic and routine behavior which are compatible with normal freedom.

Undoubtedly also among normal individuals there are wide differences. Highly creative and adaptive persons have much greater freedom in their life-style than normal, but limited, unimaginative, rigid people who operate best only in routine situations. Even here there is a question whether therapy, for example, of the Jungian type may open up such people to greater freedom. Modern therapy has tended to move from the treatment of sexual neuroses common as a result of the Victorian refusal to recognize basic biological needs to the treatment of anxiety common in our century as a result of the excessive demands of a work-oriented society which failed to recognize human needs for leisure and human intimacy. Hence, therapy deals more and more with neuroses of emptiness or lack of meaning as a result of our society's failure to recognize the creative and spiritual sides of man. In all these cases, psychological therapy can only go so far to awaken the person's full capacity for freedom.

12.3 ETHICAL PROBLEMS OF PSYCHOTHERAPY

Punishment

On the basis of the distinctions which we have just made, the first point about the ethics of psychotherapy is to reject any use of psychotherapy as a *punishment*. Punishment and reward (in the proper sense of the terms) belong only to *ethical* acts, that is, free, responsible acts. This, of course, requires that we have penological reforms by which the courts decide first on the facts of a criminal action and then separately on the *moral* responsibility of the person who has committed the act. In this second decision, expert testimony from psychiatrists should be admitted, but it should be directed toward determining whether the defendant's freedom was so limited by psychological factors as to remove his or her freedom with regard to this particular class of acts. This expert testimony should be fully subject to the adversary process so that the lay jury can determine whether there is solid grounds to doubt the freedom of the defendant (Gaylin, 1965; Robitscher, 1966; Katz, Goldstein, and Dershowitz, 1967; Szasz, 1968a; Stone, 1971).

David L. Bazelon (1974a), in "Psychiatrists and the Adversary Process" (cf. Robitscher, 1975) has reviewed legal developments on this question. According to him, the M'Naghten Rule of 1843 held that a lawbreaker can be held as not responsible only if he is suffering "from a defect of reason, from disease of the mind so as not to know the nature and quality of the act he was doing or, if he did know it, that he did not know he was doing what was wrong." The Durham Rule of 1954 changed this to "if the defendant's unlawful act was the product of mental disease or mental defect," and the Brawner case, 1972, to "if at the time of such conduct he lacks substantial capacity either to appreciate the wrongfulness of his conduct or to conform this conduct to the requirements of law" (a formula recommended by the American Law Institute). In the Brawner case, Bazelon, himself, proposed this formula: "If at the time of his unlawful conduct his mental or emotional processes or behavior controls were impaired to such an extent that he cannot justly be held responsible."

Bazelon says that in the use of all these rules the difficulty is that the psychiatric profession (1) does not like to take the time to gather the necessary data to apply the criterion and (2) confines itself in court to stating its *conclusion*. What is necessary is (1) that it gather the data on which a judgment can be made by the lay jury, and (2) that it present this data to the jury in such a way that the jury can make its own judgment of the validity of the expert conclusion. Only in this way can the adversary process be applied so that juries can decide between conflicting expert opinions.

It would seem that when a defendant is acquitted on the basis of lack of responsibility, then in an entirely different process the quest of commitment for involuntary treatment should be decided by a court on the grounds of whether this treatment is necessary and helpful. The question of whether defendants are likely to injure themselves or others is of course relevant to this question, but if confinement is necessary it should not be viewed as a punishment.

The question then arises whether psychiatrists should play any role in the process of punishment itself. It seems that their role should be limited to two functions. (1) Psychiatrists could diagnose prison inmates who develop mental illnesses and require occasional treatment exactly on the same basis as for medical ills. It would be highly desirable if inmates who require hospitalization for either medical or mental health reasons should receive it outside the prison, and that such time should not count for the fulfillment of their term of punishment. (2) Psychiatrists could act as consultants to penologists in setting up prison routines that make for good mental health and discipline, but they should not be engaged in staffing these services.

At present there is much controversy about proposals to rehabilitate prisoners by behavior control programs which in effect are action therapy designed to recondition the criminal to social behavior by a planned series of rewards and punishments (Ferster, 1968; Gaylin and Blatte, 1975; Rothman, 1975). This can be conceived in three ways: (1) as voluntary education, in which case it is certainly ethical to give prisoners an opportunity to engage in it as they would in any type of education program that is socially acceptable; (2) as therapy; and (3) as part of prison discipline. In the last case, it is part of the prisoner's punishment and should have some supervision from the courts who ought not to permit cruel or unusual punishments, that is, something other than prescribed by law as appropriate to the crime. As therapy which the prisoner must undergo involuntarily, it should not be permitted without a court order committing the prisoner to such therapy.

In actual practice at present these matters are very much confused, but the psychiatric profession has a responsibility to work to have them cleared up and to refuse cooperation with gross violations of the distinction between therapy and punishment. This, of course, is even more true if therapy is used as a means of suppression of political or social dissent, which amounts to a punishment for political crimes (Ayd, 1974; Shore and Golann, 1973; Reidlich and Mollica, 1976).

Granted that therapy has been carefully distinguished from punishment (which is no part of the therapeutic profession), what of the problem of informed consent on the part of the patient? Clearly, here as in other medical questions the informed consent of the patient is required if this is possible, for reasons already made clear in 3.4. The special problem, of course, is that mentally disturbed patients (1) may be unable to understand the purposes or risks of the treatment and (2) may not be truly free to make a decision even if they understand, either because personal freedom is removed by irrational fear of the treatment or of the consequences of refusal, or because of masochistic tendencies which lead a patient to submit to treatment out of a desire to suffer or be humiliated, or simply because of a narcissistic desire to be the center of attention.

This does not mean, however, that we should assume that such patients have no freedom. Every effort should be made to assist patients to arrive at a truly free decision if there is some hope that this can be achieved by giving them time to think it over, become calm, work through their fears, or discuss the matter with others. Any kind of therapy is much more likely to be successful and is at much less risk of traumatizing side effects if patients enter it voluntarily. Consequently, there is a responsibility to take the time and make the effort to permit patients to make their own free decisions if possible. If they freely decide *against* therapy, it should not be given, and if at any time during treatment they freely withdraw consent, it should not be continued.

Risks

Ken Kesey's novel and film *One Flew Over the Cuckoo's Nest*, already referred to, makes clear how patients self-committed to a hospital may then find themselves in a situation where in fact freedom to withdraw from highly traumatizing treatment is no longer practically possible. Yet every psychiatric institution must be dedicated to the proposition that it is therapeutic only to the degree that it really respects and seeks to enlarge the patients' capacity for freedom. If it more and more weakens this capacity, it is countertherapeutic; it is making ill rather than well.

On the other hand, where it is rightly judged that free consent, at least in the area of treatment, is impossible, then commitment must be made by the patient's guardian, and with scrupulous observance of due legal process. It is obvious that the guardian (usually a member of the family) may be biased, either because of selfishness, ignorance, and more often through unconscious factors which may very well be part of the client's own breakdown.

If the treatment is carried out without the consent of the patient, then a primary objective of this treatment must be to bring the patient as soon as possible to the level of mental integration where at least some self-determination becomes possible. This means of course that the use of drugs or psychosurgery simply as a method of controlling patients or tranquilizing them cannot of itself be a legitimate therapeutic objective. There is undoubtedly a strong temptation for those who have to care for patients who are out of control to try to pacify them so that they "don't make trouble." This, of course, is permissible in order to defend the patient against harming him or herself or harming the therapist or others, but such self-defense is not *therapy*. It can only be a preliminary to therapy. Unfortunately, some mental hospitals have become in fact hardly more than custodial. It is for this reason that recently a number of patients or guardians have successfully brought to the courts cases based on the right of treatment. It is essential, however, that in such matters the courts really require genuine therapy and not merely more tranquilization.

Is merely custodial care ever permissible? It must be granted that in some cases no therapy proves beneficial. In such cases there is no ethical responsibility to give more than ordinary care to the patient. We should be much more reluctant, however, to admit this state of affairs in the case of mental illness than of organic illness, because mental patients remain conscious and probably retain some minimal freedom. Consequently they still need human communication and interaction, as well as spiritual care.

It would seem that even very psychotic patients who have only such minimal freedom are still capable of treatment through active therapies. Although they are not free, they still can learn. Hence, it is possible to replace more destructive patterns of behavior by those which are more constructive and more compatible with freedom (Cotter, 1967; Carrera and Adams, 1970). Again the aim here must not be primarily to control patients so as to make them less troublesome, since it is possible that we might make some patients less troublesome by making them still more bottled up or increasing their rigid behavior. The aim must be to prepare the way for freedom.

For patients whose psychosis is less all embracing and for neurotic patients not only action therapies, but also the insight therapies are feasible. However, the use of insight therapies raises a whole series of ethical problems.

The first of these is raised by the process of *transference* (Menninger, 1958). Psychodynamic therapy depends in some measure or other upon patients becoming dependent for the time of treatment upon the therapist. This dependency repeats the child-parent relation and involves not only trust, but often at least also an element of erotic love. Without this profound dependency, patients are not freed from their anxieties and inhibitions sufficiently to let themselves become conscious of their true motivations. The termination of therapy is marked by the fact that patients have become sufficiently autonomous and under self-control that they no longer need the therapist. Like matured human beings such patients may still love their parents, but do not need them.

This vulnerability of patients obviously invests the therapist with special ethical responsibilities (Birmingham and Cuneen, 1964b; West, 1969; Braceland, 1969). The first of these is that therapists must not violate the trust placed in them. This requires that a therapist carefully maintain professional secrecy, be truly concerned for the patient, prompt in appointments, and reasonably available for consultation. It means also that therapists are honest with patients and do not lie to them nor break promises. Furthermore, the therapist must avoid all manipulation of the patient in the sense of seeking personal gratification from the treatment rather than the patient's benefit. This does not demand, of course, that the therapist have a superhuman objectivity; rather it simply means that the therapist is worthy of trust.

Clearly, this excludes the therapist having sexual relations with the client (although some have defended this as possibly therapeutic). The idea that the therapist could engage in such relations merely for the patient's sake seems unrealistic, and the risk that the patient will then or later view it as exploitation is all too real (Van Hoose and Kottler, 1977).

Some have raised the question as to whether it is permissible for patients to enter into therapy if they risk falling in love with the therapist. It should be emphasized that the danger here seems no greater (and perhaps more consciously avoided) than the danger of patients falling in love with their medical doctor. The relation is rather that of parent to child than of lover to lover, and its excessive erotic investment is the mark of the illness from which the patient is already suffering rather than its consequences.

A second issue sometimes raised by Catholics is whether the process of abreaction is not dangerous, since the patient in free fantasy revives the memory of former temptations or sins, of illicit sexual activity, or of hostility and destruction. Is it legitimate thus to again put oneself in the "occasion of sin" where sinful consent is possible? Similarly some object, especially in the case of nondirective therapy, that the therapist may permit the patient to engage in at least objectively wrong actions, even to commit suicide. It is true that such dangers may occur in therapy, but if they do, they are usually the result of poor therapy. The purpose of psychoanalytic abreaction is precisely to return to some sin or mistake of the past where the patient failed to resolve a problem correctly and to help the patient now face it in a clearer light. It is a freeing from the effects of sin, rather than a revival of the sin. It is not likely that patients engaged in the therapeutic process will actually consent to what they consciously reject just because their rejection now becomes fully conscious. Nor do good therapists permit their patients to act out their neuroses. Even in psychodrama or venting of feelings, the reenactment is precisely a dramatic one, that is, a make-believe in which it is essential to the therapeutic process that it not be a real, freely willed activity. It is generally recognized that if the patient acts out a neurosis this reinforces the neurosis, rather than liberates the patient from it.

Value Systems

Perhaps the biggest issue of psychotherapy is whether the therapist is permitted to change the value system of the client (Buhler, 1962; Hartman, 1960; Farber, 1965; Rokeach, 1973). The common answer is that a therapist should not change this system, but should try to adjust the patient to the system. However, this answer is somewhat disingenuous. As the existentialist psychoanalysts have pointed out, it is often distortions in the patient's value system which underlie the disorder. Furthermore, the source of many problems is the patient's superego which is nothing else but the value system of the parents or society which has been incorporated in the unconsciousness of the child. This is the source of all the issues raised by the antipsychiatrists. Is therapy simply the adjustment of patients to the disordered value system of the society in which they live?

On the other hand, it is clear that if the psychological and ethical dimensions of human personality are distinct then it cannot be the role of the therapist to indoctrinate the patient in a value system.

In answer to this difficulty we must say that there are certain values upon which the very relation of patient to the therapist depend and they must be reinforced by therapy. Thus, the therapist must teach the client to be more trustful, more honest, more hopeful, more courageous, more patient, more realistic. Such values, of course, are common to most recognized ethical systems whether religious or philosophical. The therapist must adhere to these values and should not be reluctant to strengthen them in the client. If clients are submitting voluntarily to therapy, they are *freely* accepting these values, no matter how unfree they may be in other respects. This is the small area of mental health and moral virtue which must become the basis of recovery. Therapists teach these primarily by their *example* in their relations to patients as they attempt to establish satisfactory therapeutic transferences.

The effort of the therapist then is to extend the area of freedom for patients. As patients become freer they must make some free ethical decisions and will do so according to their own *conscious*, rational system of values. At this point the therapist is nondirective in the sense that it is not the therapist's task to give the patient ethical advice, but only to help the patient be free of illusion and neurosis in making decisions. This requires great delicacy and objectivity on the part of the therapist. It may mean the therapist sometimes thinks that the client's decisions are not ethically good, objectively speaking. In such a case, the therapist may point out that the client's decisions are questionable, or refer the client to an ethical counselor (a clergyman or lawyer or a friend), but the therapist should be careful not to take any responsibility for the person's decision. Thus, the therapist ought to refer the client to ethical or spiritual advisers if it becomes apparent that the client's value system is inconsistent or inadequate.

However, a deeper problem is raised by Philip Rieff in his book *The Triumph of the Therapeutic* (1968) and by others. Is it possible that the whole system of insight therapy as it originated with Freud has a built-in system of values or ideology which it inculcates? Thus many have accused psychoanalysis of being essentially a product of the middle class in opulent capitalist countries. They argue that it has taken on the political function of adjusting this middle class to a social system riddled with inherent contradictions. Freud (1930) himself saw all of civilization as the imposition of social controls on man's infinite and even contradictory drives. Consequently, every social system is a delicate balance between the repressive controls necessary for social life and work and the explosive drives of the id. In Capitalist countries, as Rieff shows, the abundance of goods and the impersonal shape of social organization are making possible a much greater permissiveness, a society in which all kinds of behavior (between "consenting adults") is tolerable. Others, such as the proponents of radical sexual therapies, argue that as this permissiveness spreads it will lead to social revolution.

Rieff predicts that we are embarking on a "therapeutic society" in which the "therapeutic man" will become typical. Such a person, whom Rieff pictures as the type which successful psychoanalysis actually produces, is one who lives for a constant succession of intensely satisfying experiences, without any drive to realize some plan of life or some ultimate goal. He is highly autonomous in the sense that he feels no guilt over seeking his own satisfaction in every situation, leaving the others involved to take care of themselves. He is capable of satisfying intimate relations, but is not dependent upon any particular person for achieving these, so that he can move from one relation to another without any sense of loss or guilt for infidelity.

If Rieff is correct, and certainly very different interpretations of the goals of psychoanalysis are given by Erikson (1968), Rollo May (1969), Fromm (1975), and others (see also Ackerman, 1969), the inherent ethic of psychoanalytical theory is to produce autonomous, hedonistic, goalless, consciousless persons — the very sort of which ethicists have always condemned as selfish, loveless, and empty. Obviously, such persons are individualistic in the extreme, uncommitted to any social goals except the achievement of freedom to do what they please. Rieff's interpretation of psychoanalysis emphasizes Freud's belief that civilization, that is, social life, is always repression, not fulfillment, of fundamental human needs — a necessary evil. If this be the whole story, then it is hard to see how a Freudian ethics could ever be compatible with either a Christian value system or a Marxist one. It is essentially an ideological defense of the style of life of those who profit from Capitalism and who use their analysts to quiet their guilt.

These accusations are very serious ones. They demand (1) on the part of the community of therapists a serious examination of social conscience and a purification of the theory, training, and practice of therapists who must become conscious that the goals of therapy must be related to higher social and spiritual goals and (2) on the part of clients that they trust their therapists not as omnipotent fathers, but only for their limited skill, and that they also receive guidance at the ethical (political and social) and spiritual levels from others as soon as they become sufficiently free emotionally to do so (Rosenthal, 1955; Shör, 1961; London, 1964; Shakow, 1965).

Thus persons undergoing therapy ought not to change their system of values, divorce their partners, give up their religious vocation, or change their religion or their professional vocation merely under the influence of psychotherapy. Such changes should be made only when a real degree of psychological freedom has been reached and then under guidance that acts as a countervailing force to the possible ideology of the psychotherapeutic tradition. Thus the tendency to erect one of the many forms of therapy (including the various mystical cults now so popular) into a religion is a violation of the lines between the psychological level of personality and the ethical and spiritual levels doomed to end in disillusionment.

In recent years, some of the Protestant and Catholic clergy and the members of religious orders have discovered the value of psychotherapy and have come to place an excessive faith in it to meet all the needs of people for counseling, to the detriment of their confidence in the value of their own special roles as ethical and spiritual guides (Browning, 1976). They have become preoccupied with getting in touch with their feelings, getting freed up, or developing a capacity for intimacy, and some have deserted the celibate life, the priesthood, or the ministry to become psychotherapists themselves so that they might really help people. A similar phenomenon has been experienced by the Jewish community in the United States where psychotherapy has become a widespread substitute for the religious discipline of the Torah and the therapist has taken the place of the rabbi and Freud the place of Moses.

Undoubtedly, religious people and the clergy in particular have sometimes been in real need of therapeutic experiences to correct an excessively repressive religiosity which disregarded their human emotional needs. However, profound self-understanding and choice of one's life vocation require an exploration of the self that goes even deeper than depth psychology can penetrate and where ethical and spiritual guidance is of great value. What is needed are ethical and spiritual guides who have a genuine appreciation of the contributions of psychotherapy for human wholeness, but who pursue their own roles with a sense of their own mission (Duffey, 1950). There is an important analogy between psychotherapy and spiritual purification, but it is an analogy, not an identity (Browning, 1966).

However, it would be very unfair to blame either Freud or his disciples for these unfortunate consequences of an excessive faith in the power of psychotherapy in its present state of development. Freud's great contribution to our understanding of human behavior is established, and a fruitful historical development has already taken place, building on his work and giving it greater balance. Current psychoanalytical theory is concerned with the social as well as the individualistic aspects of human personality and is making a contribution to other models of human maturity than that depicted by Rieff. Consequently, there is no reason to doubt that in the future psychoanalysis can be of great service in helping Christians to be more truly Christians, or of Marxists to be more truly Marxists, in helping them to become freer to choose their own systems of values and to interpret them in a way consistent with the facts of human experience.

12.4 BEHAVIOR CONTROL

Modes

In addition to insight and active therapies, it is possible to alter human thought, feeling, and behavior by means of drugs, surgery, and psychological conditioning. All are considered forms of behavior control. Behavior control might be described as "getting people to do someone else's bidding." In this sense, behavior control has existed since the beginning of time. In the more restricted sense, however, the sense in which we shall use the term in this section, *behavior control* is any medically indicated treatment, procedure, or process which is intended, with or without a person's consent, to cause a person to discontinue an activity which is personally or socially undesirable (Gardner, 1967; Bandura, 1969; London, 1969; Ulrich, Stachik, and Mabry, 1974; Gaylin et al., 1975). As this description indicates, behavior control is not necessarily contrary to a person's intention or desires, but it signifies that some force over and above internal human motivation has been utilized in the interest of changing an activity pattern.

For example, a person trying to overcome the habit of alcoholism may use Antabuse (disulfiram) to help conquer the habit. Though the use of this drug is in accord with his desire, it is still a form of behavior control. From an ethical point of view, behavior control has become a serious problem in our time because of the increased efficacy of surgical procedures in controlling behavior, the vastly increased panoply of psychoactive drugs which modify emotional responses, and the increased tendency to impose conforming societal norms (Halleck, 1971, 1974). These procedures are not only comparatively new; they are swift and efficient and their effect upon a human person can be deep and lasting. Hence, they have greater potential for good or evil than many of the techniques of scientists and physicians in the past centuries, and there is a temptation to attempt the solution of problems by altering the person rather than attempt to transform the social environment (Bazelon, 1974b).

Principally there are three forms of behavior control prevalent today which are associated, either closely or remotely, with medical care. They are shock therapy and psychosurgery, psychoactive drugs, and psychological conditioning. Though the news media — radio, newspapers, and television — exercise an important influence in forming opinions and thus influence human activity, they are not treated in this section because their effect upon behavior control is only indirect and they are not much utilized by health care personnel, although films are beginning to have important uses in preparing patients for surgery and in reeducating alcoholics. After describing the three forms of behavior control associated with medical care, we shall present some ethical principles which may be used to evaluate their use.

1. *Shock Therapy and Psychosurgery*. Since the 1930s, there have been experiments with many types of treatment of psychological dysfunctions by means of profound stressing of the central nervous system through chemicals or electricity. Generally, this form of treatment is known as shock therapy, and because of the undesirable side effects of some of these treatments, the only one generally retained is electroshock. Many therapists and therapeutic instituions reject electroshock, but it is still considered by others as worthwhile therapy, especially for involutional depression where it often has dramatic results in patients who otherwise require protracted hospitalization. Electroshock and other treatments have been justified on various theoretical grounds, but all we really know is that these procedures produce temporarily a marked loss of memory and general state of psychic disorganization. Apparently, this makes it possible for some patients to break out of fixed patterns of fantasy and feeling and to begin to respond in a more normal way.

Psychosurgery is surgical destruction of certain parts of the brain for the purpose of treating psychiatric conditions. Arguments on the ethics and merits of psychosurgery vary from severe condemnation to considerable enthusiasm (Black and Szasz, 1977). The psychosurgery procedure that attracted the most attention was the prefrontal lobotomy performed upon people with severe psychotic disorders in the 1930s and 1940s. This procedure, which in some cases could be performed under local anesthesia, consists essentially in severing the white nerve fibers that connect the frontal lobes of the brain with the thalamus. The results of this surgical procedure is a blunting of human emotional responses.

Because lobotomy is an irreversible and drastic procedure, it was performed only on persons with severe behavior problems such as acute aggression or severe despondency. Often the results of this procedure were an almost complete lack of emotional response on the part of the patient. According to some experts, the emotional response could be restored to some degree, especially if proper treatment were given after the operation (Holden, Itil, and Hofstatter, 1970). But emotional responses would never be as strong nor as disturbing as before the operation. Because of the dramatic effect of this form of behavior control, the procedure fell into disuse when psychoactive drugs became more effective for the treatment of severe psychosis. In recent years, psychosurgery has become once again more common throughout the world. Modern procedures using, for example, ultrasound, electrical coagulation, or implanted radium seeds are more localized and less destructive.

A more sophisticated form of controlling human activity, but one which can be classified as psychosurgery, is electrical stimulation of the brain (ESB) and involves implanting electrodes in the human brain and controlling actions and responses by means of electrical stimulus. This form of behavior control was developed by a doctor, José Delgado (1969) (see Schwitzgebel and Schwitzgebel, 1973). In spite of some indications that present-day psychosurgery is helpful for severely depressed patients and in spite of the potential use of ESB in helping people with organic brain disease, there are many scientists and physicans who denounce all forms of psychosurgery ("Debate Over Psychosurgery," 1973; "Physical Manipulation," 1973; Pines, 1973; Cornish Rogers, 1973; Gustafson, 1975b). Chief among the critics is Peter Breggin (1972, 1973) a practicing psychiatrist whose scathing denunciation, based mainly on ethical considerations, was reprinted in the *Congressional Register* (Mar. 30, 1972). Legislators became so involved in this medicomoral issue that two bills to prohibit, or limit severely, psychosurgery were introduced in Congress. On the other hand, those who argue for the use of this form of therapy do so for the following reasons: (1) it has sometimes proved very successful in the treatment of patients with epilepsy or Parkinson's disease for whom drugs do not satisfactorily control the disorders (Mark, 1973), (2) it sometimes is the only remedy for intractable pain, and (3) it may be necessary in treatment of certain violent, uncontrollable seizures (some of which are epileptic) since otherwise the patients injure themselves or have to be confined in isolation (Mark, 1970; Winter, 1971; Sweet, 1973; Valenstein, 1973).

2. *Psychoactive Drugs.* A drug is psychoactive when it has some psychological effect: alters thoughts, imagination, perception, or emotions; causes alertness, drowsiness, feelings of anger; and so forth. Such drugs are also called psychotropic, and the study of these drugs is called psychopharmacology. Some psychotropic drugs have proved effective in psychotherapy (Uhr and Miller, 1960): (1) in tranquilizing patients in manic states or in uncontrollable anxiety, (2) in reducing the condition of mental confusion and dissocation, especially in schizophrenia, and (3) in lifting certain types of depression. These effects are symptomatic, rather than truly curative, but they may hasten the natural recovery from an episode. Moreover, they may help return a person more quickly to a more normal way of life and thus prevent the regression often resulting from prolonged institutionalization. Also, they make it possible for other types of therapy to be utilized. The fact that such remarkable results have been obtained by drugs strongly suggests that the physiological factors in the causation of mental illness are very important.

This raises the hope that as we come to understand these underlying organic causes we can develop much more successful therapies and preventives for mental health illness than we now have. However, it is also clear that drugs can never be the total answer to the problems of mental health which also involve the factors of social environment and psychological development.

Some forms of psychoactive agents have been used since the beginning of civilization. Alcoholic beverages were invented at the same time as the invention of cereal agriculture. Heroin in one form or another has been used as a pain reliever for centuries. Aspirin, the first of the wonder drugs, has been used for well over one hundred years as a pain and anxiety remover.

Extreme ethical concerns over the use of psychoactive drugs, however, did not develop until recent years. In the last thirty years, several pharmacological compounds have been developed or synthesized which alter mental and/or emotional functioning and are readily available to the public at large. Some of these drugs have demonstrated value to treat specific mental illness, but some others like lysergic acid diethylamide (LSD) are not associated with therapeutic use (Blum, 1964; Koestler, 1968). Given the wide range of known drugs, there seems to be one available to suppress or evoke any emotional state or symptom.

The extent to which psychoactive drugs are used in our society is itself an ethical concern (Parry et al., 1973). Antipsychotic, antidepressant, and antianxiety drugs are used not only by people who are severely ill and unable to manage their emotion without medication, but also by relatively normal people attempting to control anxiety, tension, depression, insomnia, and other states arising from the stress of life in modern society (Uhr and Miller, 1960). Prescriptions for psychoactive drugs account for twenty-five percent of all prescriptions written in the United States. Studies made in the 1970s indicate that about twenty to twenty-five percent of adults use one form of psychoactive drug or another, and women are twice as likely as men to use these forms of behavior control (Parry, 1973). In addition, many use nonprescription or over-the-counter drugs for relief of headache, backache, tension, insomnia, anxiety, and other "lesser" maladies of life (Balter et al., 1974). Much anxiety among parents has been caused by the controversy over the use of drugs in public schools to control hyperactive children (Wender, 1973, 1974; Wells, 1973, Aaronson, 1974). Though the psychotropic drugs available for behavior control at present comprise an impressive array, the potential for the future is even more awesome (McGlothin, 1971; West, 1974). Klerman (1970) says, "As knowledge of the relationship between brain and behavior increases, it is likely that we will develop knowledge of the neurochemical and neuropharmacological bases of memory, learning, mood, aggression, appetite and sexual lust" (p.312). Hence, not only must psychoactive drugs be evaluated as therapeutic agents, but also future ethical evaluation must consider their potential to improve capabilities and enhance personal pleasure and enjoyment of life (Evans and Kline, 1971).

3. *Psychological Conditioning.* We have already discussed operant conditioning (12.2) as a mode of psychotherapy. It can also be used as a form of behavior control for normal persons. In fact B. F. Skinner (1971, 1974) argues that in the future it will replace all other forms of ethical education and social control. Here we need only point out two aspects of his proposal which have important ethical implications.

First, we should note that Skinner denies that human beings possess the power of choice of alternate mode of activity, since he is convinced his experiments have demonstrated that all human behavior is deterministically shaped from birth by environmental forces. According to Skinner (1971), "Freedom and dignity are myths that are preventing us from seeing how continually and subtly we are being shaped by our environment" (p. 30).

Second, in the process of operant conditioning there is no need to let people know their behavior is being changed. Moreover, changes in behavior will be determined for the masses by an elite group of managers (Packard, 1977). As Gaylin (1973b) has pointed out, it is evident that Skinner assumes without question that his own Humanist values will be inculcated. In other hands, of course, anti-Humanistic values might just as effectively be enforced. For Skinner, all education is operant conditioning. As Bernard Häring (1975) observed, "Skinner seems absolutely unable to distinguish between manipulating persons and their minds and, on the other hand, engaging in genuine liberating dialogue. The categories of freely acquired convictions and respectful dialogue are totally absent in his technical manipulative world view" (p. 121).

Nevertheless, it may be reasonably argued that conditioning techniques may be preferable to the use of overt force when social control must be exercised over persons of defective intelligence who lack the capability of free choice or over those who incorrigibly resist necessary control (e.g., prisoners, violent mobs). However, much more research is necessary to determine the real effects of such methods (Neville, 1971, 1973; Michels, 1973; Mabe, 1975; Dworkin, 1976).

Ethical Guidelines

Given these examples of behavior control and modification methods which are prevalent and are becoming every day more common, we suggest several ethical principles which should govern their use, all of which are applications of the more general Principle of Human Dignity in Community (1.5; 8.2-1) which requires that social control enhance the dignity of the members of the community, not reduce them to mere means of political manipulation.

1. No form of treatment may be utilized which will destroy human freedom. Pius XII (1952) stated this well when he wrote:

> In exercising his right to dispose of himself or his faculties and organs, the individual must observe the hierarchy of the scale of values and within an identical order of values the hierarchy of individual goods to the extent demanded by the laws of morality, so, for example, man cannot perform upon himself or allow medical operations, either physical or somatic, which beyond doubt do remove serious defects or physical or psychic weaknesses, but which entail at the same time permanent destruction of or a considerable lasting lessening of freedom, that is to say, of the human personality in its particular and characteristic function. (n. 361).

Thus, any form of psychosurgery, personality manipulation, and use of psychoactive drugs which would remove or severely limit human freedom or destroy human personality could not be permitted and may need legal control (E. B. Brody, 1973; "Symposium on Psychosurgery," 1974).

2. If the purpose of the behavior control is therapeutic, then the benefit to the patient must be proportionate to the damage or risk to be endured. A frontal lobotomy, for example, should be performed only as a last resort and with some indication that there will be an overall benefit for the patient. Above all, lobotomy and ESB should not be considered as ordinary treatments for prisoners and others who have displayed antisocial behavior. As a general rule, a sign of organic brain pathology should be present before psychosurgery is approved.

3. If the purpose of the treatment is therapeutic, the long-range effect of the treatment must be considered as well as the short-range

alleviation of some particular difficulty (Kline and Milton, 1973; Klerman, 1974). Simply because a particular therapy alleviates or eliminates a symptom does not mean that it is ethically acceptable (Veatch, 1974). Most of the drugs currently available for the relief of anxiety and tension carry some danger of dependency, habituation, and addiction (Klerman, 1970). Such dependency diminishes human freedom and dignity and hence is to be avoided. Thus, the very theory prevalent in our country of using psychoactive drugs to treat psychological difficulties must be questioned. Would it not be better to treat the causes of anxiety or depression through counseling or increased self-awareness rather than to depend upon pills which merely treat the symptom? Questions such as this are fundamental in developing a philosophy of health care, and they are too often neglected in search of easier, but less beneficial, solutions.

4. If behavior controls are utilized, the rules of free and informed consent apply (Spoonhour, 1974). Thus, operant conditioning, psychoactive drugs, and psychotherapy should not be inflicted upon people nor imposed upon them. This requirement would limit the use of operant conditioning as it is practiced in many of the institutions of our country (Katz, 1972). Moreover, children, prisoners, and people with a limited sense of awareness should not be subjected to experimental behavioral control, nor should proxy consent be given unless the treatment is truly therapeutic for them.

5. If behavioral control forms are used for experimental purposes, the norms explained previously in the section on human experimentation (9.4) must be followed.

6. Use of behavioral control procedures to improve human capabilities such as memory, intelligence, and sexual abilities would seem to be licit if free consent is given, if there is no other way to achieve the same goal, and if the action is in accord with the finality of the human person. In itself, human betterment, or human improvement, is ethically acceptable and beneficial. Care must be exercised, however, to make sure that the basic integrity of the human person is not violated and that addiction does not result in the course of seeking self-improvement.

7. Using psychoactive drugs for relaxation or pleasure is not in itself ethically wrong provided that freedom is not notably restricted. Like alcoholic beverages, psychoactive drugs may provide needed and legitimate relief from everyday strain and tension of life. However, because there is a greater tendency to abuse the use of drugs, even to become dependent upon them or addicted to them, and because of the potential bodily harm resulting from some drugs, great care would be required in the use of drugs for recreational purposes.

12.5   ADDICTION OR CHEMICAL DEPENDENCY

Generally speaking, addiction is habituation to some practice harmful to the subject (Stedman, 1976).   Though the term *addiction* is usually used in our day in reference to habituation to drugs, one can also be addicted to other substances or activities deterimental to the person using them: for example, one can be addicted to alcohol, tobacco, coffee, and excessive food and also to too much sleep, too much work, and pursuit of sexual pleasure (Van Kaam, 1966; Peele, 1975).   Though many people use all these things in ways that do not destroy human equilibrium, some persons, for a variety of reasons not fully understood, become addicted to them so that their whole life is more and more absorbed by a single activity which distorts the personality, consumes physical and psychic energy, and often results in an intense self-centeredness, personality deterioration, and inability to communicate with others.   Addiction or dependency upon drugs and alcohol are more likely to result in such extreme symptoms.   Hence, our considerations will be addressed mostly to these addictions, which are often referred to as chemical dependency.

One component, the most obvious, of chemical dependency is its hedonistic character. In the face of every difficulty of life, every tension or frustration, the chemically dependent person runs away from the loss of normal satisfaction and achievement by indulgence in the physical pleasure, relaxation, and euphoria of the addicting experience. Vernon E. Johnson (1973), however, argues that this search for pleasure alone does not constitute addiction, but rather the increasing sense of guilt and helplessness which begin to accompany each overindulgence, with the result that the incipient addict begins to indulge not for the sake of pleasure itself, but to blot out the guilt and remorse for the consequences of previous indulgences.   Furthermore, this vicious circle is reinforced by the use of physchological coping mechanisms of rationalization and denial which victims find necessary to assist in this suppression of guilt and pain, so that they become increasingly unable to perceive the real consequences of behavior.   Alcoholics, for example, frequently suffer from blackouts, repression, and delusional euphoric recall which so distort their memory that they actually have a very incomplete picture of what is happening to them.

Persons of very different personality types can become addicted, but a common feature is excessive *dependency* needs, not infrequently masked by outward aggressiveness and competitiveness.   Moreover, as addiction progresses it tends to produce a pattern of behavior which overrides all temperamental differences.

At one time addicts were thought to come mainly from the poorer classes (Barber, 1967), and undoubtedly addiction is very common among some socially depressed groups (Suchman, 1963). Recent research demonstrates, however, that chemical dependency can affect people of all backgrounds. Often the gifted, talented, wealthy, and successful succumb to this severe personality problem.

Chemical dependency or addiction may be classified as physiological or psychological. Physiological addiction, which causes a modification or need in the addict's physiological system, usually requires increasing doses of the addicting substance in order to obtain the same physiological effect. Moreover, in physiological dependence withdrawal from the object of dependency, for example, heroin, results in severe physiological disturbance, even death, because the body has become so adapted to the presence of the substance in the system. Peele (1975), however, marshals extensive evidence to show that in physiological addiction the psychological component remains essential, so that persons who lack this component can sometimes use even so highly addictive a drug as heroin without exhibiting the typical features of addiction. Psychological dependency itself results from a learned conditioned behavior pattern which leads the victim to anticipate the pleasure and release of tension, even when the substance does not notably modify the physiological system.

Chemical dependency, especially drug addiction, is one of the most highly publicized and most morally condemned social problems in the United States (Young, 1964; Barber, 1967; Szasz, 1974a). But there are some important facts and questions that are sometimes overlooked because of the widespread moral condemnation of the such abuses. First of all, is chemical dependency more a personal or a cultural problem? Studies have shown that chemical addiction is not as serious in other countries as in the United States (Clausen, 1961). Is this because chemical addiction is merely a symptom of some larger American problem (Young, 1964) such as poverty (Barber, 1967), anomie (Lindesmith and Gagnon, 1964), or spiritual deprivation (Moraczewski, 1973)?

Second, do the strict government control of addictive substances, especially drugs, the special moral disapproval, and the severe penalties for sale or use foment rather than solve the problem? A recent study assessing the effect of the severe drug laws in New York State seems to demonstrate that these laws have been ineffective (Committee on Drug Law Evaluation, 1977). Moreover, as another authority (Clausen, 1968) states, "There is no evidence that addiction to drugs is favorably regarded in any society or culture, but the status accorded the addict varies markedly. In the United States, he has been defined as a criminal and stereotyped as a 'dope fiend.' In much of Europe, on the other hand, the addict is regarded as an unfortunate person whose problem is primarily psychological and medical" (pp. 298-299).

Would chemical addiction be less of a problem in this country if it were considered a medical or social problem rather than a moral and legal one (Suchman, 1963; Szsaz, 1977)? Removing the moral stigma from addiction to alcohol has been helpful in assisting many people overcome this addiction (Szasz, 1971b, 1974a, 1977a; Murray, 1974). Would a similar response to the use of drugs, plus legalization of narcotics for sustaining treatment of addicts, be beneficial over a long period of time? While avoiding a naive optimism about easy solutions for chemical dependency, we must seek to learn from the experience of other nations in this regard, and above all we must consider these problems in the total context of American culture and its socialization process (Duster, 1970).

Is this to say that the sense of moral guilt felt by the addict is merely neurotic? On the one hand, therapists speak of addiction as a "disease" in order to reduce its moral opprobrium and to achieve a more sympathetic attitude on the part of nonaddicts, and on the other, an important part of therapy is to get addicts to accept moral responsibility for the harm they have done themselves and others through addiction (Johnson, 1973). This ambiguity can be cleared up if two points are kept in mind. First, chemical dependency is always a psychological disease since it involves an abnormal behavior pattern accompanied by the neurotic coping mechanisms already described. It is also a physiological disease because it sometimes produces physiological dependency and usually produces widespread organic changes which greatly aggravate the condition. Second, we need to distinguish between *voluntary* and *free* acts. Addictive behavior is voluntary in the sense that it proceeds from an inner compulsion, but it always involves a restriction of freedom, since the addict becomes less and less able to perceive alternatives of action or to choose among them. In times of addictive need the practical conscience of the addict is concerned totally with the need for a drink or a fix. He or she acts voluntarily, compulsively, but without free choice.

Hence, actual consumption of addictive substances by addicts is seldom in itself a morally culpable act, and the guilt felt afterward is unrealistic and neurotic. Even the acquisition of the addiction often proceeds so gradually and subtly that it is difficult to judge that the addict knowingly and deliberately chose addiction (Johnson, 1973). Nevertheless, it would be a mistake to think that the *whole* guilt felt by addicts is illusory. If it were, it would be hard to explain why admission of responsibility has proved so important a part of therapy. The truth seems to be that the real moral responsibility of the addicted person lies in the obligation to ask and receive help from others when this is offered, since therapy cannot be effective until the addict accepts help. Johnson (1973) says that even this acceptance does not take place all at once, but passes through stages (1) of *admission* into treatment, (2) of *compliance* with treatment (with hidden defiance and resistance), (3) of *acceptance* or recognition of real need for help (with unrealistic anticipations of cure), and (4) of *surrender*, that is, realistic acknowledgement and acceptance of the responsibility for a life long change. Hence, it is a mistake to reduce this complex situation either to a purely moral question or to a purely sociological or medical one. To deny all moral responsibility or capacity to change is to degrade addicts as persons, yet to pass judgment on their degree of responsibility is to misjudge the many ways in which they are victims of forces beyond individual control.

Therapy for addiction can be highly successful. Some centers for the treatment of alcoholics (who are commonly also dependent on other drugs) report the achievement of permanent *control* in seventy-five percent of the cases (Johnson, 1973). The term *control* rather than *cure* is used because addicts must permanently abstain from any use of alcohol. There seems to be no reason that similar rates of success are impossible with all forms of chemical dependency, provided that drug addicts do not return to the social circumstances which have been part of their problem.

Here it is not necessary to describe therapeutic methods in detail. They involve detoxification and at least a month of intense group psychotherapy, accompanied by a thorough indoctrination in the nature and effects of addiction. This intensive treatment must be accompanied by at least two years of outpatient follow-up. It is important that the family of the addict share to some degree in the therapy, and that both the addict and family members participate in support societies such as Alcoholics Anonymous and Alanon (for spouses). The element of mutual help involved both in group therapy and in these support groups seems to be one of the most important features of any treatment, because the addict is able to face painful reality and yet to recover a good self-image only through support of others who have experienced the same problems.

Students of addiction emphasize that the earlier in the addiction therapy takes place the better, but they also point out that family and employers commonly contribute to the problem by covering up, excusing, or attempting to endure addictive behavior, hoping that the addict will finally come to his or her senses. In fact this spontaneous self-insight on the part of addicts is very rare, and family, friends, and employer have a serious ethical responsibility to face the facts realistically and intervene decisively and persistently until the addict accepts treatment. Intervention is best done by those who can be supportive rather than judgmental, but who can also face the addict with detailed evidence of the seriousness of his or her condition.

Health care professionals sometimes are impatient and contemptuous of alcoholics and other addicts whom they regard as delinquents rather than as victims of illness. Such attitudes are intensified by unwarranted pessimism about the effectiveness of therapy. This is especially unfortunate because health care professionals themselves have an especially high rate of chemical dependency, due not only to their relatively easy access to drugs but perhaps also to the *ethos* of the profession which maximizes guilt feelings over breach of professional standards while doing little to support persons who may have high dependency needs which they mask under professional self-assurance and pride.

Therefore, it is important for professionals to acquaint themselves thoroughly with the nature and therapy of addiction, the ways of intervening to get addicts to accept treatment, treatment centers to which they can be referred, and ways to support them in their new life.

Perhaps an even more effective way for health care professionals to combat chemical addiction is through preventive measures. They can play an important role in combatting the drug culture mentality in the United States (Bernstein and Lennard, 1973; Landau, 1974; Veatch, 1974). According to this mentality, every pain, every sorrow or frustration, can be overcome with a pill, potion, or injection of some kind. Pharmaceutical firms constantly push drugs through advertising, and health care professionals often are used by such agencies to promote unnecessary drug use (Brecher, 1972; Steinfels, 1972; Pekkanen, 1973; Silverman and Lee, 1974). Christian professionals will not share in this promotion, because they realize that human pain, frustration, and sorrow cannot be simply suppressed. Human beings grow as persons by facing the difficulties and struggles of life realistically, "bearing one another's burdens" (Gal. 6:2) as free people, not as slaves to a pleasure ethic (Illich, 1976b). In saying this, we are not proposing an exaggerated stoicism as the Christian ideal, but a realistic effort to overcome the real causes of suffering, rather than an escape into unconsciousness. Alcholics Anonymous, which has led the way to the most successful methods of therapy for chemical dependency, has always emphasized that the addict cannot recover without a reaching out for a Higher Power and a willingness to repair damage done to the neighbor and to be of service to the neighbor.

12.6 SEX THERAPY AND RESEARCH

Therapy

One authority (Green, 1970) estimates that in seventy-five percent of marital discord the inability to engage in satisfactory sexual expression is a contributing factor, although perhaps it is as often an effect as a cause. What should be not only an expression but also a source of deepening love and commitment, rich in tenderness and joy, can be a source of profound depression and alienation. Couples frustrated and puzzled by sexual dysfunction are sometimes exploited by marriage counselors or sex therapists who are unqualified or irresponsible, because these disciplines are relatively new, rapidly expanding, and lacking in well-established professional or legal controls (Van Hoose and Kottler, 1977). Health care professionals can be of great help in preserving and improving family life if they are well informed about the goals and effectiveness of sex therapy and the availability of reliable practioners to whom couples may be referred.

According to Masters and Johnson (1976) the most common forms of sexual dysfunction for men are premature ejaculation, retarded ejaculation, and impotency; for women, the most common forms are vaginismus and orgastic dysfunction. Contrary to the beliefs of some psychoanalysts, sexual dysfunction need not be a sign of a deep or severe physic pathology, but can be the result of various relatively superficial maladjustments which impede spontaneity. As Kaplan (1974) states, sex therapy "differs from other forms of treatment for sexual dysfunction in two respects: first, its goals are essentially limited to the relief of the patient's sexual dysfunction and, second, it departs from traditional technique by employing a combination of prescribed sexual experiences and psychotherapy" (p. 86). Thus sex therapy has a more limited objective than psychoanalysis or marital therapy. These latter two forms of assistance seek to help people with sexual dysfunction, but they concentrate more on the underlying conflicts and destructive interpersonal behavior which may give rise to such dysfunction. In sex therapy, however, the dysfunction is treated directly, and the therapy is complete when the couple are able to achieve a satisfactory sexual response.

During the past twenty years, centers for sex therapy have been widely established in the United States, but the original and most renowned center was founded in 1959 at Washington University in St. Louis by William H. Masters and Virginia Johnson. In 1974, this center, which offers therapy and trains professional therapists, was named the Reproductive Biology Research Foundation. Other well-known centers for treatment of sexual dysfunction exist at Cornell University and several other university hospitals. In addition, many health care professionals, psychiatrists, psychologists, and special therapists offer sex therapy in private practice, not to mention the practioners of dubious competency already referred to.

At the larger centers, the common sexual dysfunctions of married people are treated through an integrated combination of instruction and actual sexual experiences in which the couple explore a more relaxed, personalized approach to sexual relations freed from anxieties about "performance." The instructions are usually given by a man-woman team, while the actual experiences are engaged in privately by the couple in their home or a hotel near the therapy center. At the beginning of therapy a thorough history is taken and a complete physical examination given. After therapy, which commonly consists of about ten days of instruction, a follow-up is made to see if the couple has successfully integrated the new approach to sexual relations into their ordinary living. Over eighty percent success is commonly reported by such centers, which is remarkable considering the relatively short period of therapy compared to that required to meet other types of marital problems in marriage counseling.

As a general rule, most centers and private therapists accept only married couples for treatment. However, some sex therapists, Masters and Johnson included, will accept single persons. At one time Masters and Johnson made use of paid surrogate partners for single persons and in special cases for married persons, but have discontinued this much-criticized practice.

The Principle of Personalized Sexuality (8.3-2) indicates the importance for married couples to be able to express and deepen their love by satisfying sexual relations. The clinical experience of sex therapists today seems to show that when couples have good interpersonal relations and a positive and anxiety-free attitude toward bodily intimacy and sensual enjoyment sexual dysfunction is rare and special training unnecessary. However, in our culture many men and women find interpersonal communication, even at nonsexual levels, difficult and are inhibited in the spontaneous expression of their feelings both by inhibiting fears and by exaggerated competitive attitudes. Hence, much of the need for sex therapy could be obviated by adequate sex education before marriage.

From a Christian point of view this education ought to stress the intimate relation between the various meanings of sexuality as sensual satisfaction, as love and completion between man and woman, and as the source of the continuing life of the family and society and should show how permanent self-giving is the heart of the matter. At the same time such education cannot be merely abstract but must include an experiential growth which enables persons to understand their own sexuality and to learn to relate to others as sexual persons through encounters appropriate to their age and personal maturity. However, persons also need help so that these growth experiences do not lead them down the dead-end paths of autoeroticism or a depersonalized search for satisfactions unrelated to the deeper meaning of sexuality as marital commitment.

There is no doubt, therefore, that sex therapy may be necessary and ethically acceptable for married couples who need to overcome difficulties of miseducation or personal sexual development, provided that the prescribed sexual actions are performed with the married partner and in view of the expression of marital love through complete sexual union and not as a substitute for it. It is desirable that a sufficient number of Christian health care professionals prepare themselves to provide such therapy in the context of a truly personalized attitude toward sexuality lest in our culture such technical knowledge should be abused so as to further weaken family life rather than to promote and strengthen it.

At present, there is no definite set of ethical standards for professionals involved in sexual therapy, although a group of prominent practitioners are working to develop such guidelines (Masters and Johnson, 1977). Given the importance of the human activity involved, the need for definite moral standards is obvious. First of all, the same confidentiality required of anyone offering therapeutic treatment must be observed. Second, the persons involved should not be asked to perform actions which are immoral or which are contrary to their conscience. Hence, use of surrogate partners as well as activities which are intentionally and exclusively masturbatory must be rejected. Third, therapists must not engage in sexual activity with patients. Unfortunately, studies show that these moral standards are sometimes violated (Masters and Johnson, 1977; Van Hoose and Kottler, 1977). Violations of these principles will not only harm the patients, but will also destroy respect for sexual therapy and those who pursue it as a profession.

It is unfortunate also that sex therapists often seem to approach their task from a purely scientific-technological point of view. One noted psychiatrist (Kaplan, 1974) completes her study of some of the literature with the lament, "There is a conspicuous absence of the word *love*." We cannot help but wonder, therefore, whether this approach may still further the depersonalization of human sexuality from which our culture suffers. Christians working in this field should exert leadership in the opposite direction.

Research

What has just been said of sex therapy also applies to sexual research and experimentation, including diagnostic procedures which may be used to determine the normality of sexual response, for example, to diagnose homosexual tendencies. Such research is legitimate and necessary in order to understand better the nature of human sexuality and the physiological or psychological pathologies to which it is subject. However, such research must be in accord with the principles already laid down in 9.4 for psychological experimentation with human subjects, which means that the experimental experiences must be designed to be therapeutic or truly educational for the subject and not depersonalizing or reinforcing of patterns inconsistent with the total health, moral and spiritual, as well as biological and psychological, of the human person.

Such conditions exclude sexual acts between unmarried partners and especially the use of prostitutes. They would seem also to exclude the use of subjects who are immature or otherwise lacking in mature control of their sexual impulses and behavior unless the experiment itself tends to strengthen this control. The type of experiment, often reported, which exposes subjects to viewing photographs to measure sexual arousal is highly questionable because it involves risk of consent to illicit acts. However, since there could be a proportionate reason for such a risk, this type of experiment is not absolutely excluded. For example, the use of pictures for diagnostic purposes or with some benefit to the patient in conditioning experiments and therapy (for example, in some operant conditioning therapies for homosexual orientation) may be justified if the temptation involved is moderate and the subjects are warned that the purpose is not pornographic but simply to test initial reactions.

Thus, sexual therapy and sexual research can be carried on in an ethical manner. Basically, both sexual research and sexual therapy aim at helping people to express their love for one another more fully. But great care and sensitivity must be observed in the practice of sexual therapy and in the experiments prompted by sexual research. In either case, the fundamental integrity of the persons involved must be respected. Hence, actions which are in themselves immoral are not justified. Moreover, the activities involved in either research or therapy should be carried on in view of the fact that human love is not accomplished or developed through technique or knowledge alone. A deeper awareness and mutual communion must be present in order to enhance human love. Not only are these admonitions derived from an integral view of human nature and human love, but they also take into account a long-range view of human dignity. What have we gained if we learn everything there is to know about sexual activity but in the pursuit of pleasure learn less and less about fulfilling human love?

CHAPTER 13 SUFFERING AND DEATH

13.1 FEAR OF DEATH

In chapter 8 we formulated the Principle of Growth Through Suffering (8.3-1) as one of the norms of hope. In the course of this formulation, we considered the mysteries of suffering and death, their Christian meaning, and in what sense death is a culmination of life. In this chapter, we will consider how this principle understood in a Christian way can serve to help health care professionals deal with the suffering and death which they meet each day and in which they, themselves, share, although we can only touch on some of the issues raised in the phenomenal number of recent publications on such topics (Kalish, 1970; Kutscher, 1969).

Because health care professionals are human, they have a tendency to retreat from any phenomenon which causes fear or wonder. Death is such a phenomenon; it involves awe, fear, mystery. For this reason, health care professionals, just as other people, are tempted to avoid facing the evil of death. The result of this fear has been catalogued by perceptive physicians and psychologists (E. Becker, 1973; Cassell, 1976). When fear controls the actions of health care professionals, patients often are deceived as to their true condition, and the need for a person's understanding or comfort is neglected. Moreover, the occasion for personal spiritual growth for both the patient and the health care professional is lost as well as the opportunity to help another human being prepare for death and eternal life. Studies show too many health care professionals retreat and cut themselves off from the dying patient completely (Strauss, Glasser, and Quint, 1964). To put it another way, dying is not only a biological process, but is also a psychological process which involves the health care professional as well as the patient.

In order to overcome fear and to help people die well, the health care professional must learn to handle the emotional strain that accompanies suffering and death. Though many helpful books on this topic are available, some clinical training in this art is also necessary. In every hospital there should be people who specialize in the care of the dying. The purpose is not only to help the dying patient work through fear, anger, and depression, but also to help the members of the healing team participate in the event of death in a way that is healthful for themselves (Freireich, 1972; Ingelfinger, 1973). Otherwise, health care professionals, no matter how well educated or technically expert, will suffer psychological harm from their constant involvement in death. Is the high rate of alcoholism, suicide, and divorce among health care professionals in some way connected with emotional tensions which result from their inability to express the grief and sadness which the constant sight of death engenders in them?

Those who must deal with the dying have three options: they can ignore the dying patient and thus become hardened and jaded; they can relate to the dying patient in a sincerely personal manner without knowing how to deal with their own feelings; or they may relate to the dying patient in a healthy way, realizing the psychological strain that patient and professional undergo together. When this last option is taken, a professional can learn to value the experience of helping another fellow human being suffer and die in Christ, either with explicit Christian faith or perhaps simply with an openness to the mysterious future which is the effect of Christ's grace in those who do not know him except under some other name or symbol. However, few health care professionals will be able to achieve this healthy and healing attitude without special training in the art of working with the dying.

In learning this art of the care for the dying, three points (already explained at more length in 8.3) should be kept in mind. First, because suffering and death are obstacles to the fullness of life which Christians affirm, we have not only the right, but also the duty to try to overcome or mitigate them. Hence, Christians should strongly favor medical research to conquer disease and to preserve and prolong life, for example, the crusade to eliminate heart disease and cancer or to make our environment more healthful. Medicine as a profession, as a science, and as an art has a Christian birthright.

Second, efforts to overcome the evils of sickness and suffering by medical science have not eliminated the healing role of prayer which is also a part of the Christian heritage. Jesus gave physical as well as spiritual healing and commanded his followers not only to preach, but also to heal and drive out demons (Mark 3:14-15). The reference to demons indicates that the forces of evil which must be overcome for complete human healing in all the dimensions of the human person, spiritual and ethical, as well as psychological and physical, are greater than merely human intelligence, even with the aid of science, can ever hope to achieve. Hence, to complete human healing we always need to turn to Jesus Christ, who has conquered sin and death and who is the source of all healing powers, even those provided by modern medicine. Therefore, health care professionals striving to help the suffering and the dying need to pray for and with them (MacNutt, 1974, 1977).

Third, we need to remember that although sickness and suffering have entered our human world through sin they are not themselves sinful, nor can we assume that the one who is suffering is the same one who has sinned. Jesus suffered because of the sins of others and that

368 HEALTH CARE ETHICS

is also true of innocent persons today. Because we are all part of one human community we bear not only the consequences of our own personal sins, but also the consequences of others' sins. Thus we live in a world in which we often injure our own health and have to suffer the consequences, but we also suffer from a bad environment produced by others, and through the neglect of others we may lack the means to maintain and recover health. Hence, in caring for the sick, we should see them as victims, rather than as responsible for their own condition, unless in fact this responsibility is obvious. Even if they are in fact responsible, we must then help them understand the forgiving mercy of God by which the road of hope is always open. Hence, the real problem of caring for the suffering and dying is to help them realize that they can bring good out of evil by making their painful and frightening experiences a means of personal growth and a witness of courage to others who someday will have to meet the same test.

A fourth point to heed is that Christian health care professionals will best succeed in this difficult task if they themselves understand suffering and death in terms of the suffering, death, and resurrection of Jesus Christ, which provides a real answer to this mystery. Many health care professionals feel utterly defeated by the death of patients for whom they have cared and by the helplessness of even their best efforts in many cases to restore normal health. Only Christian hope has an answer for that despair.

But it is also clear that it takes more than words to accomplish this transformation of suffering and death. One must be willing to surrender to God through the person of Jesus Christ every day if one wishes to give new meaning and power to suffering and death. In short, one must enter into a lifelong love affair with God. The small deaths one dies every day prepare a person for the larger and more important deaths and finally for the ultimate moment of meaning and power.

The perfection of Christian suffering and death is to accept it with joy. This is not even possible unless one works at it faithfully, relying upon the unfailing grace of God. To communicate to patients effectively the meaning and power of death, health care professionals must have some experience of its reality themselves. Thus, health care is more than a job, more than knowledge and technique. Basically, in its fullness it is a way of life which sees beyond the hurt, the sickness, the anguish; a way of life which enables one to look beyond the drudgery of daily reality, beyond the suffering in the hospital ward and the emergency room; a way of life which centers in God's love for his children, the suffering of Christ for all human beings, and his victorious resurrection.

13.2 DEFINING DEATH

When biologists speak of the death of any living organism, they refer to that inevitable and critical moment when an organism ceases to function as a specific, unified, homeostatic system and becomes disorganized into a mere collection of heterogeneous chemical substances. Sometimes, however, even after this moment, some tissues or cells of the former organism may continue temporarily to carry on some minimum of life functions before they cease to live or are artificially sustained in the laboratory.

From a biological point of view, the death of a human organism is like any death and is determined in much the same way, by various signs that the unifying life functions have ceased, but few of us believe that it is nothing more. Human death has a mystery about it, because at death we seem irrevocably to lose touch with a person who previously was able to communicate with us and to share our human community of thought, of love, of freedom, and of creativity. Human death is not merely a decay of an organism, it is the departure of a member of the human community.

The world over, people have interpreted this departure of someone known and loved as the separation of a spiritual soul from its body. Certainly, science is unable to close the door on such an explanation (Moody, 1975). Christians are convinced that the departed will return in their fully, bodily personhood in a transformed existence, as Jesus did. In any case, while we remain in our present existence we often have the painful responsibility of determining when the death of another has occurred, because the time of death influences many other human decisions such as inheritance, legal and moral rights possessed by the dying person, spiritual care for the dying person, and possibility of organ transplantation.

Dying is a process, but death is an event (Morison and Kass, 1971). We can be certain this event has not yet occurred as long as a person can communicate with us through speech or gesture. When such communication ceases, we can only judge by signs which are no longer distinctly and specifically human. Yet we do not dare to conclude that death has occurred merely because such specifically human signs are no longer evident, as becomes very clear when we observe someone awake from sleep or coma.

Consequently, we are morally obliged to treat anybody who is apparently human (even in the fetal state) as a human person with human rights until we are sure that this body has become so disorganized that it no longer retains its human unity. To know this we must be reasonably sure of three things: (1) that the body does not now exhibit specific human behavior, (2) that it will not be able to function humanly in the future, and (3) that it no longer has even a radical capacity for human functions because it has lost the basic structures required for human unity. This third condition is required because medical experience has shown that persons who have been in prolonged, apparently irreversible coma nevertheless have sometimes recovered full human consciousness. Such resuscitation is possible as long as the radical structures of the human organism remain and the causes which inhibit their normal function can be removed. This is why some speculate that in the future we may be able to freeze the human body and revive it centuries later.

At the same time there is no reason to deny that after true human death some cells or even organs of the human body may for a time (perhaps indefinitely if artifically supported) continue to exhibit some life functions which are not those of the human organism as a unified entity, but merely a residual life at a level of organization comparable to that of plants and lower animals. Hence, the essential point about determining human death is to not decide whether any life is present, but whether human life in the most radical sense of a unified human person is still present even if that person is in deep coma.

Certainly, some signs of human death were always easy to identify. If rigor mortis or putrefaction occurred, then even nonprofessionals were able to recognize that the human organism was irreversibly destroyed. Other less conclusive signs of human death were the absence of breathing and heartbeat, although it was known that these might sometimes be revived by such methods of resuscitation as were then available. When such efforts failed, death was judged certain. Physicians were required to pronounce the patient dead on the basis of such evidence and certify the time of death for legal purposes such as inheritance. Thus cessation of spontaneous heart and lung function became known as the *clinical* signs of death.

In recent times, two developments have led to the proposal of a new set of clinical signs for determining the fact of human death (Cassell and Kass, 1972; Walker, 1977). First of all, machines have been perfected which artificially aid the function of the heart and the lungs. Often people recover full and spontaneous heart and lung function as a result of being temporarily assisted by such machines, proving that the radical structures of the unified human organism had not been destroyed. On the other hand, it seems possible that such machines may be able to maintain heart and lung action, at least temporarily, even after this unity of the organism has ceased to exist, since the heart completely separated from the body can continue to beat, and tissues in a test tube can continue to exhibit some residual life if nourished by an appropriate solution.

Thus, such artificially sustained heart and lung action are not proof that human life still remains, yet as long as they are sustained it is impossible to verify the traditional signs of human death. Therefore, the question arises: Are there other clinical signs that can be used, not to constitute a new definition of death, but rather as an alternative means to establish the same essential fact, namely, the irreversible cessation of spontaneous heart and lung function?

The second, and perhaps more important, reasons for seeking new clinical signs of death has been the recent advancement of techniques of organ transplantation, especially of the kidney and heart. Such transplantations are more likely to be successful if the organs are freshly harvested from a body through which blood is circulating, although this is not absolutely necessary. Hence, surgeons prefer to keep the body of a "dead" donor "alive" on a respirator. How then is it possible to be sure that the donor is in fact dead (Biorck, 1967; Halley et al., 1968a, 1968b, 1968c; Bleich, 1973; Joseph Fletcher, 1974b)?

First, we should retain the traditional clinical signs as basic and sufficient and make use of the new brain death criteria only when such signs cannot be used because of the dependence on a respirator or other form of artificial maintenance. If we permit brain death to become the exclusive definition (as is the increasing tendency in some states), we may end with the absurd result that no one can be certified as dead without first being taken to an elaborately equipped hospital. Our present moral dilemmas about how to determine death have been created in large part by an excessive reliance on technology, and we need to moderate, rather than encourage, that excess.

Second, the new signs must be ascertained by well-trained professionals. Human error and even carelessness must be anticipated and avoided, since a number of examples of such human error in determining brain death have already been reported in this country. How to prevent such errors when human life is at stake? The Harvard criteria envision a process of observation for no less than twenty-four hours. Moreover, the persons using the electroencephalogram (EEG) must be trained to recognize such conditions as hypothermia and drug-induced coma which may produce a flat EEG in a patient who can recover, since the flat EEG is not alone an infallible sign of death (Bird and Plum, 1968; Alderete et al., 1968; Korein, 1969; Silverman et al., 1969; D. P. Becker et al., 1970). Other safeguards require the physician who certifies death should not be a member of a transplantation team which might be over-anxious to pronounce the donor dead. In some cases, the opinion of more than one physician is required. One way or another then, fail-safe procedures must be built into the process of using the new clinical signs to ascertain human death.

Third, and perhaps most serious, is the question about the nature of brain death itself. Does brain death mean the death of the *total* brain, with the cessation of discernible central nervous system activity or merely of some *part* of the brain, that is, of the higher or neocortical centers on which it appears specifically human thought processes are dependent (Brierley, 1971; Braunstein, 1973)? Some are willing to defend this latter view. Thus the philosophers Rizzo and Yonder (1973) state:

> We must ask whether the death of the cerebral cortex or neocortex signals human death, even though other parts may be still functioning

for a time . . . We offer the hypothesis that human death should be related to the cessation of functions distinctly human since breathing, heartbeat and circulation are vegetative processes shared by other animals . . .

From all clinical evidence the death of the neocortex marks the end of the physiological basis for human consciousness, that is, a consciousness unique in its powers of reflection. It signals the end of the brain as a dynamic integrated whole and presages in most cases the imminent death of other cerebral systems. (p. 226)

Those physicians who have accepted the idea that the fetus although alive is not a person also conclude that the cessation of personhood can take place with the cessation of cortical function even when total brain function has not ceased (Moore, 1968).

In spite of the support for the position that cortical death constitutes human death, there are several difficulties inherent in this position. First of all, if we are willing to say that people who have spontaneously functioning heart and lungs, but no other vital signs, are dead, what will we say in the near future about people who have weak signs of "human life" (Veatch, 1975)? If we wish to declare that those in a deep and irreversible coma are dead insofar as human life is concerned, then what about people who are mentally retarded or senile? Do they show sufficient signs of human life to be kept alive? or should we give minimal care only to those who do not seem to have the functioning signs of human life that we associate with activity of the cortical center of the brain? The Euthanasia Educational Council of America and other persons who argue for the elimination of the retarded, senile, infirm, and debilitated in certain circumstances are interested in having partial brain death accepted as a proper clincial sign for human death. But we must go very slowly in accepting such a definition unless we are willing to bury people when they are still breathing and their hearts are pulsating spontaneously.

If the criteria of *partial* brain death were to be used as a sufficient evidence of death, ethical responsibility would require that we were reasonably sure about three matters of fact. First, we would have to be convinced that the radical structures necessary and sufficient to constitute the unified organism of the human person are to be found in the human brain separated from the rest of the body. This certainly is plausible from what we now know. Second, we would also have to know that most of the brain is unnecessary for the specifically human functions of thinking and willing, but exists only to maintain and move the body and supply the higher brain centers with nourishing materials. This also is plausible, but in the present state of our knowledge is far from certain. It is generally recognized today that the brain is a system of subsystems which are intimately interdependent. Although it is possible to localize such functions as speech and sight in particular parts of the brain, this is not proof that only one such part is involved in the function or even that it is its primary center, since inhibition of a merely secondary or auxiliary part of a system may impede its function. As Arthur Benton (1975) writes:

> [science has found that] the nervous system *is* a system and that the neural loci in it that had been identified as centers subserving behavioral functions are simply crucial links in a complex chain and not the seat of the functions. This is a conception with which all students would agree, but it is one that apparently needs to be kept constantly in mind because . . . there is a tendency even now to slip back into the simplistic notion that a specific part of the brain is distinctively responsible for a particular function or characteristic, e.g., Wernicke's area in the left temporal lobe for the understanding of language, the frontal lobes for the "awareness of self," etc. (p. 42)

Thus at present such localization of human functions is merely tentative. Third, even if we could exactly define these higher centers as sufficient for the radical unity of the human organism, it would be very difficult to determine their exact condition without an autopsy. The mere absence of function would not establish their condition. Perhaps some day (as we suggested in 9.1) we may be able to determine in special cases that such centers are totally destroyed, but this is not the case at present.

Hence, while we accept total brain death as a sufficient criterion for human death, we do not believe that partial brain death is sufficient. Thus, we should not certify death as long as patients are able to spontaneously maintain breathing and heartbeat since this constitutes strong evidence that the brain as the seat of the radical unity of the human body is still living, even if it is not evidencing its higher functions. Although even then there may be reasonable doubts, the benefit of the doubt should be given to the rights of the person.

13.3   TRUTH TELLING TO THE DYING

"What to tell the patient" has been considered one of the more difficult and delicate ethical questions for health care professionals. We formulated in 8.1-7 the Principle of Professional Communication which is relevant here. In the not too distant past, some physicians and other health care professionals thought that the less patients knew about their condition, the better would be the chances of recovery (Oken, 1961). Moreover, some health care professionals would even withhold information of impending death, fearing that such knowledge might lead a person to despair (Cope, 1968). Due to an awakened moral sense on the part of health care professionals and a sharper realization that patients have legal and moral rights that must be respected (AMA, 1972), today there is a much greater tendency to be open and honest with patients concerning their condition. In general, patients have the right to the truth concerning their condition, the purpose of the treatment to be given, and the prognosis of the treatment. "The Patient's Bill of Rights" of the American Hospital Association (1972) states:

> The patient has the right to obtain from the physician complete current information concerning diagnosis, treatment, and prognosis in terms the patient can be reasonably expected to understand. (n. 3)

And the *Ethical and Religious Directives* (United States Catholic Conference, 1971) declare:

> Everyone has the right and duty to prepare for the solemn moment of death. Unless it is clear, therefore, that a dying patient is already well prepared for death as regards both temporal and spiritual affairs, it is the physician's duty to inform him of his critical condition or to have some other responsible person impart this information. (n. 8)

Clearly, the information concerning serious sickness or impending death is to be furnished even if the individual does not ask for it. Legal precedent as well as moral concern prompts this realization. Hence, physicians and other health care professionals may not defend their lack of communication by pleading that the patient did not wish to know and did not ask questions. Many moral and legal rights put the burden of fulfillment upon the other person, and the right to information concerning one's health is an example. In some hospitals, a patients' representative helps patients understand their situation, especially when surgery is anticipated. Whenever possible, the leader of the health care team, the physician, should be involved in explaining the situation to the patient.

Though health care professionals usually respect the rights of patients insofar as providing the proper information is concerned, difficult situations often arise and health care professionals hesitate to tell patients their true condition. For example, patients with serious cases of cancer might become despondent and lack the desire to live, thus contributing to their illness, if their true condition is known. People who are dying might become despondent, morose, and even suicidal if they know their true situation. With this in mind, "The Patient's Bill of Rights" states:

> When it is not medically advisable to give such information to the patient, the information should be made available to an appropriate person in his behalf. (n. 8)

Though it is well intentioned, this statement is unsatisfactory and incomplete. It seems to indicate that when health care professionals feel that harm might result if the patient knows the truth, they fulfill the obligation by telling some friend or member of the family about the patient's condition and the prognosis. But the statement does not indicate what the member of the family or the friend is supposed to do once the information has been communicated. In order to ensure Christian treatment for the patient then, another dimension of the situation must be explored.

Even though the medical personnel might fear untoward results if patients are informed of their true condition, it does not mean that patients should never be told the true facts. Indeed, health care professionals should remember in these cases the words of Dr. Eric Cassell (1976), "The depression in patients that commonly occurs after the diagnosis of a fatal disease seems to stem in part from the conspiracy of silence. The physician can be a great help by simply making it clear to the patient that he is available for open and direct communication" (p. 197). Hence, the medical team, along with a friend of the patient or a member of the family, should work together and dispose the patient so that he or she will be able to accept the truth. Interviews with people who are seriously ill or with dying patients reveal that they do not wish to be kept continually in doubt about their condition; on the other hand, they do not want it revealed to them in an abrupt or brutal manner, according to Kübler-Ross (1969):

> When we asked our patients how they had been told, we learned that all the patients know about their terminal illness anyway, whether they were explicitly told or not, but depended greatly on the physician to present the news in an acceptable manner. (p. 183)

Howard Brody (1976) assesses the practical situation aptly when he states:

> . . . telling a patient something takes place over a span of time and is not a one-shot affair. Thus, the shading of phrases used, whether the truth is delivered all at once or in small doses, and the kind of follow-up are all important parts of the ethical decision, as well as "tell" or "don't tell." A decision to reveal a grave prognosis, which may be "ethical" in itself, may become "unethical" if the physician tells the patient bluntly and then withdraws, without offering any emotional support to help the patient resolve his feelings. In fact, the assurance that the physician plans to see it through along with the patient, and that he will always make himself available to offer any comfort possible, may be more important than the bad news itself. In many of the "sour cases" that are offered as justification for withholding the truth, it may well be the absence of this transmission of compassion, rather than the telling of the truth, that produced the unfortunate result. (p. 40)

Because physicians are not always able to convey information concerning serious illness or impending death in a fitting manner, a person who is trained in the dynamics of accepting sickness and death is a necessity in the present-day hospital setting. The value of pastoral care people trained in helping the sick and dying accept their suffering in a Christian manner and in working closely with the health care professionals is evident. Every health care facility that is responsible concerning its moral obligation should have people available who are adept at helping people accept the truth of their situation during the crisis situations of sickness and death. Crisis counseling of this nature is not an arcane art, but on the other hand, one must be prepared competently in order to perform it well. Well-meaning but untrained people can do more harm than good when trying to help in crisis situations.

Kübler-Ross maintains that in order to help others face death, one must be at peace with death oneself. The normal training for priesthood or ministry does not prepare a person for this specialty. Several hospitals in the country have training programs to help people become adept at helping people accept suffering and death. The need for this service in hospitals is clear and has been recognized, but help in facing sickness and death is also necessary for people in a noninstitutional setting. The poor and elderly, for example, should be helped in working through the acceptance of suffering and death so that the truth to which they have a right might be communicated safely to them.

In summary, it is clear that because of our increased knowledge of psychology and greater regard for the subjective process that accompanies sickness and dying, the ethical question in regard to truth telling has changed. As Kübler-Ross declares: "The question should not be 'should we tell?' but rather, 'How do we share this with the patient?' "

13.4 CARE FOR THE CORPSE OR CADAVER

When a human being dies, the body is no longer unified by the life-giving principle or soul by which it is a human person. The cadaver of a person, then, is not a *human* body in the proper sense of the word. Insofar as is possible, we should avoid referring to the remains of a person as though the human person existed *in* the human body or was, so to speak, limited by the human body. Language of this nature is misleading because it implies a duality in human existence; in a certain sense, the living human person is the living human body. When persons die, they exist in a new form, in a sense incomplete, because they no longer have a body (Rahner, 1968c). While existing in this life, the human person is a substantial unity of spirit (form) and body (matter), not an accidental juxtaposition of two distinct entities. Though the remains of a human body may resemble the body of a living person, and though this resemblance may be prolonged through embalming, the remains are not a *human* body, but a mass of organic matter, decomposing into constitutive, organic elements.

If the corpse of a human person is not a human body, then why are people so concerned about proper care for the remains of the deceased person? Why treat it with the respect and reverence which it usually receives? Respect and reverence are due the remains of a human being because of the sacredness of human life which once informed the now inert mass still bearing the image of the one we know. In order to mourn and express sorrow for the fact that the person will no longer be present in the same human manner as before, certain reverential spiritual actions are performed which express the love of the people who remain. Respect for the dead body, then, signifies respect for human life, respect for the Author of life, and respect for the person who once subsisted with this now corrupting corpse, and who now exists in a different modality. Hence, the actions, the ritual that people follow when caring for the body of a deceased person, have a meaning beyond their apparent signification.

Though the ritual of wake, funeral, and burial has been criticized in our American culture for its gross and inhuman excesses (Mitford, 1975), fundamentally this process has a meaning and worth in accord with the Judeo-Christian Tradition. Having friends share the burden through liturgical services is also a source of strength and support for bereaved people. Hence, the legitimate customs of people at the time of death are not signs of superstition or blind fear; rather they bespeak a noble belief about life, its purpose, and the enduring strength of human love.

In accord with the respect due to the remains of a human person, no organs should be removed from a corpse nor should the body be dimembered in any way unless there is a sufficient reason which would justify such an action. Usually the next of kin or the person to whom the corpse is committed for care has the legal right to determine if organs may be removed from the body and if an autopsy may be performed (Pierce v. Swan Point, 1872). The right of the next of kin in regard to caring for the human body is not absolute. It may be superseded by statements made by the person while still alive, for example, through the Anatomical Gift Act, or by the needs of society, for example, when an autopsy might help stave off a contagious disease.

The Anatomical Gift Act is "designed to facilitate the donation and use of human tissues and organs for transplantation and other medical purposes and provide a favorable legal environment for such activities" (Sadler et al., 1968). At present, all fifty states have enacted the Anatomical Gift Act, thus enabling persons who are of sound mind and eighteen years of age or more to give all or part of their body to persons or institutions authorized to practice or perform research medicine or to engage in tissue banking, the gift to take effect upon death. This law also recognizes the right of the next of kin to donate the body or any part for the same purpose, but in most states the law declares that if there is a conflict between the donor and the next of kin that the wishes of the donor have precedence. The person or institution to whom the donation is made need not accept the gift. If the gift is accepted, following removal of the part named the body is transferred to the next of kin or other persons under obligation to dispose of the body. If the whole body is retained for research at a medical school, it will often be cremated upon completion of the research. In such cases, there might not be a wake, but a funeral service; a mass, for example, is usually held without the corpse being present.

Protection from civil and criminal proceedings which might result from the removal of organs or experimentation upon the corpse is granted to all persons concerned including physicians, next of kin, funeral directors, and medical examiners. Persons interested in donating a part or all of their body upon death should contact the particular person or institution to whom the donation will be made so that all required legal stipulations will be followed.

From a Christian point of view, the practice of donating organs and one's body for scientific research is ethical and even to be encouraged if a true need exists. As Pope Pius XII (1956a) stated:

> The public must be educated. It must be explained with intelligence and respect that to consent explicitly or tacitly to serious damage to the integrity of the corpse in the interest of those who are suffering, is no violation of the reverence due to the dead. (n. 646)

However, another ethical question does not admit of such easy solution: Is it immoral to accept or solicit payment for the gift of certain organs? While some have defended such practices, other authors, notably Paul Ramsey (1970b), maintain that abuses could spring up very quickly if cadaver organs were sold or contracted for money. He points out that blood replaces itself, while human organs do not. With this latter opinion we agree. If our society is to live in a humane manner, then generosity and charity, rather than monetary gain and greed, must serve as the basis for donation of functioning organs.

Autopsy is the examination of a cadaver after death performed in order to provide greater medical knowledge concerning the cause of death. Occasionally, the benefit of an autopsy will be to provide knowledge about a rare or contagious disease. In such cases, the good of the community would overrule the rights of the next of kin, and if the next of kin were not willing, the court could order that an autopsy be performed. In cases of violent death or unattended death an autopsy is required by law, no matter what wishes are expressed by the next of kin.

Usually, however, the purpose of an autopsy is not to trace the etiology of a rare disease nor to discover unknown or violent causes of death. More frequently, autopsies are performed in order to help health professionals achieve a higher level of efficiency in the care of the living. The autopsy rate of a hospital is usually a good sign of concern for excellence and offers a gauge of professional integrity and interest in scientific advancement. Through autopsies, the diagnosis and treatment a person received can be evaluated and staff members encouraged to observe a high level of proficiency. For this reason, autopsies should be encouraged and people should be encouraged to look upon them as an ordinary part of the medical care process. Needless to say, the human remains of a person should always be treated with utmost respect during an autopsy.

In the Judeo-Christian Tradition, respect for the dead was usually displayed through interment of the corpse in the ground or in a mausoleum. Cremation of the remains, while not a common part of this

Tradition, has never been considered as disrespectful treatment. However, for a long time cremation was forbidden in the Catholic Church because anti-Christian groups in the eighteenth century advocated cremation as a means of denying externally the immortality of the human person and the Resurrection. Thus, not because it was immoral in itself, but rather because of what it might signify, cremation was not an acceptable form of caring for the remains of a person in the Catholic Church.

Because cremation is no longer associated with a denial of religious truth today, while burying the dead is encouraged as the usual procedure, the total remains or an amputated member may be cremated if there is a serious reason (Congregation of Holy Office, May 8, 1963): for example, if the custom of the country favors cremation, if there is danger of disease, or if suitable grave sites cannot be obtained at a reasonable cost. If there is no certain sign of disrespect for Christian dogma involved in the request, cremation may be requested by a dying person or the next of kin. Those who direct that their bodies are to be cremated, then, may be given the sacraments of the Church, as well as liturgical rites of burial, provided that the latter are not performed in the actual place of cremation.

Because of what it represents, the remains of a human person should be shown respect and reverence. Health care professionals should never allow their frequent experience of human death to inure them to the great mystery and sacredness of human life. The danger in the practice of medicine at any level of its experience is that people become blasé or insouciant about suffering, death, and human remains in order to cover their own feelings of fear, inadequacy, or lack of faith. Though such feeling is often motivated unconsciously, it is nonetheless destructive of humane Christian health care. Moreover, it bespeaks a personality defect on the part of the health care professional that requires a new orientation toward the act and experience of death.

13.5   EUTHANASIA

Suicide

The word *euthanasia* is derived from two Greek words which mean "good death" or "happy death." For centuries, the accepted meaning of the term referred to an action by which a person was put to death painlessly usually to avoid further suffering from an incurable disease or to end an irreversible comatose condition (J. B. Wilson, 1975; Gruman, 1973; Triche and Triche, 1975; Clouser and Zucker, 1974; Euthanasia Educational, 1970). *Webster's New International Dictionary* (3rd ed.), for example, defines *euthanasia* as "a mode or act of inducing death painlessly as a relief from pain." Euthanasia in this sense is often called "mercy killing" or even "death with dignity." In the more traditional meaning of the term, it could be performed with or without the consent of the person to be put to death. In the Judeo-Christian Tradition, euthanasia without the consent of the patient would be murder and with consent of the patient would be both suicide and murder. Today, the proponents of euthanasia generally defend it in this latter form where the patient's consent is given or at least presumed. Thus, our ethical analysis needs to begin with the question of whether suicide is ever permissible, or whether it exceeds the limits of our rightful control over our own lives. The high rate of suicide in the medical profession (Steppacher, 1974) gives this question a special significance for bio-ethical reflection.

It is important to be clear, as David Novak (1971) has pointed out, that the issue here is not whether persons who commit suicide are to be morally condemned. No doubt the great majority of persons who take their own life do so because they are so emotionally disturbed that they act compulsively, or at least their perception of objective reality is so distorted by their anguish and depression that their freedom of choice is greatly restricted. Consequently either their act is not to be evaluated ethically at all, or at least it may be assumed that they act in good faith and are subjectively guiltless. Indeed many experts in suicidology today seem to take it for granted that all suicides are compulsive and irrational (Menninger, 1938; Durkheim, 1951; Farberow and Schneidman, 1961; Douglas, 1967; Schneidman, 1967, 1969, 1970; Resnick, 1968; Lester, 1971; Alvarez, 1972; Perlin, 1975). However, can we really make this assumption, or must we face the possibility that the decision about whether to live or to take one's life may be a genuine ethical issue for some people who have the capacity to make a free and sane choice? Only in such cases does it make any sense to talk about the *morality* of suicide.

Among the Greeks and Romans suicide was both condemned and defended (Choron, 1972; Noyes, 1973), as they were also in Eastern cultures (Holck, 1974). The Epicureans, who considered pleasure and peace of mind the highest human goods, argued that it was better to kill oneself than to endure life if it had become more painful than pleasurable or peaceful. The Stoics, who believed that virtue or self-control was the highest good, argued that it was permissible to kill oneself if suffering or torture might force one to lose self-control or act ignobly, or where a choice had to be made to perish in a shameful way or "die with dignity." Dualists, like some Platonists (but not Plato, himself), agnostics, and Manichaeans taught that the soul, which is the real man, is burdened by the body in this life or in many reincarnations; hence suicide might be justified as a laying down of this burden. Even in Christian Europe men and women have been regarded as heroic if they committed suicide for the sake of honor. Recently some Catholic Irishmen and Buddhist Vietnamese have used sucide by self-starvation or self-immolation as a protest against injustice.

However, the monotheistic religions of Judaism, Christianity, and Islam have always opposed suicide because they regard life as God's gift which his children are to use as faithful stewards. Moreover, these monotheistic religions, unlike others, hold that eternal life is not the survival of a disembodied soul, nor endless reincarnation, but resurrected life with God. Consequently, we cannot escape accounting to God for our stewardship of this one life which is given us on earth, nor can we reject the body which will always be part of us. This view was already anticipated by the great Greek philosopher Plato who argued that suicide is a rejection of our duty to our body, to the community of which we are a part, and to God Who gave us life. In a very different way, another great philosopher, Kant, argued that suicide is the greatest of crimes because it is man's rejection of morality itself, since man must be his own moral lawgiver (cf. 7.3). For a person to kill himself or herself is to treat himself or herself as a thing (a means) rather than as a person (an end in himself or herself).

However, today this classical stand is being reexamined (Pretzel, 1968; Szasz, 1971a; Mays, 1973; Noyes, 1973; Kluge, 1975). The Protestant moralist Joseph Fletcher (1960) has said, "The real issue is whether we can morally justify taking it into our own hands to hasten death for ourselves (suicide) or for others (mercy killing) out of reasons of compassion" (p. 140). Fletcher answers this in terms of his own situationism according to which the only command of God is to "act lovingly." This leads Fletcher to an ethics of intention which justifies any means if it is effective for achieving loving ends because "If we will the end, we will the means." Consequently, it appears to him that there are many situations in which persons can will their own death for the good of others (as a war prisoner fearing torture that may cause him to reveal the hiding place of others) or in which we may put others to death out of compassion for their sufferings, assuming that they would want this to be done for them (cf. also Leeman, 1968; McEllhenney, 1973).

Catholic theologians generally reject situationism, but those who hold for the principle of proportion as developed by Peter Knauer and others, are arguing that the moral law against suicide and euthanasia is not absolute. Thus Daniel Maguire in *Death by Choice* (1974a) maintains:

> What he [Knauer] means is that the taking of innocent life is wrong if there is no commensurate reason for taking it . . . At the theoretical level, then, Knauer's ethical theory allows for euthanasia, suicide, or abortion under his dominant rubric of "commensurate reason." He slips out from under the old rule against intentionally taking human innocent life and comes up under the position that commensurate reason is what counts. (p. 69)

Maguire admits that Knauer and Richard McCormick "are not willing to go as far as their theories," that is, they consider mercy killing and suicide to be wrong because no proportionate good could come from allowing exceptions. But Maguire is willing to follow the theory to its ultimate conclusions, as are others (Curran, 1970a; Dedek, 1975), and he states, "The morality of terminating life, innocent or not, is an open question although it is widely treated as a closed one" (p. 112). Maguire believes termination of life can be moral or immoral according to the circumstances that give it moral meaning.

In general these Christian thinkers believe that to make an absolute rule against suicide is under some circumstances to fail to respond compassionately to useless human suffering or to draw subtle distinctions which indicate the Pharisaic legalistic mentality repudiated by Christ. Humanists, emphasizing the autonomy of the individual, tend to favor the right of all persons to determine when their own life shall cease (Russell, 1975; Koh, 1975; Downing, 1970), and their arguments have proved very disturbing to Christians (cf. Bok, 1973; Trowell, 1973; Trubo, 1973). What, then, are the values and countervalues which need to be balanced if we are to decide in particular circumstances whether it is permissible? The usual advantages often mentioned can be summarized as follows:

1. Suicide gives the human person full autonomy since he or she can choose to live or die, to be part of society or reject it.

2. It enables someone to leave life with dignity, instead of endure useless suffering, be a useless burden to others, and so forth, or suffer mental disease or unjustified disgrace and dishonor.

3. It may enable one to avoid temptation to treacherous or ignoble acts which destroy one's personal integrity, or which may be harmful to others, such as the revelation of secrets under torture.

4. It relieves society of burdens and also one's family, so that their resources can be used for something better.

5. It can be an act of heroic sacrifice for others, such as the Kamikaze pilots in World War II.

6. It can be a protest against social injustice, such as the Buddhist monks who burned themselves in protest against tyranny in Vietnam.

The following disadvantages are also frequently mentioned:

1. It is an intrinsic evil for a person to reject living out life to its full, since as long as conscious suffering or conscious endurance is possible, there is opportunity for personal growth.

2. It is contradictory to the very basis of morality since by this act the person gives up all other moral responsibilities.

3. Suicide is not a road to immortal life, since that life is mysterious, and we do not know whether this is the proper way to enter it.

4. By suicide the individual withdraws himself from the community

which has given him life and deprives it of a unique member.

5. Suicide is a rejection of God because it is a rejection of God's gift of life.

6. Suicide deeply hurts those who love us and discourages them in their own task of living.

When we attempt to weigh these various values one against another in concrete cases, we notice that the reasons given to justify suicide are either social or personal. As regards the social reasons that persons might feel they have a duty in justice or charity to kill themselves for the good of others, we have already argued in chapters 8 and 10 that society has no right to require some of its members to directly sacrifice their life for others, although it can require that they perform some positive action for the common good which may involve the risk or even the certainty that they may incur death. Thus those who kill themselves because they believe this will benefit others are following an exaggerated sense of moral obligation, while at the same time they are failing to fulfill their social obligations to continue to participate in the life of the community.

It is probable that the personal reasons for suicide often underlie the social arguments. Basically persons kill themselves because "life is no longer worth living." The question, therefore, is whether this can ever be reasonably said to be true. There is no doubt we can *feel* this way easily enough, but can we conscientiously judge that it is really the case? Of the very essence of the human person is that we are historical beings oriented to the future. As long as there is hope for a future, suicide is clearly unreasonable. Because hope in the future is closed off, suicide may look like a rational thing to do. In a Christian scheme of values, however, our hope in God grounds our future. We know that by God's providence even the most painful situations not only can be endured, but also may be extremely important events in the completion of our earthly life. In secular and other Humanist systems this may not be true, but as Christians, we ought to wait on the God Who gave us our life, because He knows best how to prepare us for the mystery of eternal life with Him.

Hence, attempts to balance the various values of suicide lead us back to the conclusion that suicide is intrinsically and always wrong, because in all circumstances it constitutes an abdication of our responsibility to live out our life in community with other persons and with God.

Active Euthanasia

Granted that suicide is intrinsically wrong, it also becomes clear that euthanasia is also wrong (Baelz, 1972; to the contrary, Worden,

1972). When sufferers freely choose to die and ask to be killed, they are not only commiting the crime of suicide, but are also compounding it by making another a partner in the crime. To yield to such a request because of compassion is false compassion (Sullivan, 1952). If we have true compassion for the person who has made such a decision, we will realize that it must be because that person is hopeless, alienated from community, and doubtful of God's love. Our mercy should lead us to stay by such a person's side and by our friendship help him or her recover hope. The mercy killer in such a case is really adding a final rejection to the many rejections which have already driven the person to this point of despair.

On the other hand if the sufferer is no longer really free to make a truly human decision, but is pleading to be put out of the pain or depression that has taken away the sufferer's capacity to think straight, then the mercy killer is simply a murderer putting to death someone no longer able to protect himself or herself.

If we ask ourselves honestly what are the motives of mercy killers, we will not accept easily their claim that they did it for the sake of the victim. May it not well be that the real motive was that the relative did not want to accept the responsibility of helping the dying person to the end? Often the killer says, "I loved my mother, I couldn't bear to see her suffer!" It is true in such a case that the killer could not bear to see her suffer, but it is not so certain just what the quality of that love was. However, no doubt sometimes mercy killers are themselves not free enough from tortured feelings to make a sane decision. Medical personnel hardly have such excuses. By consenting to help their patients die they may simply be evading the painful and threatening task of adequate care for the dying which we will discuss in chapter 14.

As for euthanasia of the type used by the Nazis in which patients were put to death without their consent because they were senile, insane, or defective or as genocide, few in the United States would at the present defend such a practice, but some are again beginning to discuss the morality of such acts as part of lifeboat ethics (cf. 9.3).

Generally the medical profession has rejected euthanasia absolutely, as is evidenced by the Hippocratic Oath as well as by the more recent codes of medical ethics such as *The Declaration of Geneva* of the World Medical Association. Generally the Christian churches have also rejected it. Thus, Pope Pius XII (1952), wrote with reference to Nazi horrors:

> The direct destruction of what they call "worthless life," born or unborn, practiced a few years ago on many occasions, can be no way justified. For this reason, when this practice began, the Church formally declared that the killing, even by order of public authority, of those who although innocent are not useful to the nation on account of physical or psychic defects but also a burden upon it, is contrary to positive natural and divine right and therefore illicit. (n. 368)

The Second Vatican Council also declared in *The Church and the Modern*

World (1965c):

> Whatever is opposed to life itself, such as any type of murder, geno-
> cide, abortion, euthanasia or willful self-destruction, all these things
> and others of their like are infamous indeed. (n. 51)

Recently, however, the term *euthanasia* (as well as such terms as *death with dignity*, *mercy killing*, and *right to die*) have become ambiguous because they are used to cover not only direct killing but also letting die or indirect killing. Consequently several writers have distinguished between euthanasia in the ordinary sense of killing (which they call "active") and letting die which they call "passive euthanasia."
Thus, passive euthanasia refers to an action which from an ethical point of view is entirely different from active euthanasia. Passive euthanasia means allowing oneself, or another person, who is terminally ill to die when there is no hope that the person will recover. Though the terms are somewhat similar, the actions are different entirely. As one study (Amulree et al., 1975) states, "For a doctor to take measures deliberately to kill the patient . . . involves a definite and in its implications a mo-
mentous change of policy. There is a clear distinction to be drawn between rendering someone unconscious at the risk of killing him and killing him in order to render him unconscious" (p. 9). From an ethical or moral point of view, it makes a difference if one causes something to happen when it can and should be prevented as opposed to allowing something to happen when there is no need to prevent it.

Because of the fact that active and passive euthanasia are distinct ethically, some authors point out that the term *passive euthanasia* is confusing and might even foster the acceptance of active euthanasia (Marx, 1974). Others wish to substitute the term *benemortasia* or *aganathasia* for the type of care given to people who are allowed to die when terminally ill (cf. Ramsey, 1970b). For our part, while we realize that the terms do present some difficulty, we feel that the difficulty can be avoided if it is borne in mind that these two actions involve different ethical judgments.

Letting Die in Peace

Although some argue against the relevance of the distinction (Rachel, 1975; cf. Dinello, 1971), most people recognize the difference between active and passive euthanasia, even though they do not always use these terms. Passive euthanasia is approved by ethicists of varied viewpoints. For the Christian, human life is a gift from the Creator over which our control is one of stewardship not of absolute autonomy (Principle of Stewardship and Creativity, 8.3-3; Cooper, 1973). It is like the talents given by the master to his servants which he expects them to invest to gain him a proper return on his investment (Matt. 25:14-30). Hence, we must use this gift of human bodily life in this existence to a good purpose. Such life, however, is not the ultimate value for the Christian which is to be found only in serving God and living with Him forever. The time may come, therefore, when someone is reasonably convinced that life is coming to an end, and a prolongation of dying by additional complicated medical treatments is not the best investment the person can make of what remains. It would be better, he or she judges, to use my remaining hours to compose myself for death than to extend them in a profitless way that would only add to suffering and confusion of spirit for myself and for my relatives and friends. To reject such additional medical efforts is not to reject life, itself, or the God Who gave it, but simply to reject well-meant efforts which will not really help in completing the final task of living out life to its end.

In the same way the relatives and the medical professionals who care for the dying person may judge that any further efforts to preserve life will be of no significant benefit and may even make it more difficult for the person to finish the course of life in peace, composure, and union with God. Hence they can make the decision to terminate the supports that prolong the dying process and allow the person to die more quickly.

Finding the right words to express the judgment that must be made as death approaches and further effort to prolong life is no longer helpful is difficult. We wish to avoid saying that a person has "a right to die," as many seem to be doing today (cf. Heifetz, and Mangel, 1975; Malone, 1974; Mannes, 1974; Robitscher, 1972b; Bard and Fletcher, 1968), or that human beings exist "to get to heaven," or that one may be allowed to die if "life is useless." All these terms can lead to faulty conclusions. For example, some means of prolonging life may be useless, but human life is never useless because of the dignity of the gift and the transcendence of the Giver. Moreover, if one admits there is a right to die, then some would conclude that suicide is licit, which is not to be easily conceded. In discussing passive euthanasia, it is wise to avoid all slogans and spell out completely what one implies by this ethical terminology and to recognize that the distinction is difficult to define with legal precision (Silving, 1954; Williams, 1968; Gurney, 1972; Baughman et al., 1973; Senate Judiciary, 1973; Vodiga, 1974).

Though ethicists in general have little problem approving passive euthanasia, many physicians and nurses (Popoff, 1975; Crane, 1975; Kron, 1968; Scott, 1974; *Proceedings of Royal Society*, 1970; Travis, Noyes, and Brightwell, 1974) are not as ready to remove life-supporting means and allow a person to die. There are good reasons for this attitude and they can be summarized in the following three arguments. (1) It is very difficult to know when a patient is terminally ill. As one noted expert (Foye, 1972) declares, "We must never forget that on occasion patients, their families, and their physicians will conclude that a disease has reached the hopeless stage and death is imminent and be wrong.   If they can stop treatment on the basis of their hopelessness, the prophecy becomes self-fulfilling" (p. 24) (cf. Ayd, 1962; Modell, 1974). (2) Even though a patient may be desperately ill, some physicians will not give up hope of doing some good.   Indeed, they would identify "doing something to help" as the role of the physician (Freireich, 1976): "There is no doubt that the physician has the capability to offer treatment for and prevention of disease to anyone who seeks his help.   The modern physician is living through a period of revolution in our ability to restore man's normal physiological mechanisms.   In fact, medical breakthroughs occur everyday . . ." (p. 62) (cf. Poe, 1973).   (3) Some physicians, wishing to avoid malpractice suits, are hesitant to remove life-sustaining means, even though there are signs that the means are no longer useful (Collins, 1968; Moore, 1968; Schaefer, 1971).   In commenting on this practice, the Supreme Court of New Jersey stated in "The Karen Quinlan Case" (1976):

> The modern proliferation of substantial malpractice litigation and the less frequent but even more unnerving possibility of criminal sanctions would seem, for it is beyond human nature to suppose otherwise, to have bearing on the practice and standards as they exist.   The brooding presence of such possible liability, it was testified here, had no part in the decisions of the treating physicians.   As did Judge Muir, we afford this testimony full credence.   But we cannot believe that the stated factor has not had a strong influence on the standards, as the literature on the subject plainly reveals.

Clearly, physicians and ethicists approach the dying patient with different emphases, the ethicist being more concerned with how the person dies and the physician being more concerned with how to prolong life.   We believe that there need not be any radical disagreement between physicians and moralists, however, if three truths are understood clearly (Middleton, 1975).

1. Physicians and moralists often use the terms *ordinary means* and *extraordinary means* with different connotations.

2. While the physician has the expertness and the right to make decisions concerning the usefulness or medical effects of some particular means, the patient (and/or the family of the patient) has the right to determine whether a particular means is ordinary or extraordinary from an ethical point of view.

3. If the means are determined to be ordinary, then they must be employed; if extraordinary, they may or may not be employed, the decision being made by the patient (and/or the family) in consultation with the physician, but ordinary care should continue.   In order to explain these factors, let us say a word about the ethical meaning of the distinction of ordinary and extraordinary means and decision making concerning the use of these means (Kelly, 1950, 1951; Cronin, 1938).

Many physicians use the term *ordinary* to describe a customary or useful medical procedure; a procedure which is rarely used is called *extraordinary* or *heroic*. Thus, physicians are inclined to use these terms without reference to a particular patient. Hence, penicillin might be described as ordinary medical treatment for pneumonia, and a gallbladder operation would be ordinary because it is comparatively safe and common. The moralist, on the other hand, takes into consideration the total situation of the patient, the nonmedical, as well as the medical, factors that would influence the ethical decision. From the ethical point of view, ordinary means of preserving life are "all medicines, treatments, and operations which offer a reasonable hope of benefit for the patient and which can be obtained without excessive expense, pain, or other inconvenience," and extraordinary means are "all medicines, treatments, and operations which cannot be obtained or used without excessive expense, pain, or other inconvenience or which if used would not offer a reasonable hope of benefit" (Pius XII, 1957). Hence, ethically speaking, one cannot make a priori classifications of ordinary and extraordinary means. Simply because a means is inexpensive and readily available does not render it ordinary. Penicillin might be considered an ordinary means, but if a person is allergic to penicillin and would have a hyperactive reaction that might cause death, it would not be considered ordinary for that person. A relatively simple surgical procedure, such as the removal of gallstones, might be ordinary for a healthy person, but extraordinary for one in terminal illness due to cancer.

The rationale for this distinction was expressed accurately in the writing of Pope Pius XII in a statement (1957) that is quoted often by non-Catholics as well as by Catholic ethicists:

> Natural reason and Christian morals say that man, (and whoever is entrusted with the task of taking care of his fellowman) has the right and duty in case of serious illness to take the necessary treatment for the preservation of life and health. This duty that one has toward himself, toward God, toward the human community, and in most cases toward certain determined persons, derives from a well-ordered charity, from submission to the Creator, from social justice and even from strict justice as well as from devotion toward one's family . . .

> But normally one is held to use only ordinary means — according to the circumstances of persons, places, times and cultures — that is to say, means that do not involve any grave burdens for oneself or another. A more strict obligation would be too burdensome for most men and would render the attainment of a higher, more important good too difficult. Life, health, all temporary activities are in fact subordinated to spiritual ends. On the other hand, one is not forbidden to take more than the strictly necessary steps to preserve life and health, as long as he does not fail in some more serious duty.

Though the distinction between ordinary and extraordinary means for prolonging life is often presented as neat and orderly, in reality it is usually difficult to apply, especially if it is a case of discontinuing a means already utilized (McCormick 1974a, 1976a). As Paul Ramsey (1970b) states, "These are meaningful specifications but there is uncertainty in applying them" (p. 120). This difficulty is evidenced excruciatingly in the case of newborn babies with birth defects (Freeman and Cooke, 1972; Duff and Campbell, 1973; Smith and Smith, 1973; Lorber, 1974; Working Party, 1975). Gustafson (1975b) has urged caution in dealing with this problem, but others (Robertson, 1975; Kelsey, 1975; Heymann and Holtz, 1975; *Choices of Life*, 1975) have emphasized the urgency of finding some practical solution. Richard McCormick and Paul Ramsey have attempted to propose such a solution without falling into the quality of life ethic, while at the same time recognizing that in some cases continuing the life of the newborn "would render the attainment of the higher and more important good too difficult" (Pius XII, 1957).

The important point to recognize is that parents sometimes have the problem of distributing their resources and care between a seriously abnormal child who requires very great care, yet can benefit very little from this attention since he or she is incapable of normal development and liable to early death. Parents (and society) in such cases must apply the triage principle discussed in 9.3. Both normal and abnormal children must be given ordinary care appropriate to their stage of development. However, parents are not obliged to give to the abnormal child such care that the normal child, who in the long run actually has much greater needs, will be neglected. This means that in some cases the parents (and society) are justified in not giving extraordinary care necessary to prolong the abnormal child's life. It is essential, however, that this prudential decision should not be erected into some kind of routine by which the right of every child to at least ordinary care, no matter what it's condition, should be denied (cf. Reich and Smith, 1973; Jonsen et al., 1975; John Fletcher, 1974, 1975).

Who makes the difficult and delicate decisions that a certain means is ordinary or extraordinary? And since an extraordinary means need not but may be utilized, who decides whether a particular extraordinary means will be employed, retained, or set aside? Clearly, the physician is involved in the decision in an integral manner and has the responsibility of considering the condition of the patient and determining the medical prognosis, that is, whether the means in question will cure, help appreciably, or have no effect upon the dying patient. But there are other circumstances to be considered in addition to the medical effectiveness of the means. What about the expense, pain, and inconvenience? Only the patient or the family can decide concerning these circumstances. Hence, the radical right to make a decision as to what would be an ordinary means and what would be an extraordinary means from an ethical point of view belongs to the patient (McKegney and Lange, 1971; Cantor, 1972; Viederman and Burke, 1974; "Right of a Patient," 1974; White and Engelhardt, 1975; Platt, 1975). With the guidance of the physician, often in consultation with family members, the patient decides what actions should be performed and which should be omitted. Pope

Pius XII (1957) expressed the physician and patient relationship in this manner:

> The rights and duties of the doctor are correlative to those of the patient. The doctor, in fact, has no separate or independent right where the patient is concerned. In general, he can take action only if the patient explicitly or implicitly, directly or indirectly, gives him permission.

The statement of the House of Delegates of the American Medical Association (Dec. 1973) corresponds with the thinking of Pius XII:

> The cessation of the employment of extraordinary means to prolong life of the body when there is irrefutable evidence that biological death is imminent is the decision of the patient and/or his immediate family. The advice and judgment of the physician should be freely available to the patient and/or his immediate family.

If the patient is unconscious (Beecher, 1968) or otherwise unable to make a personal decision concerning the means of prolonging life, the next of kin should express what the patient would be supposed to decide in such circumstances, not what the family member making the decision would find more suitable for his or her own purposes. This is a recognized principle of civil law as well as of Christian ethics. "The rights and duties of the family depend in general upon the presumed will of the unconscious patient if he is of age and *sui juris*. Where the proper and independent duty of the family is concerned, they are usually bound only to the use of ordinary means" (Pius XII, 1957).

Pain

As we have seen, the basic issue in both active and passive euthanasia is the question as to what compassion requires of us in the face of hopeless suffering. This problem of suffering was treated at length in chapter 8, but a few observations are relevant here.

1. Pain is not an absolute human evil. Though suffering is truly an ontological evil to be alleviated whenever possible, it is not of itself a moral evil nor without supernatural and human benefits when rightly used. Some will scoff at this view of life, but the Christian Tradition holds that great good can come out of suffering when this is joined to the suffering of Jesus. Though Christian teaching in this regard is often misrepresented, it does not imply a masochistic desire for pain, nor does it stand in the way of medical progress. As one group of Christians who have investigated the situation (Amulree et al., 1975) maintain, "A terminal illness can be transformed into a time for which everyone concerned is grateful."

2. Alleviating pain by means of medicine or even by surgery does not constitute active euthanasia, even if the suffering person's life

might be shortened as a result of the medical or surgical procedure (Alsop, 1974). In this case, the direct object of the act is to relieve pain; if life is shortened, it is an accidental, even though foreseen, result. This view is expressed succinctly in the *Ethical and Religious Directives for Catholic Health Facilities*: "It is not euthanasia to give a dying person sedatives and analgesics for the alleviation of pain when such a measure is judged necessary, even though they may deprive the patient of the use of reason, or shorten his life" (n. 29).

The opportunity for suffering to be an opportunity for spiritual growth is not destroyed if painkilling drugs are used. Rather, the individual and those who care for him have the right to use such drugs in a way that will permit the best use of the patient's remaining energies, times of consciousness, and so forth, so that the patient can complete life with the maximum of composure.

3. In recent years, medical and psychological breakthroughs have occurred in regard to severe pain. Medically speaking, pharmaceutical and surgical procedures make it possible to control and alleviate severe pain in the hospital and at home. Severe and excruciating pain, then, is hardly a realistic cause for direct euthanasia or suicide. Moreover, an even more startling discovery in the control of pain has been made by people in the hospice movement (Lamerton, 1973). Case studies demonstrate that pain is alleviated and controlled when human concern and care are given to the elderly. The ultimate human pain seems to be loneliness and the feeling of dying alone. If these feelings are overcome, it seems that pain is not such a prominent factor, even for those who are dying of debilitating diseases (Verwoerdt, 1966; Kübler-Ross, 1969, 1974; Cassell, 1974, 1976; Westberg, 1971; Peterkin, 1975; Neale, 1973; Soulen, 1975).

In summary, the following pastoral norms can be formulated:

1. A physician may admit that a patient is incurable and cease trying to effect a cure; however, physicians should not cease trying to find a remedy for disease itself.

2. As long as there is a slight hope of curing patients or checking the progress of their illness, the physician should use the available remedies at hand.

3. The patient, considering his medical prognosis as well as other spiritual and temporal circumstances of life, determines in consultation with the physician whether a particular means is ordinary or extraordinary from an ethical point of view.

4. If the means are ordinary, then they must be utilized; if the means are extraordinary, they may be utilized but need not be. Minimal means of maintaining the patient's comfort and well-being (such as spiritual care, hygienic measures, and basic sustaining measures, for

example, minimal nourishment and water) are always considered ordinary means.

5. If the patient is unable to make the pertinent decisions, then the family, in consultation with the physician, should have the right and obligation to determine whether the means in question are ordinary or extraordinary, and whether extraordinary means will be utilized. In making this decision, the family decides as would the patient and for the benefit of the patient, not solely for the benefit of the family.

6. Such documents as the *Christian Affirmation of Life* and the *Living Will* may be utilized by patients as a means of informing family and physician and as a help in preparing for death (O'Rourke, 1974b; The Catholic Hospital Association, 1974). However, we do not favor that such documents be given legal status by natural death acts. Though such acts are not in themselves wrong, potentially they may lead to disrespect for human life and inhuman care of the dying (Lebacqz, 1977; McHugh, 1976).

PART V

PASTORAL MINISTRY IN HEALTH CARE

CHAPTER 14 PASTORAL CARE AND ETHICAL DECISIONS

14.1 RELIGIOUS MINISTRY AND THE HEALTH CARE TEAM

Overview

In this book we have dealt with persons seeking health, with the health care professionals who serve them in this search, and finally with some of the many difficult ethical decisions professionals and health seekers have to make together. In this concluding Part V, which will consist of a single chapter, we will deal with one type of health care professional whose professional status is often not even recognized in the health care team, yet who has a very special, integrative role to perform in that team and in its ethical decision making, namely, the pastoral care minister.

We will first show that pastoral care is needed in the health team not as an adjunct to psychotherapy or social work, but precisely in its service to human persons in their search for spiritual health, which we argued in chapter 2 is essential for total health and also in service to the hospital staff itself (14.2). We will then treat of the ways in which pastoral ministry can make this contribution to health care through spiritual counseling (14.3) and the celebration of Word and Sacrament (14.4). In this way, a truly caring and therapeutic community can be formed in which the crises of ethical decision can best be met. Finally, in 14.5 we will conclude by discussing the ways in which the religious minister can assist professionals, patients, and their families in the actual process of ethical decision.

Need for Pastoral Health Care

If Christian ministry is to be Christ-like, there can be no doubt that care for the sick is an essential part of it. If we look at the Gospel According to St. Mark, commonly considered to be first written of the Gospels, we discover that if we leave aside the Passion Narrative devoted to Jesus' own suffering and death at least a third of the Gospel is devoted to accounts of how Jesus healed the physically and mentally sick. His care for the sick seems to have been the clearest evidence to others of his mission from the Father and of the life-giving truth of his preaching.

Clebsch and Jaekle (1964; cf. also McNeill, 1951) in a study devoted to the history of pastoral care come to the conclusion that traditionally religious ministry has four functions: (1) to heal, (2) to sustain, (3) to guide, and (4) to reconcile. While by healing and sustaining they have in mind something broader than physical and psychological healing and encouragement in times of sickness, yet it is obvious that ministers cannot heal and sustain if they are not intimately concerned with problems of physical and psychological health. Furthermore, we will try to show in later sections that guidance and reconciliation are in some respects especially effective when they occur in times of health crisis.

The hospital as we know it in Western culture (6.3) originated in the pastoral care of the sick and only with the rise of secular Humanism in the eighteenth century began to subordinate that concern to purely medical care. Yet even in the nineteenth century, the nursing profession in its modern form was the creation of Florence Nightingale, herself inspired by the Christian ideals of the Anglican Church and in conscious continuity with the traditions of the Catholic nursing sisters. Today, however, in many hospitals, pastoral care is left to occasional visiting ministers who are treated much as any other visitor. In others, a chaplain is provided, but he is regarded by the medical staff simply as a convenience to the patients like the hospital barber or proprietor of the gift shop. It is becoming much more common, however, even for public hospitals to include a department of pastoral care as a recognized part of their therapeutic work. Yet the members of such a department are still often regarded as somewhat less than professional colleagues of the medical staff, who think of them according to outmoded stereotypes (H. L. Smith, 1975; Bane and Smith, 1975).

The first reason for this situation is the secularization of the medical profession which believes itself neutral to religious concerns. This is the case even in many, perhaps most, Catholic and other church-related hospitals where a large part of the medical staff may not be members of the sponsoring church. Even when a Catholic hospital has a largely Catholic medical staff, these health care professionals may still conceive their own tasks as rigidly separated from the concerns of pastoral care. Our interpretation of this secularization, on which we have insisted throughout this book, is that it is neither neutral, nor genuinely pluralistic, but simply fidelity to Humanism as an equivalent religion.

Thus the question arises as to whether a purely secular hospital serving principally Humanist patients (who make up probably at least forty percent of the American public) should have a pastoral care department and, if so, what its character should be. We believe that in such a health care facility a pastoral care department would still be necessary, although it probably should have a different name more in keeping with the symbol system of Humanism. The purpose of such a department would be to help patients deal with those existential (spiritual) problems which arise so acutely in times of illness or dying. The recent spate of books on death and dying, many written from a purely Humanist point of view, are evidence of this concern. Nor can this need be met adequately by psychotherapists or social workers. Some psychotherapists, it is true, have developed an existential psychology to deal with human problems at this deeper level, but for reasons we have already given in chapter 12, this exceeds the professional competence of therapists who are not ordinarily prepared to deal with philosophical issues concerning the meaning of life and with questions of ethical evaluation.

Since today most hospitals are pluralistic, a counselor working from the viewpoint of Humanism must also be prepared to assist patients of other faiths. In order to do so, the Humanist counselor must be able to take an honestly ecumenical approach, not scorning the value systems of Catholics, Protestants, and Jews. To do this adequately, a Humanist spiritual care department would probably have to include some professionals committed to the major faiths.

The same standards, on the other hand, should hold also for church-sponsored health care facilities. In a Catholic hospital, pastoral care should be thoroughly Catholic, but as Second Vatican Council has taught us, to be truly Catholic we must accept pluralism and ecumenism. Hence, Catholic hospitals should provide counseling for the large number of secular Humanists patients who say they "have no religion," are "not interested in religion," and so forth. Such counseling should respect the system of values by which Humanist patients live and should avoid proselytization or denominational pressures. At the same time, it should not neglect the need of such patients to deal with the problems of suffering, death, alienation, and loneliness in their own terms. Large church-sponsored hospitals need to provide in their pastoral departments for professional counselors able to help such Humanist patients because these counselors are themselves Humanists.

A second reason for the ambiguous situation of pastoral care in many hospitals is that in fact the chaplain or others occupied in pastoral care lack specialized professional training to work with the sick (Belford, 1968). While it is a part of all ministerial education to supply general skill in pastoral health care, assignment to a chaplaincy or pastoral care department in a modern hospital requires specialization. Catholic hospitals only recently have begun to move from the period when the local bishop supplied the hospitals of his diocese with a chaplain priest, often one unable to accept a regular pastoral assignment because of age or illness, but who could reside at the hospital and administer the sacraments. Catholic hospitals are now insisting that they will employ only chaplains certified for special training and competency in health care.

The development of clinical pastoral education (CPE) as the result of the pioneering work of Anton Boisen (1936, 1945) and its accreditration through a national association involved a shift to a more psychotherapeutic approach to the sick (Wise, 1951, 1966; Hiltner, 1958; Oates, 1962; Thornton, 1964; Clinebell, 1966; Grollman, 1967; Hulme, 1967; Faber, 1972; Cobb, 1977). This shift agreed in some respects with the traditional Protestant emphasis on pastoral counseling, but it produced a certain tension in ministerial identity for those who found it hard to reconcile the moralistic and evangelistic emphases of their tradition with modern psychotherapy's stress on guiltless self-expression.

Because of their emphasis on sacramental ministry (in which counseling was often largely restricted to hearing confessions) Catholics were slower to accept the new psychotherapeutic approach. However, after the Second Vatican Council, CPE began to be a regular part of priestly formation in many seminaries, and the National Association of Catholic Chaplains began to develop its own programs and certification in specialized pastoral ministry. Here again the tension between traditional types of ministry and psychotherapeutic emphasis has not yet been completely resolved.

While clinical pastoral education or its equivalent has served to make ministers more professional in their ministry of pastoral health care and thus somewhat improved their status with medical staffs, it has also raised the question as to whether pastoral care is simply another form of psychotherapy and social work. Until pastoral care people themselves have a clearer theology of pastoral care and a surer sense of their specific identity, it will be difficult for them to be accepted as professionals by hospital administrators and medical staffs (R. K. Smith, 1977; Curran, 1972; Nouwen, 1971).

In seeking this identity, clergy often claim that in some sense they deal with the whole person or the patient as person, while other health care professionals are more concerned with special parts of the person. On the contrary, some physicians feel that it is the doctor who is the only complete health care professional who must, therefore, head the health care team and make the final decision in all matters. Hence, it is the physician who deals with health care as a whole, while other members of the team including the minister deal only with special or incidental aspects of the health problem of the patient (cf. 6.4). Thus for such a physician, the ministry of the clergy to the patient is merely partial, auxiliary, or incidental, and any claim on the clergy's part to deal with the whole person is resented as presumptous and intrusive.

This controversy about whole and part can be clarified by realizing that different wholes are in question. If we view the patient under the aspect of *physical* health, then in that perspective the physican is the chief of any health care team and *de jure* has the ultimate decision in presenting to the patient an evaluation of possible course of treatment, although *de facto* a nurse, a dietitian, a physical therapist, or a pharmacist may actually know more about the patient. However, the ultimate decision remains with the patient or those responsible for the incompetent patient.

Patients as whole persons in making their decisions about how to use the services of the health care team must take into consideration other aspects of personality than that of physical health. Consequently, patients need the help and counsel of the psychotherapist, the ethical counselor, and the spiritual guide. In taking such counsel, it is clear that for the patients considerations of physical health are only a *part* of the problem, and in this problem the ethical and spiritual are more inclusive than the psychotherapeutic or physical (see chapters 1 and 2). From this point of view, patients after receiving the physician's advice may need to take ultimate counsel with their minister, priest, or some other equivalent spiritual guide. Sensitive physicians are quick to realize this and are happy not to stretch their responsibility beyond their professional competence for physical or, perhaps, mental health.

Nevertheless, ministers insofar as they stand for the personhood of the patient in its totality and its ultimately spiritual character have the obligation to defend the patient as a person in conflict situations, both against unjust actions of the staff and imprudence or negligence of the family or other guardians.

Thus in behalf of the whole person, the first task of the health care ministry is to help patients understand the several dimensions of any health decision which must all be taken into consideration. Hence, in a hospital it is reasonable that the pastoral department play a significant role in receiving and dismissing patients. Entering patients need to look forward to their experience in the hospital as one over which they have genuine control, and they should leave it feeling they are prepared to go on with normal life. Ministers can help patients achieve thise sense of self-control at a time when patients often feel they are helpless.

The foregoing tasks of the health care ministry, however important as they are, remain secondary in relation to its specific and central task of helping patients grow through their experience of sickness and convalesence or of death. Before discussing this principle work of health care ministry, however, we must ask about the responsibility of the pastoral care people for the other members of the health care team.

14.2 MINISTRY TO THE HOSPITAL STAFF

Not only the patients are persons, but so also are the members of the administrative and medical staffs and all the auxiliary personnel. Today, it is well recognized in mental hospitals that the mental health of the staff is an important factor in the therapy of the patients. In fact, in any health care facility the effectiveness of health care depends in large part upon the kind of interpersonal relations which exist among its staff.   Ultimately, this is a spiritual problem, because physicians, nurses, and others engaged in the very difficult vocation of caring for the suffering and confronting the crises of life and death are engaged in their own spiritual struggle (see chapter 13).

Staff members need help to maintain their sense of dedication, their courage, and their human compassion against all temptations to routine, cynicism, callousness, and ambition.   If the Christian Church from a long and often bitter historical experience has accepted the motto *ecclesia semper reformanda* ("the Church needs constant renewal"), this must be equally true of the hospital and the health care profession. Only on the basis of this constant effort to renew Christian humanism within the staff is there any real hope of sound ethical judgment in the care of patients.

A distinction needs to be made here between the *chaplain* who is most properly an ordained minister (in Catholic institutions, a priest or perhaps a permanent deacon) to whom the role of pastor of a community belongs by office and other pastoral care professionals who are not ordained, but who nevertheless have a genuine ministry, often entrusted to them by the local bishop. Where there is a fully developed pastoral care department, its *director* may be the chaplain, but this is not always the best arrangement, since the task of director of a department is administrative rather than immediately pastoral and can often be best fulfilled by a member of a religious order or a properly trained layperson.   The director has the responsibility of assigning the tasks of the department to different members, which will include the ordained chaplain's specifically priestly or diaconal functions, while counseling and other functions will be shared with nonordained members under the director's coordination and supervision.   All members of the department should be guaranteed the relative autonomy proper to their respective professional roles, including that required by the canonical duties of ordained ministers.   This does not mean, of course, that in a pluralistic hospital the chaplain can be the pastor of the hospital community or of the hospital staff in any strict sense of the word, but he will seek to minister to all insofar as they are open to his help and to provide for the others to the degree possible.

The pastoral care department as a whole will be concerned with bringing to the attention of the hospital administration issues of interpersonal relationships within the staff which affect the working of the institution and the good of the patients. Most pastoral care ministers soon learn of many of these interpersonal issues informally through members of the administrative and medical staffs who come to them for counsel and encouragement.

Although pastoral care people usually attempt to help those who come to them with such interstaff difficulties with as much tact as they can muster, accusations of interference in medical or administrative matters can easily result.   For pastoral care people to react to such criticism by confining their concern to private counseling often seems like neglect of responsibility to the institution and the patients it serves.

We would suggest this might be handled as follows.

1. The chaplain or director of the pastoral care department or some representative of that department who is especially competent should be included in the Christian identity committee of the hospital (see 6.5). This will provide a channel for ethical issues to be raised.

2. The staff should be thoroughly informed of the religious and counseling services which the pastoral care department is ready to provide to hospital personnel who voluntarily wish to avail themselves of these opportunities. It is important here, for example, that a Catholic hospital let the personnel know they are welcome at the Eucharist and for personal confession or counseling, but it is also important (and often neglected) to let non-Catholics know that the department has considered their needs, studied them, and made some kind of provision for them in a way that is convenient and free of embarrassment.

3. The director should have a recognized procedure by which is possible discussion with the administration, with the medical staff, with whatever group represents the nurses, and with the union or other representative body of the hospital employees issues of interpersonal relationships which the members of the pastoral care department may have observed are affecting patient or institutional welfare. Naturally, administrations may be reluctant to give the director this formal access to groups in the hospital with which the administration may be at odds. However, unless such recognized access exists, the director or chaplain will not be able to play that role of arbitrator and peacemaker which must be a primary and spiritual ethical concern of any truly human institution. Ethics is always concerned about the tension between justice and social harmony. It is absurd to speak of an institution's concern for medical ethics if it does not recognize the need for this kind of peacemaking as a truly ministerial function.

If the pastoral care department is to fulfill this role, its members must have a profound respect for those who dedicate their lives to the healing profession and should acknowledge that Christian ministry to the sick is not a monopoly of the pastoral care department. For Catholics, the Second Vatican Council reemphasized the ancient concept of "the universal priesthood of the believers" (*The Church*, 1965c) according to which Christ's ministry is not confined to ordained clergy, but in its threefold function of teaching, shepherding, and worshipping is shared in a variety of ways by every member of the Christian community so that all Christians are ministers along with Christ, who is the Servant of the Father (Rahner, 1968b; Küng, 1972).

Consequently, all Christians also share in pastoral ministry to the sick. Jesus made this one of the responsibilities for neighbor on which we are all to be judged (Matt. 25:31-46). In a very special way, therefore, the physicians, nurses, administrators, and all the members of a hospital staff are not merely carrying out a secular service, but a genuine Christian ministry of healing, deriving its authority from Christ's own healing work and witnessing to his continuing presence in the world. Thus, the priest chaplain and the whole pastoral care department not only should refrain from monopolizing the religious aspect of health care, but should also carry on an educational effort to help the hospital staff appreciate the spiritual and ethical values of their own professional work.

With this respect for their coministers should also come an increased sensitivity on the part of pastoral care people to the way in which many medical professionals are warped or destroyed as persons by the tensions under which they work. From such insight should come a creative effort to suggest and develop ways in which justice, charity, and peace can heal the "wounded healers" (Nouwen, 1972).

Finally, it is important that the pastoral care department itself provide a model of true humanity and good interpersonal relations (Nouwen, 1971). Not infrequently, the chaplain is the most difficult person in the staff, not because he plays the role of prophet, but because he is a warped personality constantly defending his own clerical status. Needless to say that in such cases the administration should not let respect for the clergy stand in way of seeking a reeducation or a replacement of the chaplain.

14.3 SPIRITUAL COUNSELING IN HEALTH CARE

Trust

We have discussed some of the functions which the religious minister can perform as an integrator of health care in the interests of the total health of the human person, but we have not yet discussed the specifically spiritual role of the minister. The reason that some have confused pastoral care with psychotherapy is because they are uncertain about what "spiritual ministry" really means or how it can contribute significantly to the patient's healing. To discuss this problem, we will first begin with the question as to how spiritual counseling differs from psychological counseling as these take place during a person's stay in a hospital.

Persons who are ill are faced with potentially serious problems.

1. They may fear suffering and death.

2. They face the uncertainties of diagnosis and prognosis and fear

about the pain or embarrassment of various testing or treatment procedures unfamiliar to them or all too painfully familiar.

3. They face the tedium of a long stay in the hospital under circumstances they find either boring or excruciating.

4. They suffer separation from their regular work, friends, and family and are not at home in the new situation.

5. They are worried and perhaps guilty about the various responsibilities at home that they cannot care for.

6. They suffer from a sense of deprivation of privacy and of freedom almost as if they were imprisoned.

7. They feel puzzled about Why has this happened to me? and may interpret their sickness as punishment for moral guilt. They may also anticipate further guilt through failure in courage and hope.

8. They feel alone and deserted in meeting all of the foregoing, and their sense of dignity, worth, and membership in the human community may be diminished by real moral guilt for which God's forgiveness is truly needed.

Spiritual ministers in their own proper role are called on to help patients in these struggles and may also be called on to help members of the health team who are faced with similar problems both in their personal lives and in their professional involvement with patients. As a counselor, the first task of the spiritual guide, as of any counselor and any real professional (in the sense we defined profession in chapter 4), is to establish *trust*, but this trust differs from that on which most professional relations are based because it has a kind of ultimacy. People often seek out a minister to confide in when they can no longer trust their lawyer, doctor, or even their psychiatrist!

Yet many patients do *not* even trust a minister, and when the chaplain visits them they are thinking, What is his game? Is he trying "to save my soul," to make a convert out of me? Is he looking for an offering? or for a confession? Hence, ministers must build up trust on the foundation not of words, but of behavior (Mitchell, 1966). A minister must keep promises, maintain contact, and be available to help in whatever difficulty is bothering the patient or to look for someone who can help. A minister must also be nonjudgmental, empathetic, and very careful about confidentiality. Finally, it is expected that a chaplain's care should extend beyond the patient to the patient's family.

Nevertheless, as in other counseling, this trust has its limits, and ministers must make clear to those they serve that a spiritual counselor has limited powers (Clinebell, 1966). Otherwise the trust between chaplain and patient will soon appear to be violated. Thus chaplains should make clear (1) that they cannot work miracles at will, or change the hospital structures, or get the patient out; (2) that they cannot be continuously present, and can give only limited time to any one patient, and (3) that their role is primarily that of a listener, counselor, and celebrant of the sacraments. All of this should become clear in the implicit or explicit counseling contract. It is up to counselors tactfully to set these limits and to remember that they are dealing with patients who may very well have undergone considerable psychological regression which makes them as dependent and demanding as a child in relation to its parents. The minister should give the patient permission for this dependency, but a limited permission. If such limits are not set, the minister will soon find that the patient interprets much that the minister does as a betrayal of trust.

This trust between a spiritual guide and the spiritual pilgrim, between a shepherd and the straying sheep, takes its special character first from the charisma of the minister as an *ordained* person. The spiritual guide is an "apostle," that is, one sent by the Church in the name of God upon whom the Spirit of God has been invoked by the prayers of the Christian community. Even when guides are not ordained, their ministry must somehow be authorized by the Christian community if it is to be given that special trust which should characterize it. Physicians and pyschotherapists in their white coats are often invested with an analogous charisma, as we explained in chapter 4, in speaking of the priestly character of the whole healing profession, but this is only an analogy to the charisma of the spiritual guide.

A minister, particularly if young and humble, may find the reverence showed him by a client because of this charisma very embarrassing and even unreal. The young minister would prefer simply to be on friendly terms with a patient, not to be invested with a halo of mysterious power.

Timothy seems to have had the same problem if we can judge from the advice which Paul gave him, "Do not let people disregard you because you are young, but be an example to all the believers in the way you speak and behave, and in your love, your faith, and your purity" (I Tim. 4:12). However, if ministers have set appropriate limits to their role, this charismatic function will not expand absurdly. Yet within these limits, they should accept honestly the task of speaking for God and in his name, however awesome that claim may be (Hiltner, 1969a).

This requires on the part of spiritual counselors constant reflection on two realities: first, that God is acting through them to accomplish what is quite beyond their own abilities and, second, that unless they acknowledge their own human limits, they will be placing obstacles in the way of God's work. Ministers who have this correct perception of their own role will not attempt too much, put themselves under impossible strains, or feel guilty at an inability to solve all problems of all patients. On the other hand, they will feel and communicate to patients unlimited hope in the loving power of God and a sense of each patient's dignity in God's eyes and their own (LaPlace, 1975).

Some ministers are so secularized that they feel more comfortable in a psychotherapeutic role than in a spiritual one and thus fail their patients by refusal to speak in God's name. They avoid talking with patients about spiritual issues, praying with them, or inquiring about their need for the sacraments as if these were forbidden or offensive topics. Patients may very will read this as a lack of faith on a minister's part and hence as a threat to the patient's own faith which is already sorely tried by doubts and anxieties raised by the patient's condition. Ministers who find themselves in a quandry about their own pastoral identity should attempt to resolve this ambiguity through spiritual guidance and perhaps psychotherapy if they are going to fulfill their responsibility of helping patients in *their* quandries.

Discernment

The minister, like a psychotherapist, is a listener and a reflector through whom the realities of the patient's situation become clearer to the patient and more manageable. Furthermore, like the psychotherapist, the minister listens not just to what the patient seems to be saying superficially, but to what the patient, perhaps unconsciously, is trying to say nonverbally and symbolically (Cavanaugh, 1962; Hostie, 1966). However, the psychotherapist is listening for the message that rises from the patient's subconscious emotional drives, while the minister as a spiritual therapist is listening for a message that comes from a still deeper level, from what the Scripture calls the "heart," that is, from the spiritual interior of the person's being where the person is committed to some sort of ultimate values and to some fundamental insight into reality (Johnston, 1971; Merton, 1971). In most patients, as in most of us all, this commitment and vision is dim and confused indeed, and yet it is the source of all our personal lives, where we really live and where we really die (Bugental, 1965; R. May, 1961). "Out of the depths I call to you O Lord, O Lord hear my voice" (Psalm 130). It is this voice *de profundis* to which the minister must listen. Moreover, a spiritual guide is not looking, as is the psychotherapist, for the psychic energies and motivations that flow from human instinctual needs, but for the work of the Holy Spirit in the patient, the signs of faith, hope, and charity and the spiritual forces of sin and alienation which oppose these. This is the spiritual level of human functioning which we discussed in chapter 2 (LaPlace, 1975).

The patient himself may raise these questions directly by saying, "Why has this happened to me, Father? Have I sinned? Am I going to be punished? What will happen to me if I die?" or "I don't seem to be able to pray now I am sick," and so forth. However, today in a secularized society, such questions are seldom asked *directly*. Even if they are, the chaplain may very well suspect that they do not really come from the spiritual level of personality, but are merely the pious language which some people (especially those who are from fundamentalist religious background) use in speaking of purely physical or psychological problems (Howe, 1963; Faber and Van der Schoot, 1965). Or the patient may think that this is the way you are supposed to converse with a minister, who is supposed only to talk that kind of religious language.   Therefore, the counselor has to listen to religious questions inherent in secular language or to secular problems inherent in pseudo-religious language (Greeley, 1976a). In both cases counselors must go deeper to find the really spiritual level in the patient.

This requires patience, and certainly it is usually a mistake to begin asking spiritual questions of a patient with whom the needed level of trust has not yet been established.   On the other hand, experienced spiritual counselors learn how to cut through other levels of small talk and psychological talk to the issues with which they have to deal (Isabel, 1976; Nouwen, 1975).   Simple directness is ordinarily not resented by patients.   Ordinary Catholics are not alarmed and even expect for "Father" to ask them if they want to go to confession or receive communion and to make some further tactful inquiry if they refuse. *Directness* is not bluntness or insensitivity.   It is rather a form of respect for a patient, a refusal simply to play games.

This respect for the person demands that the minister not take advantage of the patient's weak condition (Harmon, 1958). It is unethical to try to force conversion of patients, to accuse them of sin, to make demands for prayer or faith, and so forth. It may seem incredible that some ministers carry on such a preaching attack on patients, but many patients will report unpleasant experiences of being confronted by zealous ministers in a hospital and being embarrassed or pressured. Reports of such experiences have done much to prejudice doctors and nurses against the ministerial profession.

The minister who exerts this kind of pressure fails to trust in God's providence by which God is using the patient's experience of illness as an occasion of possible spiritual growth. The Spirit of God is already at work in the sufferer in ways that are not labeled religious.   The minister must recognize this growth process and cultivate it, helping patients to understand this in their own terms (Gannon, 1975).

A specific responsibility for ministers is not only to deal with the patient's spiritual problems, but also to help him become vividly aware of the real presence of God and of Church as the People of God in the patient's life in this very event of sickness where the patient may feel abandoned and isolated.   Ministers are themselves a visible sign or sacrament of this presence, incarnating God, as it were, in a tangible, human, imperfect, but real form.

Nor is it enough that ministers provide this witness of God's presence only to members of their own church (Zumbro Valley, 1975).   Too many ministers assume that they have responsibility only to their own parishioners or to those of their own denomination, and that others will resent their presence. Usually, however, this is not the case. Most laity are less ecclesiastically defined than we think. For them any minister, even a rabbi, is still a "man of God" and as such ought to have some interest in them as "children of God." Even the Humanist is seldom content with the silence of Humanism in the face of the ultimate questions and is resentful if the religious minister writes him off as a nonbeliever.

Thus as a spiritual adviser the minister's primary task is really a very simple one (Gleason, 1968; Carter, 1972). It is to say, as much or more by presence, attitude, and nonverbal symbols as by the exhortatory Word, that God is present to sick persons in their fear or suffering, that God as loving, caring Father, as cosuffering Lord Jesus, as Healing Spirit is present and acting, but this presence is in *mystery*, that is, it exceeds our human rational empirical comprehension because it is leading us into an open future (DeArment, 1975). This implies, of course, a spiritual awe before the *mysterium tremendum*. The sick person, like Job, feels guilty and yet is not clear how he is guilty. There is a sense of *judgment*. The minister should not deny this. Indeed, a minister symbolizes this judgment. But the minister also overcomes judgment by being a sign of mercy and reconciliation.

Sickness may be the time of genuine conversion in which persons truly find God for the first time in their life or after a long time of forgetfulness and separation. The minister must affirm the reality of this invitation of divine mercy, but that is not the whole of the minister's responsibility. Conversion is the beginning of a new life, but that life has to be lived authentically or it will be lost again. Consequently, one of the chief aims of spiritual counseling is to assist converts to begin to grow daily in the Christian life and to plan practically to continue that growth once they have returned to the routine situations of everyday life.

It is important also that the minister in helping sick persons realize God's presence should also make vivid to them that the minister is also a sign of the concern of God's people, of the Christian community or church, for a suffering brother or sister. Sickness is in Old Testament terms a kind of "uncleanness," and the patient may experience the "leprosy" of loneliness, alienation, and "excommunication" of the outcast from life and the human community. The minister removes this excommunication and reunites the lonely one with the community that is praying for him or her. We may recall how Jesus, healing a leper, sent him to a priest to be readmitted to the Jewish community (Mark 1:44).

14.4 CELEBRATING THE HEALING PROCESS

Word and Sacrament

The specific spiritual task of pastoral care, however, is not exhausted simply by the counseling situation, it must not be confined to talking about the Presence of God, but it must deepen into an *experiencing* of that presence in prayer, worship, celebration, and communion (Cooke, 1968; Champlin, 1973).

Today when most chaplains and other ministers as well are training in clinical pastoral education, they sometimes feel a tension between the model of the chaplain as a pastoral counselor whose main task is to engage in a therapeutic psychological process with the patient and the older model of the pastor as the one who reads the Scriptures, prays with and exhorts the patient, and administers the sacraments (Hulme, 1973; Quesnell, 1976). These two models seem opposed to each other. In particular, one seems aimed at removing feelings of guilt and giving feelings of interpersonal warmth and confidence and getting clients "in touch with their feelings," while the other tends to generate guilt and to impose a formalized religious response which covers up a patient's real experience (Gleason and Hagmaier, 1959; Hiltner, 1969b).

Actually the two models when they are well understood are complementary and can reinforce each other. We have already shown how pastoral counselors by their own presence are already a *sacrament*, that is, a sign of the presence of God. The Word of God first came to man, not in the text of the Bible which records his coming, but in the incarnation of Jesus Christ, the man who came to the sick and suffering, shared their suffering, and healed them by his contact (Schillebeeckx, 1963; O'Neill, 1964). Ministers, by the fact that they are sent by Jesus, are the living witness, "another Christ" as a sign of Christ's care for the patient. Therefore, everything that the minister does to witness this tender concern, this ability to empathize, to listen, and not to judge, is a sacrament of Jesus' presence. Even humor and light banter, if its purpose is precisely to establish real communication, is like the wit which Jesus constantly displayed in his preaching and parables. Above all, the down-to-earthness, the freedom from stuffiness, self-righteousness and elitism which can be the curse of the clerical state are in imitation of Jesus who did not hesitate to eat with sinners in simple fellowship.

Thus when ministers read the Scripture with patients they should already have placed the Scripture in the kind of human relational context in which the Word of God can be truly understood. Prayer also must grow out of this living context where it is natural for two people who have come to share a common concern to give it prayerful expression. A minister should not be praying in front of an embarrassed patient who feels as if something is "being laid on him" in which he has no part. An opening for prayer will come, however, only if the patient senses that the minister's concern for him goes *deep*, deeper than the mere professional interest.

The Scriptures which are used should be chosen just because they help to make real the presence of Jesus especially in his power to forgive, heal, and lead on into the fullness of life (Navone, 1967; Adams, 1975; Crabb, 1975; Bower, 1974; Oates, 1953).

The Catholic priest is more likely than the Protestant minister or the rabbi to be concerned about the administration of the sacraments. But these, too, must be understood not as some ritual intruding into a real situation, but as a ritualization of a process of healing which is already going on. The primordial sacrament is the touching which Jesus used when he healed the leper. It indicates the intimate presence, the care, the community, the power of life between Jesus and the sick and outcast. When a chaplain does what is so natural, namely, to hold the hand of sick persons to give them reassurance that the minister is there, that they are not alone, that is the primordial sacramental rite on which all the other sacraments are based — *human bodily contact* as a sign of *spiritual presence*.

Anointing the Sick and Reconciliation

In administering the sacraments using the new rites which have been improved precisely for this purpose, ministers must try to enhance this character of human contact already present in the counseling situation. What ministers have done as good pastoral counselors, they now deepen and intensify by a sign which combines the verbal word of Scripture with the nonverbal sacramental act.

The new rite of Anointing of the Sick brings this out clearly (cf. Paul VI, *Apostolic Constitution on Sacrament of Anointing the Sick*, 1972; Ling, 1973). It is not merely for the dying, as formerly, but for any person seriously ill. *Serious* should be judged here not merely in physical terms, but also in psychological terms. Thus when anyone is sick enough that we suspect the thought of possible death with its deep anxiety has entered his or her mind and produced fear and the threat of despair, then the spiritual and perhaps physical healing of the sacrament is needed and should be given. Whenever there is question of major surgery or of any disease which patients know sometimes leads to death and thus raises this fear in their own mind, we can anoint. We should not anoint when the illness is one in which recovery is assured and which consequently does not appear to contain any serious threat.

What is the meaning of this rite? First of all, it is not merely something done by a priest to a patient. Even when ministers are alone, they are there to represent not only God, but also the Christian community (Rahner, 1963). In fact, God is the center of the Christian commnity, so we can simply say that the minister is there to represent the Trinitarian community into which all Christians are incorporated in the Second Person Incarnate by their baptism. The anxiety of sick persons is that by their illness they are outcasts, aliens to this community. Patients experience this by their isolation from usual daily life and by the threat of death which might take them away forever. What such patients need is the reassurance that their people and their God are still with them. The priest supplies the sign of this by *touching* a patient. This touch means "presence," "acceptance," and as such is common to all the sacraments. But it is a special kind of touch in this case, a *healing* touch because it is the "anointing with oil," a common kind of healing remedy that has the sense of soothing pain and infusing life and movement. Its significance as a spiritual healing is given by the words which are spoken.

But this actual form of the sacrament is also preceded by brief Scriptural passages which can be expanded, in keeping with the general principle of the new rites that each sacrament should begin with a proclamation of the Word of faith, since it is faith that opens the person to God's work and this faith itself is the beginning of God's gifts.

While the sacrament is valid with only the priest and the recipient present, this is not the ideal way to perform it. A recent study made in several public hospitals shows that the doctors and nurses frequently resent the visit of the priest to perform "the Last Rites" (Nolin, 1972). There are several reasons for this. One is the notion, now out of date, that these rites seal the fate of the patient and therefore mark the failure of the medical profession, something that health care professionals hate to face. Again, professionals think the rites may frighten and depress the patient. However, another reason is that the priest seems like a medicine man who has been brought in as competition to the medical profession because the family has given up on the doctor's efforts. A third reason is the exclusive character of the rite. Even in Catholic hospitals when the priest comes, the doctors, nurses, and family often leave the room. Finally, there is sometimes a simple objection to an outsider coming in to do something for the person as if the hospital were not all-sufficient.

These misunderstandings thus have a source in what is really poor pastoral theology and practice. If the purpose of the sacrament is to help patients escape their sense of isolation, then obviously it is best if family and friends can be present, and that would include if possible the nurse and the doctor. Furthermore, if the sacrament is not to mark the end of life, but to help in the healing process, physical and spiritual, then it is certainly not separated from or in competition with the medical work of the hospital. Rather, it is part of that healing process. In fact, it is a celebration of the healing work of God which God performs not only through the ritual, but also through the *ministry* of the doctors, nurses, and administration. Priests are not the only ministers of health; they are part of a healing team every member of which is called by God to a healing work and empowered by Him through their natural gifts and education. The priest's special role in this team is to make explicit and Eucharistic (thankful) the work of all.

It is essential to realize that the sacraments are not performed merely in the ritual moment. Rather, they are the celebration of a culminating moment (not necessarily the last) of the saving work of God that has gone on for sometime through what are apparently merely secular events. Therefore, it is fitting not only that doctors and nurses be present at the anointing, but also that they participate in it by reading the Scriptures, or saying some of the prayers and by imposing hands on the patient or signing with the cross. Priests in their instruction and commentary and by additions to some of the prayers, if necessary, should thank God for the healing gifts and work of the medical staff. It would be very appropriate for patients also at this time to express their thanks to the doctors and nurses.

This expansion of the ritual can best be done, of course, when the sacrament takes place at mass in the hospital chapel, but it can also be done in the hospital room or ward when the doctor can be present. The confession of the patient when this is necessary would, of course, be done privately before the ceremony begins.

The proper rite for the dying patient is not the Anointing of the Sick but the reception of Viaticum, or final communion. This is the expression of the sick person's communion and unity with the Church on earth which prays for his or her swift passage to the eternal banquet. Hence this communion should be shared with others present if possible.

When in an emergency there is the problem of anointing someone who has not yet received the sacrament in an illness, it is necessary of course to perform it quickly, but if the patient recovers consciousness it is possible to hold a healing service of prayer so that the patient can more fully participate in the fruits of the sacrament. In the case of a person who is doubtfully alive, the Sacrament of Anointing should be administered, but the new ritual forbids it to be given to someone who has already died.

Previously priests were advised to administer it to someone who had recently died — up to two or three hours — if the death had been sudden. The ritual no longer prescribes this. However, in the present liturgical transition when many people are still poorly instructed with regard to the Sacrament of Anointing, a Catholic family may be very disconsolate to hear that the sacrament was not received. Priests, therefore, may prudently judge in given circumstances whether they might better administer the anointing conditionally where there is still some doubt (even minimal) that life still remains for the sake of the family. Perhaps a better procedure is to assure the family that the patient received the proper rites of the Church, meaning by this that the priest has prayed for the departed and blessed the body, since these are the proper rites according to the present discipline. It is important we begin to instruct people that the Church prays daily for all its members and no one departs this life without the powerful intercession of the Church. In our ecumenical times, chaplains should not hesitate to administer anointing to non-Catholics who might present themselves at a general anointing service since they probably are baptized and in good faith. If not, the sacrament still constitutes a prayer for their healing.

What is to be done with ministers who are not priests? These days religious sisters and brothers and lay people may be exercising some of the ministry of priests. It is theologically disputed whether it might be possible for the Church to delegate to a deacon the Anointing of the Sick, as confirmation has been delegated by bishops to priests (Palmer, 1974). At present, however, this is not legal nor valid. However, it is perfectly possible for deacons and nonordained persons, sisters, and lay persons to hold a service of healing (MacNutt, 1977b; Sanford, 1976). This can consist of Scripture readings, prayers, and the laying on of hands for the sick. It can even make use of blessed oil as a sacramental. It would seem, however, that in such services it should be made clear to all that what is taking place is not a sacrament in the strict sense. By this is not meant that it is inefficacious (all true prayer is efficacious), but that it is *preparatory* to the full public visit of the priest to the sick as a representative of the Christian community. Just as the arrival of the doctor completes the care given to patients by nurses, although in fact the doctor does nothing additional except to approve and confirm what has already been done, so the priest approves and confirms the healing prayer of a local group and of auxiliary ministry. This is not a mere formality but an expression of the unity and public witness of the Church.

The Sacrament of Reconciliation (*Rite of Penance*, 1975; Sottocornola, 1975) for the sick can also take place in the form of a penance service in the hospital chapel or even in the ward, with the invitation to all who wish to make individual confession and receive absolution. Such a service is an opportunity for the priest to deal with the question of sin and guilt and the meaning of suffering and to alleviate neurotic guilt. When confession is made on a ward, it should be remembered that if it is difficult to achieve sufficient privacy the penitent can be instructed simply to make a general acknowledgement of sins and to speak of them in detail in a future confession.

It should be remembered too that deacons, sisters, brothers, and other visitors, although they cannot give absolution, can truly help a sick person to conversion and reconciliation with God and neighbor in an efficacious way. We are not proposing we revive the "confession to a layman" which was common enough in the Middle Ages when a priest was not available, but are emphasizing that today in pastoral counseling such confession often takes place spontaneously. When it does, the ministers who are not priests should help such patients make an act of contrition and then encourage them to go to the sacrament when it becomes possible, but should also assure them here and now that the mercy of God is truly present in prayer, and that with this trust in God's mercy they should be at peace. The reason for confession later is to ratify and complete by the public acknowledgement of the priest as a representative of the Church of a conversion which has already taken place. There is no reason that nonordained ministers should feel that because they are not ordained they cannot help patients achieve this reconciliation here and now.

Baptism and Eucharist

If the patient is unbaptized and wishes to become a Catholic Christian, the new ritual should be followed (Rite of Christian Initiation, 1974). When patients have been certainly baptized as Protestants, but wish to be Catholic they should be received as members of the Catholic community and confirmed (Kiesling, 1974). What about the infant in danger of death or the unconscious dying person? Today, there are some Catholics who are raising doubts about infant baptism. This, however, seems to have Pelagian overtones because it implies that the grace of God can only be received on our initiative. Baptism, however, is a sign of the pure gift of God, the gift of faith and justification which comes to us without any merit on our part merely because we do not reject it. Before the infant is born it is already subject to the grace of God through the prayers of the Church. Infant baptism is the public ratification of this drawing of the infant, alienated from God through no fault of its own by the sins of society (original sin), who is now being drawn by the Holy Spirit through Jesus Christ and his redeemed community of the Church into union with the Father. This act of incorporating the infant into the life of the human community begins biologically and sociologically from the moment of conception and birth. Why then should not the infant also be incorporated into the redeemed community of the Church? Consequently, it is certain that baptism can be validly conferred on the child from the moment of conception and probable that it can be conferred on any unconscious adult (although not certain, because the person may have positively rejected the grace of God).

From this some theologians in the past concluded that it is essential that all children, even *in utero*, should be baptized in danger of death and encouraged the baptism of all doubtfully baptized adults who had not actually refused baptism. This was based on the idea that salvation without baptism (at least *in voto*, i.e., "baptism of desire") was impossible, since it is a matter of faith that we can only be saved through Christ, and this must be applied to us through his Church. Augustinian theologians came to the inescapable but embarrassing (to a Christian believing in God's mercy as Augustine strongly did) that unbaptized children are damned. St. Thomas found a way out of this embarrassment by pointing out that it is possible (1) for unbaptized children to enjoy a natural happiness (Limbo) even if they are not admitted to the inner mystery of God, the existence of which they have never even been aware, and (2) for unbaptized adults to be saved by an implicit desire for baptism if they have conscientiously followed what light God has given them.

Today theologians (Fortman, 1976) still maintain the principle that we can only be saved by Christ through the Church, but they see the *prayer* of the Church as efficacious even when it cannot be ritually expressed in the sacraments (cf. I Cor. 7:14). Thus it is very probable that the infant dying before baptism has already been justified through the prayer of the Church (especially of the child's family) and will enter into the intimate mystery of God. Nevertheless, it still is important to administer baptism, not so much because the child absolutely needs it, but in order to manifest the concern of the Church and thus to keep alive the consciousness of the dignity of the human person from the first moments of existence (*Rite of Baptism for Children*, 1971). Consequently nurses and doctors should baptize infants who are in danger of death and even miscarried fetuses which exhibit human form. They should pour water on the child (on the head, if possible) so as actually to touch the skin and should say, "I baptize you in the name of the Father, Son, and Holy Spirit." In this way they have expressed Christian reverence and fellowship with this little person who will forever be part of the Trinitarian community.

For the dying unconscious person, it is permissible also to perform such a baptism with the condition, "If you are not baptized, I baptize you." Clearly this is not a grave obligation unless the person has asked to be baptized before lapsing into unconsciousness, and should not be done in a merely mechanical manner (trying to baptize everyone in the hospital, and so forth), but as part of nurses' care for particular persons in their charge whom they believe have given some indication that they might wish such an administration. Again, the reason is to show the Church's concern for a person who has providentially come under the care of the Catholic community.

The Eucharist is the supreme sacrament and sign of the Christian community, indicating that such patients remain a part of that community, even when absent from the public worship assembly, and that they are destined for eternal life with the community (*Selected Documentation*, 1974). It is a life-giving, health-giving sacrament, since the eating of bread and drinking of wine are the basic symbols of the power to live. After Jesus raised the daughter of Jairus, "He told them to give her something to eat" (Luke 8:55). Again St. Paul believed (I Cor. 11:27-31) the unworthy reception of the Eucharist leads to sickness and death because this empty formalism cuts a person off from the God of the living.

Today the Eucharist is often distributed by auxiliary ministers, not by the priest. This is wholly appropriate since in the earliest days communion was taken from the public assembly to the homes of the sick. In a hospital it would be appropriate when possible (and the current leniency with regard to the fast before communion makes this easy) to have the patients who wish to listen to the mass in the chapel on closed circuit radio or television then to be brought communion immediately after the mass. Ambulatory patients who attended the mass could be the auxiliary ministers. In this way the union between mass and communion would be emphasized. It is essential in any case that communion in the hospital should not be reduced to a routine in which someone pops in and out of a room to place a wafer in a sleepy patient's mouth. We would suggest at least a card containing Scripture reading and prayers that a patient can use while preparing for communion.

What we have been saying may sound liturgical rather than ethical, but it sums up the ethical message of this book, namely, that medical ethics has to do not with certain rules about forbidden procedures, but with a healing process by which the dignity of every human person in all its dimensions is respected by the community and the sick person is restored to full life in community. Unethical behavior is that which tends to exclude persons from the deepest sharing of communal life centered in the Trinity. Ethical behavior is that which fosters this communion. This ethical vision with its perception of the true scale of values is summed up and expressed in the sacraments, especially in the Eucharist. A Catholic hospital which really understands the healing character of the sacraments will have a perfect model for an ethical treatment of the patients. The sacraments represent for us how Jesus went about treating sick people.

What makes a Catholic hospital different from all other hospitals? That its vision of the sick is a Eucharistic vision, carried out in all details of the treatment of the patient and the mission of the healing team.

14.5 ETHICAL COUNSELING AND PASTORAL CARE

Respecting the Patient's Value System

Don S. Browning in *The Moral Context of Pastoral Care* (1976) ably argues for renewed stress on the ethical dimension of pastoral care. He believes that the Christian emphasis on our spiritual relation to God by grace must never be allowed to eradicate the memory of our Jewish origins in Torah, in the Law understood not as a death-dealing Pharisaism, but as a true discipline of life through which the seeds of grace can be cultivated. A Christian spirituality which neglects moral obligation, or which speaks of love but forgets justice, is foreign to the teaching of Jesus who came not to destroy the Law, but to fulfill it (Matt. 5:17-19). Systematic theologians have the task of relating and balancing law and grace, but pastoral counselors have to live with the tension, neglecting neither grace nor discipline.

We have been arguing in this chapter that the primary task of pastoral care is *spiritual* guidance and celebration, yet the purpose of this book has been to deal with *ethical* questions confronted by health care professionals and their patients. Certainly, ministers frequently have to be of help to professionals and patients in their struggles to make such ethical decisions. What is the relation between *spiritual* and *ethical* guidance? In 2.3 we showed that the spiritual and ethical dimensions of the human person although interrelated are not identical. Spiritual counseling deals with the ultimate, existential questions, the problems of commitment to certain fundamental values or life goals. Ethical counseling in the strict sense, on the other hand, deals with the decisions that have to be made about actions that have to be taken to achieve these goals. In brief, the former deals with *ends*; the latter, with the *means*.

Some theologians, especially of the Lutheran tradition (Søe, 1965), question whether ethics in this sense is relevant for a Christian. Are we not in danger of self-righteousness and legalism the moment we begin to measure our actions by some ethical system? For such theologians Christian life is a spontaneous grateful response to God's gracious forgiveness, a loving response that can only be distorted by any ethical calculation of ends and means. Nevertheless, others, including Lutherans like Thielicke (1969) and Althaus (1972) recognize that although our ethical decisions must be motivated by faith and love yet they also require a rational decision-making process. Thus, although the main task of pastoral care is spiritual, it must also extend to assisting professionals and patients to live out their spiritual commitments by prudent decisions about concrete actions.

This book has been devoted to providing ethical guidance for health care decisions, but in concluding we still have to ask, What is the responsibility of a minister or a pastoral care department in medicomoral decisions?

In answering this question the first difficulty to be met is how a minister can be an ethical counselor to persons who in our pluralistic culture are committed to such different value systems? As spiritual counselor a minister may have to deal with someone who is struggling with a strictly spiritual problem which involves commitment to a value system, but as ethical counselor the client's value system is not in question. The problem is its application. How are counselors to help if they do not share the client's value system?

In chapter 7 we argued that different value systems cannot be simply reduced to some common denominator, but are *analogous* to each other, that is, really and fundamentally different, yet have much in common. Consequently, we believe that in pastoral care it is possible to proceed ecumenically to find a common ground for ethical decision between different value systems, whether these differences separate pastor and patient or members of the health team. Such an ecumenical method depends (1) on clarity about one's own set of values and fidelity to it, (2) on respect for the values of others and their fidelity to these, and (3) on a common effort to find a basis for mutual dialogue and action. Since at a time of sickness patients are seldom in any condition to rethink their whole outlook on life, an ethical counselor should in general not disturb the patient's basic commitment unless it becomes apparent that such issues at the spiritual level have to be faced because the patient is already struggling with them. Consequently, the counselor must deal with a Jew within the Jewish ethical tradition, a Baptist within the Baptist tradition, a Humanist within a humanistic set of values. Efforts at proselytization to one's own faith are an unfair exploitation of the sick.

Next we must ask: What is the goal of ethical counseling? How can we help patients within the context of their value system to achieve a free and informed conscience and to arrive at prudent ethical decisions (Brodsky, 1968; Pruyseur, 1976)? Human decisions to be ethical must first of all be free. The sick suffer from various limitations of their psychological freedom. When their illness is mental, obviously this freedom is severely restricted or even eliminated by neurosis or psychosis; but when it is physical, the sick still suffer some degree of unfreedom because of the weakness, mental confusion, depression, and so forth, consequent on their physical condition, and also because they are confined to a narrow and unfamiliar social situation. Hence the sick patient is often not able to think clearly and realistically.

Ethical counseling, therefore, must first of all aim at creating an atmosphere in which the patient's freedom is maximized. Until some area of genuine freedom opens up for the patient, ethical discussion is useless. When such an opening is achieved, the counselor must strive to keep ethical discussion confined to just that area of freedom and not waste time with what seem to be ethical arguments but which in fact are only the expression of emotional conflict. The means to achieving this increased freedom are essentially the techniques of psychotherapy which the minister needs to understand and use in a modest way, referring more difficult problems to members of the health team who are professionally skilled in such therapy. However, religious ministers have something special to contribute to this freeing process, because they can help to lift the burden of existential fear or hopelessness which may be one of the chief obstacles to freedom. Patients who are confident of God's loving and forgiving care have a peace of mind even in the face of suffering and death that makes it possible for them to face difficult decisions with serenity and sanity.

Once the counselor is assured that the patient is sufficiently free to deal with an ethical decision, the counselor's next objective should be to help the patient arrive at a decision which is prudent and hence at least *subjectively* good, that is, according to the patient's honest conscience, even when the counselor is not convinced that this decision is *objectively* good. There are three reasons why such a gap between subjective and objective morality may occur or may seem to the counselor to exist (3.4): (1) the patient may have a different value system than the counselor, (2) the patient's decision may appear inconsistent with the patient's own value system, and (3) the patient's decision may be inconsistent with the facts of the situation as the counselor perceives these facts.

In the first case, as we have already said, the counselor generally should not attempt to convert the patient to the counselor's own value system, but should help the patient to make decisions consistent with the patient's own values. In the second case, the counselor should do what is possible to help the patient to make a self-consistent decision, since only then will the decision be conscientious and subjectively right. In the third case, the counselor should try to help the patient perceive the facts of the situation correctly. Nevertheless, in this last case the counselor should remember that our perception and interpretation of facts is influenced by our value system and by our personal experience, so that it may not be possible for patient and counselor to come to an agreement on the facts.

The reason that the counselor should be first of all concerned to help the patient come to a subjectively honest decision is twofold: first, because the patient always retains primary responsibility for health decisions (3.1) and, second, because the proximate norm of all moral decisions is the conscience of the agent (3.4; 8.1-3). Ethically it is more important that persons do what they sincerely believe to be right at a given stage of their moral development than that they do what is objectively right. Because we live in a sinful world, and each of us suffers from the darkness of mind and hardness of heart resulting from our own sins, the Word of God is received by us in obscurity. Only little by little do we move forward into the light, as is so eloquently witnessed in the Old Testament by the history of the Chosen People. What is most essential is that we keep moving forward, even if our steps are frequently missteps. For those who make mistakes in good faith, experience is self-corrective. In the New Testament we see how Jesus (unlike the Pharisees) is more concerned with the faith and goodwill of sinners than he is with their conformity with a Law of which they are often ignorant and to which they do not know how to comply.

St. Paul (I Cor. 8) also urges us to respect the consciences of others, even when we perceive they are mistaken and immature in their moral understanding.

However, the task of the counselor does not stop with helping a patient arrive at a subjectively prudent and conscientious decision. The fact that a decision is honest does not prevent it from being harmful to others or even to the one who makes the decision when in fact it is an *objectively* wrong decision. Our honest mistakes do not injure our moral integrity, nor destroy our spiritual relations to God and neighbor, nor prevent our spiritual growth, but they do have consequences from which we and others suffer. Moreover, Christian morality is creative. It is a response to God's call to us to move forward toward Him and to share in his redemptive work. This divine call is often present in the crisis of sickness or dying. Consequently, the counselor cannot be simply content to ratify, as it were, decisions made by a patient within the narrow limits of the patient's routine morality.

On the one hand, if the counselor sees that the patient's decision may in fact be clearly injurious to the patient or to others (e.g., if the patient is thinking of suicide or abortion), then the counselor has to do what is possible to prevent this harm, even when the counselor is convinced of the moral honesty of the decision (5.2). On the other hand, the counselor may judge that it is necessary in particular cases to confront the patient with the challenge inherent in the decision that has to be made. Hence the counselor must raise disturbing questions which ultimately go beyond the ethical level to the spiritual level of the patient's value system. Obviously, counselors must be very cautious about disturbing sick people in this manner, yet they should have the courage to do so when the patient's own behavior gives signs that such probing and confrontation is necessary. The wonderful scene of Jesus and the Samaritan woman (John 4:4ff.) shows us how the Spirit of God can be at work in the human conscience, revealing itself by the uneasiness, the denial, the defiance, and the disguised cries for help which a spiritually sensitive and experienced counselor can recognize. In these cases the apparent subjective honesty of the client masks a hidden conflict of conscience which cannot be resolved without probing that goes beyond the subjective to a new and deeper perception of reality.

It is no simple matter for a counselor to balance these two counseling aims of subjective and objective conscience. Formerly, it would seem that the clergy were too quick to impose objective moral standards on the people, with little sensitivity to the moral development or experience of different individuals. Today, with the growth in psychological understanding of individual differences and of the developmental aspects of morality, it would seem that the opposite temptation prevails. The axiom People must make their own decisions has often been pushed so far that ministers have lost interest in objective morality.

A disturbing example of this was provided by the way in which many clergyman who had been active as draft counselors during the Vietnam War then went on to become "abortion counselors" (Moody, 1971). In both cases they believed they were serving the cause of human rights, and they probably contributed significantly by reason of their clerical prestige both to ending the war and to liberalizing the anti-abortion laws. Yet when we read the accounts given by some of them concerning their experience as counselors in the latter cause, we are struck with the fact that they seemed to have felt that compassion for the woman was the only ethical issue involved in abortion. We do not find that they saw any inconsistency in their concern for the napalmed children of Vietnam and their lack of concern for the salined fetuses of the United States.

If we ask why this apparent inconsistency was so little discussed, we are inclined to believe that it was because these counselors saw their task purely in terms of the individual subjective conscience of the client. When the client was a conscientious objector, the counselors supported his decision to refuse service in the war. When the client was a pregnant woman who honestly believed it would be wrong for her to bear her child, they supported her decision and were ready to help her find a good clinic and to help her overcome any sense of guilt. The concern for the subjective conscience of the client in both cases was certainly proper, but we have to ask whether it was enough. Does not the counselor also have to face the question of the objective justice or injustice of the war and also the question of the rights of the unborn child? While counselors cannot impose their personal judgment about the objective justice in either instance, they cannot simply avoid the issue. Rather, the minister must do what is possible to prevent objective harm and to challenge the judgment of the patient when signs indicate that such challenge may be an opportunity for successful moral growth.

Christian Discernment

An important aspect of this moral growth for the Christian is the deepening of the vital relation between the conscience of the individual and the conscience of the Christian community. The Holy Spirit guides us not merely privately, but also through diaglogue within the historical Christian Church. Ethical counselors frequently find great immaturity in Catholic clients with regard to the relation between personal conscience and what they understand to be the official teaching of their Church. What is a counselor to do when confronted by patients who express such dilemmas as the following? (1) I know the Church condemns this, but I don't think God will condemn me. (2) I think I have to do this, but I am afraid I will have to go to hell for doing it. (3) I know this is supposed to be wrong, but why can't you as a priest give me permission to do it? (4) I have made up my mind, but I want to know what you think. (5) I am not going to confess this because I know the confessor will argue with me. (6) I guess I will just have to go ahead and do this and then go to confession afterwards. (7) I am going to do what I think is right, but I guess this means I will have to leave the Church. (8) I did what I thought was right, but I still feel guilty about it.

Moreover, counselors find such difficulties not only in patients, but also dealing with the professional staff (1) who may separate their professional opinions and their obedience to Church teachings into separate mental compartments, making no effort to reconcile their professional and their Christian lives or (2) who complain that the bishops and priests are ignorant of medical problems and always behind the times in the ethical regulations they impose on the medical profession or (3) who complain that there is too much variation in the guidance given by different priests or in different dioceses and lack of clear enforcement of Church teachings or (4) who object to taking time from their work to discuss moral issues because such discussions come to no clear conclusions.

Finally such difficulties are compounded by the fact that the members of the pastoral care department itself may have widely different ethical views and may themselves be struggling with the tension between official Church teaching, the diverse views of theologians, and their own pastoral experience.

We have argued previously (3.4) that such difficulties are not abnormal in the Christian community, because it is a historical catholic, pilgrim people in which the pastors must struggle to keep the flock unified and continuously on its march; yet the diversity of experiences and talents must play their complementary and sometimes conflictual roles. The pastoral role in the situation of a health care facility is not to deny tension and conflict, but to help the persons involved make a contribution to the growth of all. Jesus welcomed into his following a great variety of people at various levels of moral growth, providing for the weak and challenging the strong. St. Paul followed this pattern, with special emphasis on helping the Christians of each community mature in conscience.

In carrying out this educative task ministers should first of all emphasize as we have attempted to do in this book, the primary values and principles of Christian living as they apply to the healing process. These principles should not be presented as rules, but as goals to be creatively achieved in a loving and generous response to the grace of God, after the pattern of the Good Samaritan (Luke 10:25-37) who saw in the injured man in the ditch the call of God. The professional or the patient who has these goals at heart and uses the knowledge and imagination available to reach these goals will act in a truly humane and Christian way, enlightened by the Holy Spirit.

Christians open to the Spirit in this way are not negligent of or ungrateful for the guidance given by the pastors of the Church, whether that guidance has the certitude of the Gospel or simply the authority of pastors doing what they can to apply the Gospel in a given time or place according to the lights they possess. On the other hand, mature Christians know that God requires of them personal decisions based not only on pastoral guidance, but also on their own gifts and experience.

The final task of ethical counselors, therefore, is to help those they counsel mature in conscience and live in peace with the responsbility for their own decisions, content with the assurance that God calls us to share in his own task of healing a wounded world.

BIBLIOGRAPHY

Included in the Bibliography are the works cited and
sources consulted.

For works of historical interest the original date of
publication is provided (in brackets) as well as the
current date of reissue.

Aaronson, Stephen. "Treating the Hyperkinetic Child: Isn't There a Better Way?" *Medical Dimensions* 4 (1974): 23-28.

Abell, Aaron I., ed. *American Catholic Thought on Social Questions.* Indianapolis: Bobbs-Merrill, 1968.

Abelson, Raziel, and Nielsen, Kai. "Ethics, History of." In *The Encyclopedia of Philosophy*, edited by Paul Edwards. New York: Macmillan and The Free Press, 1967. Vol. 3, pp. 81-117.

Ackerknecht, E. W. *Short History of Medicine.* New York: Ronald Press Co., 1955.

Ackerman, Nathan W. "Ethical Issues in Psychotherapy." *Conservative Judaism* 23 (1969): 1-15.

Adams, Jay. *Use of Scripture in Counseling.* Nutley, N.J.: Presbyterian & Reformed Publishing Co., 1975.

Adler, Mortimer J. *The Difference of Man and the Difference It Makes.* New York: Holt, 1967.

_____. *The Time of Our Lives: The Ethics of Common Sense.* New York: Holt, 1970, chap. 17, pp. 185ff.

Agress, Hyman. *"Why Me?"* Carol Stream, Ill.: Creation House, 1974.

Agus, Jacob B. *The Vision and the Way: An Interpretation of Jewish Ethics.* New York: Ungar, 1966.

Alcock, John. *Animal Behavior: An Evolutionary Approach.* Sunderland, Mass.: Sinauer Associates, 1975, pp. 432-504.

Alderete, J. F., et al. "Irreversible Coma: A Clinical, Electroencephalographic, and Neuropathological Study." *Transactions of American Neurological Association* 93 (1968): 16-20.

Alexander, Leo. "Medical Science Under Dictatorship." *New England Journal of Medicine* 241 (1949): 39-47. Reprinted in *Child and Family* 10 (1971): 40-57.

Alford, Robert R. *Health Care Politics: Ideological and Interest Group Barriers to Reform.* Chicago: University of Chicago Press, 1975.

Allan, D. J. *The Philosophy of Aristotle.* London: Oxford University Press, 1952, pp. 63-100.

Allen, James E. "How Catholics Are Making Up Their Minds on Birth Control." *Christian Century* 87 (1970): 915-18.

Allport, Gordon W. *Personality: A Psychological Interpretation.* New York: Henry Holt, 1937, pp. 24-50.

Alsop, Stewart. "The Right to Die with Dignity." *Good Housekeeping*, August 1974, pp. 130ff.

Althaus, Paul. *The Ethics of Martin Luther*. Philadelphia: Fortress Press, 1972.

Altman, Stewart H., and Weiner, Sanford L. "Constraining the Medical Care System: Regulation as a Second Best Strategy." Paper delivered at the Federal Trade Commission Conference on Competition in the Health Care Sector, Washington, D.C., June 1977.

Alvarez, A. *The Savage God: A Study of Suicide*. New York: Random House, 1972.

American Hospital Association. "The Patient's Bill of Rights (November 1972)." In *The Rights of Hospital Patients* by George J. Annas. New York: Avon Books, 1975, pp. 25-27.

American Medical Association. "Extending the Scope of Nursing Practice." Report of the Secretary's Committee to Study Extended Roles for Nurses. *Journal of the American Medical Association* 220 (1972): 1231-1236.

————. "Report of the Judicial Council on Death." Adopted by the American Medical Association House of Delegates, December 1973. (Mimeographed.)

American Psychological Association. "Ethical Principles in the Conduct of Research with Human Participants." *American Psychologist* 28 (1973): 79-80. Reactions by Baumrind, Diana, *Am. Psychol.* 27 (1973): 1083-1086.

Amos, Bernard, et al. "ACS/NIH Organ Transplant Registry." *Journal of American Medical Association* 226 (1973): 1211-1216.

Amulree, Lord, et al. *On Dying Well: An Anglican Contribution to the Debate on Euthanasia*. London: Church Information Service, 1975.

"An Appraisal of the Criteria of Cerebral Death: A Summary Statement of a Collaborative Study." *Journal of American Medical Association* 237 (1977): 982-986.

Anderson, Bernard W. "Human Dominion Over Nature." In *Biblical Studies in Contemporary Thought*, edited by Miriam Ward. Somerville, Mass.: Green, Hadden, 1975.

Anderson, Odin W. *Health Care: Can There Be Equity?: The United States, Sweden and England*. New York: Wiley, 1972.

Annas, George J. "The Patients Have Rights: How Can We Protect Them?" *Hastings Center Report* 9 (1973): 8-9.

————. *The Rights of Hospital Patients: The Basic American Civil Liberties Guide to a Hospital Patient's Rights*. New York: Avon Books, Discus, 1975.

————, and Coyne, Brian. " 'Fitness' for Birth and Reproduction: Legal Implications of Genetic Screening." *Family Law Quarterly* 9 (Fall 1975): 463-489.

————, and Healey, Joseph. "The Patient Rights Advocate." *Journal of Nursing Administration* 4 (May/June 1974): 25-32.

Appleton, William S. "The Importance of Psychiatrists' Telling Patients the Truth." *American Journal of Psychiatry* 129 (1972): 742-745.

Aquinas, Saint Thomas. *Summa Theologiae*. Edited by Thomas Gilby, O.P. New York: McGraw-Hill, 1976. On the body: Vol. 11, I, 75, 4 ad. 2; 76, 1 ad. 6; on the principle of totality: Vol. 38, II-II, q. 65 1 c.

Ardrey, Robert. *The Territorial Imperative*. New York: Atheneum, 1966.

Arieti, Silvano. "Creativity and Its Cultivation." *American Handbook of Psychiatry* 3 (1966): 722-741.

_____. *The Intrapsychic Self: Creativity and Its Cultivation.* New York: Basic Books, 1967.

Armstrong, R. A. *Primary and Secondary Precepts in Thomistic Natural Law Teaching.* The Hague: Martin Nijhoff, 1966.

Arnold, J. D., et al. "Public Attitudes and the Diagnosis of Death." *Journal of American Medical Association* 206 (1968): 1949-1954.

Arnold, Magda B. *Emotion and Personality.* 2 vols. New York: Columbia University Press, 1960.

Arnold, Mary F. "Philosophical Dilemmas in Health Planning." In *Administering Health Systems: Issues and Perspectives,* edited by Mary F. Arnold, L. Vaughn Blankenship, and John M. Hess. Chicago: Aldine-Atherton, 1971, pp. 208-225.

Ashley, O.P., Benedict M.
    1972. "A Psychological Model with a Spiritual Dimension." *Pastoral Psychology* 23: 31-40.
    1973. "Change and Process." In *The Problem of Evolution: A Study of the Philosophical Repercussions of Evolutionary Science,* edited by John N. Deely and Raymond Nogar. New York: Appleton-Century-Crofts, pp. 267-294.
    1975. "Ethics of Experimenting with Persons." In *Research and the Psychiatric Patient,* edited by Joseph C. Schoolar and Charles M. Gaitz. Proceedings of the Eighth Annual Symposium, Texas Institute of Mental Sciences, October 16-18, 1974. New York: Brunner/Mazel, pp. 15-30.
    1976. "A Critique of the Theory of Delayed Hominization." In *An Ethical Evaluation of Fetal Experimentation: An Interdisciplinary Study,* edited by Donald G. McCarthy, and Moraczewski, O.P., Albert. St. Louis: Pope John XXIII Medical-Moral Research and Education Center, pp. 113-133.

Ashley, O.P., Benedict M., et al. *Focus on Social Justice: An Outline of Catholic Social Teaching.* Department of Religious Education, Archdiocese of Dubuque, Iowa, 1976.

Ashley, Jo Ann. *Hospitals, Paternalism and the Role of the Nurse.* New York: Teachers College Press, Columbia University, 1976.

Augenstein, Leroy. *Come, Let us Play God.* New York: Harper & Row, 1969.

Ayd, Frank J., Jr. "The Hopeless Case: Medical and Moral Considerations." *Journal of American Medical Association* 181 (1962): 1099-1102.

_____, ed. *Medical, Moral and Legal Issues in Mental Health Care.* Baltimore: Williams & Wilkins, 1974.

Ayer, A. J. *Language, Truth and Logic.* London: Gollancz, 1936.

Baelz, P. R. "Voluntary Euthanasia." *Theology* 75 (1972): 238-251.

Bajema, Clifford E. *Abortion and the Meaning of Personhood.* Grand Rapids: Baker Book House, 1974.

Balint, M. *The Doctor, His Patient, and The Illness.* New York: International Universities Press, 1964.

Balter, Mitchell B., Levine, Jerome, and Manheimer, Dean I. "Cross-National Study of the Extent of Anti-Anxiety/Sedative Drug Use." *New England Journal of Medicine* 290 (1974): 769-774.

Bandura, A. *Principles of Behavior Modification.* New York: Holt, 1969.

Bane, J. Donald; Kutscher, Austin H.; Neale, Robert E.; and Reeves, Robert B., Jr., eds. *Death and Ministry: Pastoral Care of the Dying and Bereaved.* New York: Seabury Press, 1975.

Bane J. Donald, and Smith, Elizabeth Dorsey J. "The Minister as Part of the Health Care Team." In *Death and Ministry: Pastoral Care of the Dying and Bereaved*, edited by Donald J. Bane, et al. New York: Seabury, 1975, pp. 192-201.

Barber, Bernard. "Some Problems of the Sociology of Professions." In *The Professions in America*, edited by Kenneth S. Lynn. Boston: Houghton Mifflin, Daedalus, 1965, pp. 647-865.

_____. *Drugs and Society*. New York: Russell Sage Foundation, 1967.

_____. "The Ethics of Experimentation with Human Subjects." *Scientific American*, February 1976, pp. 25-31.

_____, et al. *Research on Human Subjects: Problems of Social Control in Medical Experimentation*. New York: Russell Sage Foundation, 1973.

Bard, B., and Fletcher, J. "The Right to Die." *Atlantic*, April 1968, pp. 59-64.

Bardwick, Judith M. "Psychodynamics of Contraception with Particular Reference to Rythm." In *Proceedings of a Research Conference on Natural Family Planning*, edited by W. A. Urrichio. Washington, D.C.: Human Life Foundation, 1973.

Barnhouse, Ruth Tiffany. *Homosexuality: A Symbolic Confusion*. New York: Seabury Press, 1977. On psychiatric classification, pp. 43ff.

Barnlund, Dean C. "The Mystification of Meaning: Doctor-Patient Encounters." *Journal of Medical Education* 51 (1976): 716-725.

Barr, O. Sidney. *The Christian New Morality: A Biblical Study of Situation Ethics*. New York: Oxford University Press, 1970.

Baughman, William H., et al. "Euthaniasia: Criminal Tort: Constitutional and Legislative Questions." *Notre Dame Lawyer* 48 (1973): 1202-1260.

Bayer, Charles H. "Confessions of an Abortion Counselor." *Christian Century* 87 (1970): 624-626.

Bazelon, David L. "The Right to Treatment: The Court's Role." *Hospital and Community Psychiatry* 20 (1969): 129-135.

_____. "Psychiatrists and the Adversary Process." *Scientific American*. June 1974, pp. 18-23. (a)

_____. "The Perils of Wizardry." *American Journal of Psychiatry* 131 (1974): 1317-1322. (b)

Becker, D. P., et al. "An Evaluation of the Definition of Cerebral Death." *Neurology* 20 (1970): 459-462.

Becker, Ernest. *The Denial of Death*. New York: Macmillan and The Free Press, 1973.

Becker, Howard S. "The Nature of a Profession." In *Education for the Professions*, edited by Nelson B. Henry. 61st Yearbook of the National Society for the Study of Education, 2nd ed. Chicago: University of Chicago Press, 1960, pp. 27-46.

_____, and Geer, Blanche. "Medical Education." In *Handbook of Medical Sociology*, edited by Howard E. Freeman, Sol Levine, and Leo G. Reeder. Englewood Cliffs, N.J.: Prentice-Hall, 1963, pp. 169-186.

_____, Geer, Blanche; Hughes, Everett C.; and Strauss, Anselm. *Boys in White*. Chicago: University of Chicago Press, 1961.

Becker, Laurence C. "Human Being: The Boundaries of the Concept." *Philosophy and Public Affairs* 4 (Summer 1975): 334-359.

Beckhard, Richard. "Organizational Issues in the Team Delivery of Comprehensive Health

Care." In *Organizational Issues in the Delivery of Health Services*, edited by Irving K. Zola and John B. McKinlay. New York: Milbank Memorial Fund, 1974, pp. 97-126.

Beecher, Henry K.
1968. "Ethical Problems Created by the Hopelessly Unconscious Patient." *New England Journal of Medicine* 278: 1425-1430.
1969a. "Procedures for the Appropriate Management of Patients Who May Have Supportive Measures Withdrawn." *Journal of American Medical Association* 209: 405.
1969b. "After the 'Definition of Irreversible Coma'." *New England Journal of Medicine* 281: 1070-1071.
1970. "Definitions of Life and Death for Medical Science and Practice." *Annals of New York Academy of Sciences* 169: 471-474.

Belford, A. "The Relation of Religion to Pastoral Counseling." *Journal of Religion and Health* 7 (1968): 26-42.

Bell, Daniel. *The Coming of Post-Industrial Society: A Venture in Social Forecasting.* New York: Basic Books, 1973.

Benham, Lee. "Guilds and the Form of Competition in the Health Care Sector." Paper delivered at the Federal Trade Commission Conference on Competition in the Health Care Sector, June 1977.

Benjamin, Roger. *Nation de personne et personalisme ametien.* Paris: Mouton, 1971, pp. 11-27.

Bennet, Edward A. *What Jung Really Said.* New York: Schocken Books, 1972.

Bennet, John C., et al. *Storm over Ethics.* Fletcher's answers to critics. Philadelphia: United Church Press, 1967.

Benton, Arthur. "Historical Development of the Concept of Hemispheric Cerebral Dominance." In *Philosophical Dimensions of the Neuro-Medical Sciences*, edited by Stuart F. Spiker and H. Tristram Engelhardt, Jr. 2 vols. Boston: D. Reidel, 1976. Vol. 2, pp. 35-38.

Berdiaev, Nikolai A. *Spirit and Reality.* New York: Scribner's, 1934.

Berelson, Bernard. *The Great Debate on Population Policy: An Instructive Entertainment.* New York: The Population Council, 1975.

Berg, Paul; Baltimore, David; Brenner, Sydney; Roblin, Richard O. III; and Singer, Maxine F. "Asilomar Conference on Recombinant DNA Molecules." *Science* 188 (1975): 991-994.

Berger L. Peter, and Luckmann, Thomas. *The Social Construction of Reality: A Treatise in the Sociology of Knowledge.* Garden City, N.Y.: Doubleday, 1966.

Bergron, Henri. *The Two Sources of Morality and Religion.* New York: Henry Holt, 1935.

Bergsma, Daniel, ed. "Advances in Human Genetics and Their Impact on Society." *Birth Defects.* Original Articles Series, VIII, no. 4 (July 1972). White Plains, N.Y.: National Foundation of March of Dimes, 1972.

_____, et al. "Contemporary Genetic Counseling." *Birth Defects.* Original Articles Series, IX, no. 4 (April 1973). White Plains, N.Y.: National Foundation of March of Dimes, 1973.

Berlant, Jeffrey Lionel. *Profession and Monopoly: A Study of Medicine in the United States and Great Britain.* Berkley: University of California Press, 1975.

Bernfield, Simon, ed. *The Foundations of Jewish Ethics.* New York: KTAV Publishing House, 1968. Vol. 1: *The Teaching of Judaism.*

Bernstein, Arnold, and Lennard, Henry L. "The American Way of Drugging: Drugs, Doctors and Junkies." *Transaction/Society* 10 (1973): 14-25.

Bernstein, Dorothy M., and Simmons, Roberta G. "The Adolescent Kidney Donor: The Right to Give." *American Journal of Psychiatry* 131 (1975): 1338-1343.

Bertalanffy, Ludwig von. *General System Theory: Foundations, Development, Applications.* New York: Dover, 1968.

Bertocci, Peter. *The Person God Is.* London: George Allen & Unwin, 1970, p. 20.

Bidney, David. *Theoretical Antrhropology.* New York: Columbia University Press, 1953.

Biorck, G. "On the Definition of Death." *World Medical Journal* 14 (September-October 1967): 137-139.

Bird, Thomas D., and Plum, Fred. "Recovery from Barbiturate Overdose Coma with a Prolonged Isoelectric Electroencephalogram." *Neurology* 18 (1968): 456-460.

Birk, Lee, et al. *Behavior Therapy in Psychiatry: A Report of the American Psychiatric Association Task Force on Behavior Therapy.* New York: Jason Aronson, 1974.

Birmingham, William. *What Modern Catholics Think About Birth Control.* New York: New American Library, Signet Books, 1964.

———, and Cuneen, Joseph E., eds. *Cross Currents of Psychiatry and Catholic Morality.* New York: Pantheon, 1964.

Birnbaum, Morton. "The Right to Treatment." *American Bar Association Journal* 46 (1960): 499-505.

Black, Peter, and Szasz, Thomas. "The Ethics of Psychosurgery: Pro and Con." *The Humanist* 37 (1977): 6-11.

Blanshard, Paul, and Doerr, Ed. "A Glorious Victory." *The Humanist* 33 (May-June 1973).

Bleich, J. David. "Establishing Criteria of Death." *Tradition* 13 (Winter 1973): 90-113.

Bloch, Ernst. *Philosophy of the Future.* New York: Seabury, 1970.

———. *Man on His Own: Essays in the Philosophy of Religion.* New York: Seabury Press, 1971.

Bloom, Samuel W. "The Process of Becoming a Physician." *Annals of the Academy of Political and Social Science* 346 (1963): 77-87.

———. "The Sociology of Medical Education: Some Comments on the State of the Field." *Milbank Memorial Fund Quarterly* 43 (April 1965): 143-184.

Blum, Henrik L. *Planning for Health: Development and Application of Social Change.* New York: Behavioral Publishers, 1974.

Blum, Richard H. *A Commonsense Guide to Doctors, Hospitals and Medical Care.* New York: Macmillan, 1964. (a)

———. *Utopiates: The Use and Users of LSD.* Chicago: Aldine-Atherton, 1964. (b)

Böckle, Franz. *Fundamental Concepts of Moral Theology.* New York: Paulist Press, 1968.

Boisen, Anton T. *Exploration of the Inner World.* New York: Harper & Row, Torchbooks, 1936.

———. *Religion in Crisis and Custom.* New York: Harper & Bros., 1945.

Bok, Sissela. "Ethical Problems of Abortion." *Hastings Center Studies* 2, no. 1 (1974): 33-52. (a)

_____. "The Ethics of Giving Placebos." *Scientific American*, November 1974, pp. 17-23.
(b)

_____, and Lappé, Marc. "The Threat of Hemophilia." *Hastings Center Report* 4 (1974):
8-10.

_____. *Lying and Moral Choice in Public and Private Life.* New York: Pantheon Books,
1978.

Bok, Sissela, et al. "The Dilemmas of Euthanasia." *Bio-Science* 23 (1973): 461-478.

Boné, E. L. "Le preoccupation bioethique dans les pays anglo-saxons." *Revue Theologique
de Louvain* 4 (1973): 340-356.

Boros, S. J., Ladislaus. *The Mystery of Death.* New York: Herder & Herder, 1965.

Bottomore, Tom. "Three Authors in Search of a Proletariat." *New York Review of Books*
18:6 (April 6, 1972): 31-34.

Boulogne, O.P., Charles D. *My Friends, The Senses.* New York: Kenedy, 1953.

Bourke, Vernon J. *Ethics.* New York: Macmillan, 1951.

_____. *History of Ethics*, 2 vols. Vol. 1: on voluntarism, pp. 147 ff. New York: Double-
day, Image Books, 1970.

Bouscaren, T. L. *Ethics of Ectopic Operations*, 2nd rev. ed. Milwaukee: Bruce, 1944.

Bower, Robert K., ed. *Biblical and Psychological Perspectives for Christian Counselors.*
South Pasadena, Calif.: William Carey Library, 1974.

Bowker, John. *Problems of Suffering in the Religions of the World.* New York: Cambridge
University Press, 1970.

Boyle, John P. *The Sterilization Controversy: A New Crisis for the Catholic Hospital?* New
York: Paulist Press, 1977.

Braceland, Francis J. "Historical Perspectives of the Ethical Practice of Psychiatry." *American
Journal of Psychiatry* 126 (1969): 230-237.

Brandt, Richard B. *Ethical Theory.* Englewood Cliffs, N.J.: Prentice-Hall, 1959.

_____. "Ethical Relativism." In *Encyclopedia of Philosophy*, edited by Paul Edwards.
New York: Macmillan and Free Press, 1967. Vol. 3, pp. 75-78.

Braunstein, P., et al. "A Simple Bedside Evaluation for Cerebral Blood Flow in the Study
of Cerebral Death: A Prospective Study on Thirty-Four Deeply Comatose Patients."
Journal of Roentgenology, Radium Therapy and Nuclear Medicine 118 (1973):
757-767.

Brecher, Edward, ed. *The Consumer's Union Report: Licit and Illicit Drugs.* Boston: Little,
Brown, 1972.

Bredell, Frank. "Ombudsman: Problem Solver in Action." *Michigan Hospitals* 12 (1976):
16-19.

Breggin, Peter R. "New Information in the Debate Over Psychosurgery." *Congressional
Record*, March 30, 1972, E3380-86.

_____. "The Return of Lobotomy and Psychosurgery." *Quality of Health Care — Human
Experimentation.* U.S. Senate, 1973, E1602-12.

Brierley, J. B., et al. "Neocortical Death after Cardiac Arrest." *Lancet* 2 (1971): 560-565.

Brim, Orville G., Jr., et al., eds. *The Dying Patient.* New York: Russell Sage Foundation,
1970.

British Guild of Catholic Doctors. "Report of Ethical Committee on *in Vitro* Fertilization." *Catholic Medical Quarterly* 24 (1972): 237-243.

Brock, Dan C.: "Recent Work in Utilitarianism." *American Philosophical Quarterly* 10 (1973): 241-276.

Brockman, S. M., Norbert C. "Contemporary Attitudes on the Morality of Masturbation." *American Ecclesiastical Review* 166 (1972): 597-614.

Broderick, O.P., Albert. "A Constitutional Lawyer Looks at the *Roe-Doe* Decisions." *Jurist* (Spring 1973): 123-133.

Brodsky, C. M. "Clergymen as Psychotherapists: Problems in Inter-Role Communication." *Community Mental Health Journal* 4 (1968): 482-491.

Brody, Baruch. "Abortion and the Sanctity of Human Life." *American Philosophical Quarterly* 10 (1973): 133-140.

_____. *Abortion and the Sanctity of Human Life: A Philosophical View.* Cambridge, Mass.: M.I.T. Press, 1975.

Brody, Eugene B. "On the Legal Control of Psychosurgery." *Journal of Nervous and Mental Disease* 157 (1973): 151-153.

_____. "Biomedical Innovation, Values and Anthropological Research." *Journal of Nervous and Mental Disease* 158 (1974): 85-87.

Brody, Howard. *Introduction to Ethical Decisions in Medicine: A Self-Instructional Unit.* Rev. ed. East Lansing, Mich.: Michigan State U. Press, 1975.

_____. *Ethical Decisions in Medicine.* Boston: Little, Brown, 1976.

Bromley, Dorothy Dunbar. *Catholics and Birth Control: Contemporary Views on Doctrine.* Old Greenwich, Conn.: Devin-Adair Co., 1965.

Brown, Esther Lucile. *Newer Dimensions of Patient Care.* New York: Russell Sage Foundation.
    1961. Part I The Use of Physical and Social Environment of the General Hospital for Therapeutic Purposes.
    1962. Part 2 Improving Staff Motivation and Competence in the General Hospital.
    1964. Part 3 Patients as People.

Browning, Don. *Atonement and Psychotherapy.* Philadelphia: Westminster Press, 1966.

_____. *The Moral Context of Pastoral Care.* Philadelphia: Westminster Press, 1976.

Brownmiller, Susan. *Against Our Will: Men, Women and Rape.* New York: Simon & Schuster, 1975.

Brunner, Emil. *The Divine Imperative.* London: Lutterworth Press, 1937.

Brzezinski, Zbigniev. "The American Transition." *New Republic* 157 (1967): 18-21.

Bucharest Report of the Symposium on Population and Human Rights. World Population Conference, Bucharest, Romania, January 21-29, 1974. New York: Unipub. 1974.

Bugental, J.F.T. *The Search for Authenticity: An Existentialist-Analytic Approach to Psychotherapy.* New York: Holt, 1965.

Buhler, Charlotte. *Values and Psychotherapy.* New York: Free Press, 1962.

Bultmann, Rudolf. *Jesus and The Word.* New York: Scribner, 1958.

Bumpass, Larry, and Westoff, Charles F. "The Perfect Contraceptive Population." *Science* 169 (1970): 1177-1182.

Burns, Chester R., and Engelhardt, H. Tristram, Jr., guest eds. "The Humanities and Medicine." Special Issue. *Texas Reports on Biology and Medicine* 32, no. 1 (Spring, 1974).

Burns, Eveline M. *Health Services for Tomorrow: Trends and Issues.* New York: Dunellen, 1973.

California Medicine. Editorial, "On a Definition of Health." 112 (1970): 63.

Callahan, Daniel
    1969a. (ed.) *The Catholic Case for Contraception.* New York: Macmillan.
    1969b. "The Sanctity of Life." In *Updating Life and Death: Essays in Ethics and Medicine,* edited by Donald R. Cutler. Boston: Beacon Press.
    1970a. "Contraception and Abortion: American Catholic Response." *Annals American Academy of Political and Social Science* 387: 109-117.
    1970b. *Abortion: Law, Choice, Morality.* London: Macmillan.
    1973a. "Abortion: Thinking and Experiencing." *Christianity and Crisis* 32: 295-298.
    1973b. Comments. In Moore et al. "Abortion: The New Ruling." *Hastings Center Report* 3 (April): 4-7.
    1973c. *The Tyranny of Survival and Other Pathologies of Civilized Life.* New York: Macmillan.
    1973d. "The WHO Definition of Health." *Hastings Center Studies* 1, no. 3: 77-87.

Camenisch, Paul F. "Abortion: For the Fetus's Own Sake?" *Hastings Center Report* 6 (1976): 38-41.

Campbell, A. V. *Moral Dilemmas in Medicine.* Baltimore: Williams & Wilkins, 1972.

Canadian Catholic Conference. *Medico-Moral Guide,* 1970. Reprinted in *Origins* 1 (December 9, 1971): 427-428, n. 25.

Cannon, Walter. *The Wisdom of the Body.* Rev. ed. New York: Norton, 1939.

Cantor, Norman L. "A Patient's Decision to Decline Life-Saving Medical Treatment: Bodily Integrity Versus the Preservation of Life." *Rutgers Law Review* 26 (Winter 1972): 228-264.

Capps, Walter H., ed. *The Future of Hope.* Essays by Bloch, Fackenheim, Moltmann, Metz, and Capps. Philadelphia: Fortress Press, 1970.

Capron, Alexander M. "Determining Death: Do We Need a Statute?" *Hastings Center Report* 3 (1973): 6-7. (a)

_____. "Medical Research in Prisons." *Hastings Center Report* 3 (June 1973): 4-6. (b)

_____, and Kass, Leon R. "A Statutory Definition of the Standards for Determining Human Death: An Appraisal and a Proposal." *University of Pennsylvania Law Review* 121 (1972): 87-118.

Cardegna, Felix F. "Contraception, the Pill and Responsible Parenthood." *Theological Studies* 25 (1964): 611-636.

Carrera, Frank, and Adams, P. L. "An Ethical Perspective on Operant Conditioning." *Journal of American Academy of Child Psychiatry* 9 (1970): 607-623.

Carter, Edward J. *Spirituality for Modern Man.* Notre Dame, Ind.: Fides Publishers, 1972.

Cass, Leo J., and Curran, William J. "Rights of Privacy in Medical Practice." *Lancet* 2 (1965): 783-785.

Cassell, Eric. "Dying in a Technological Society." *Hastings Center Studies* 2, no. 2 (May 1974): 31-36.

_____. *The Healer's Art.* New York: Lippincott, 1976.

_____, Kass, Leon, et al. "Refinements in Criteria for the Determination of Death: An Appraisal." *Journal of American Medical Association* 221 (1972): 48-53.

Cassin, René. "The Text of the Universal Declaration." *Lumen Vitae* 24 (1969): 17-30.

Cassirer, Ernst. *The Philosophy of Symbolic Forms.* Vol. 1. New Haven: Yale University Press, 1953, pp. 86-93.

Catholic Hospital Association. "A Christian Affirmation of Life." *Hospital Progress*, July 1974, p. 65.

_____. *Ethical Issues in Nursing: A Proceedings.* St. Louis: Catholic Hospital Association, 1976.

Catholic Theological Society of America. "Catholic Hospital Ethics." Report of Commission on Ethical and Religious Directives for Catholic Hospitals commissioned by the Society, September 1, 1972. *Hospital Progress*, February 1973, pp. 44-56.

Cavalier, Richard. "Ombudsman Is Middle Man Between Clinic Patients and Hospital." *Modern Hospital*, January 1970, pp. 92-96.

Cavanaugh, Denis. "Reforming the Abortion Laws: A Doctor Looks at the Case." *America* 122 (1970): 406-411.

Cavanaugh, John R. *Fundamentals of Pastoral Counseling.* Milwaukee: Bruce, 1962.

_____. *The Popes, The Pill and The People.* Milwaukee: Bruce, 1964.

Cerling, C. E., Jr. "Abortion and Contraception in Scripture." *Christian Scholar's Review* 2 (Fall 1971): 42-58.

Chakrabarty, A. M. "Which Way Genetic Engineering?" *Industrial Research* (January 1976): 45-50.

Chalkley, D. T. "Panel Discussion." In *Experiments and Research with Humans: Values in Conflict.* Washington, D.C.: National Academy of Sciences, 1975, pp. 161-163.

Champlin, Joseph M. *The Sacraments in a World of Change.* Notre Dame, Ind.: Ave Maria Press, 1973.

Chayet, Neil L. "Confidentiality and Privileged Communication." *New England Journal of Medicine* 275 (1966): 1009-1010.

Childress, James F. "Who Shall Live When Not All Can Live?" In *Readings on Ethical and Social Issues in Biomedicine*, edited by Richard W. Wertz. Englewood Cliffs, N.J.: Prentice-Hall, 1973, pp. 143-153. Reply by Frederic B. Westervelt, Jr., pp. 154-158.

_____. "A Response to 'Conferred Rights and the Fetus'." *Journal of Religious Ethics* 2 (Spring 1974): 77-84. Answers Ronald Green's article in same issue, pp. 55-83.

"Choices of Life or Death in the Case of Defective Newborns." In *Social Responsibility Journalism, Law, Medicine.* Program of Society and the Professions: Studies in Applied Ethics. Lexington, Va.: Washington and Lee University, 1975, pp. 62-78.

Choron, Jacques. *Suicide.* New York: Scribner, 1972.

Christman, Luther P. "Nurse-Physician Communication in the Hospital." *Journal of American Medical Association* 194 (1965): 539-544.

Ciba Foundation Symposium. *Law and Ethics of AID and Embryo Transfer.* New York: Association of Scientific Publishers, 1973.

Clapp, Betsey M.; Gant, Annajee R.; Nagy, Emil J.; and Strauss, James F. "Seven Steps to Setting up a Patient Representative System That Works." *Hospital Financial Management* 29 (1975): 42-47.

Clausen, John A. "Drug Addiction." In *International Encyclopedia of Social Science*. New York: Macmillan, 1968. Vol. 4: Part 3, "Social Aspects of Drug Use and Addiction," pp. 298-304.

Cleary, S.J., Francis X. "On Death and Afterlife: A Biblical Reflection." *Hospital Progress*, December 1975, pp. 40-44.

Clebsch, William A., and Jaekle, Charles R. *Pastoral Care in Historical Perspective*. New York: Jason Aronson, 1964.

Clements, Leslie C. "Abortion: The Right to Life — or to End Life." *Study Encounter* (World Council of Churches Publication) 8 (1972): 1-8.

Clinebell, Harold J., Jr. *Basic Types of Pastoral Counseling*. Nashville, Tenn.: Abingdon, 1966.

Clouser, K. Danner, and Zucker, Arthur. *Abortion and Euthanasia: An Annotated Bibliography*. Philadelphia: Society for Health and Human Values, 1974.

Cobb, John B. *Theology and Pastoral Care*. Philadelphia: Fortress Press, 1977.

Coe, Rodney M. *Sociology of Medicine*. New York: McGraw-Hill, 1970, p. 91.

Cohen, Stanley N. "The Manipulation of Genes." *Scientific American*, July 1975, pp. 24-33.

Collen, Morris; Siegelaub, A. B.; Cutler, John L.; and Goldberg, Robert. "Aspects of Normal Values in Medicine." *Annals of New York Academy of Sciences* 161 (1969): 572-580.

Collins, V. U. "Limits of Medical Responsibility in Prolonging Life: Guides to Decision." *Journal of American Medical Association* 206 (1968): 389-392.

Comfort, Alexander. "The Computer and the Doctor." Center for Study of Democratic Institutions. *Center Report* (1972): 21-23 (Feb.); 26-28 (April).

Committee on Drug Law Evaluation, 1977, Department of Justice, Law Enforcement Administration, Drug Abuse Council, June 1977.

"The Conflict over Patients' Rights." Special Issue. *Psychiatric Annals* 5 (April 1975).

Congar, Yves. *Tradition and Traditions*. New York: Macmillan, 1967.

Congregation for the Doctrine of the Faith
    1974.   May. *Declaration on Procured Abortion*. Translated in *Osservatore Romano*, December 5, 1974.
    1975a. March 13. "Doctrinal Congregational Statement on Sterilization." In *Linacre Quarterly* 44 (1977): 117-118.
    1975b. December 29. "Persona Humana: Declaration on Certain Questions Concerning Sexual Ethics." With Commentaries. Washington, D.C.: United States Catholic Conference, 1977.

Congregation of the Holy Office, May 8, 1963. "Cremation." In *Canon Law Digest*. Milwaukee: Bruce, 1969. Vol. 6, pp. 666ff.

Connell, Francis J. Articles in *New Catholic Encyclopedia*. New York: McGraw-Hill, 1968. Vol. 4: "Principle of Double Effect"; "Moral Doubt"; Vol. 9: "Systems of Morality"; Vol. 12: "Reflex Principles."

Connell, R. J. "A Defense of 'HV'." *Laval Theologique et Philosophique* 26 (1970): 57-88. Criticism by Albury, W. R. and reply by Connell, *L. Theolog. et Philos.* 27 (1971): 135-149.

Connery, S.J., John R. "Grisez on Abortion." *Theological Studies* 31 (1970): 173.

———. "Morality of Consequences: A Critical Appraisal." *Theological Studies* 34 (1973): 396-414.

_____. *Abortion: The Development of the Roman Catholic Perspective.* Chicago: Loyola University Press, 1977.

Conway, William. "The Act of Two Effects." *Irish Theological Quarterly* 17 (1951): 125-137.

Conzemius, Viktor. "Quietism." In *Sacramentum Mundi: An Encyclopedia of Theology,* edited by Karl Rahner, S.J. New York: Herder & Herder, 1970, pp. 169-172.

Cooke, Bernard J. *Christian Sacraments and Christian Personality.* New York: Doubleday, 1968.

_____. *Ministry to Word and Sacraments: History and Theology.* Philadelphia: Fortress Press, 1976.

Cooper, David. *Psychiatry and Anti-Psychiatry.* London: Tavistock, 1967.

Cooper, Eugene J. "The Fundamental Option." *Irish Theological Quarterly* (1972): 382-392.

Cooper, Robert M. "Vasectomy and the Good of the Whole." *Anglican Theological Review* 54 (1972): 94-106.

_____. "Euthanasia and the Notion of 'Death with Dignity'." *Christian Century* 90 (1973): 225-227.

Cope, Oliver. *Man, Mind and Medicine.* Philadelphia: Lippincott, 1968.

Coppleston, S.J., Frederick. *A History of Philosophy.* New York: Doubleday, Image Books, 1963. Vol. 3: part 1, "Voluntarism," pp. 115ff.

Coriden, James A. "Church Law and Abortion." *Jurist* 33 (Spring 1973): 184-198.

Corwin, Ronald G., and Taves, Marvin T. "Nursing and Other Health Professions." In *Handbook of Medical Sociology,* edited by Howard E. Freeman, Sol Levine, and Leo G. Reeder. Englewood Cliffs, N.J.: Prentice-Hall, 1963, pp. 187-212.

Costanzo, J. F. "Papal Magisterium and '*Humanae Vitae*'." *Thought* 44 (1969): 377-412.

Cotter, Lloyd H. "Operant Conditioning in a Vietnamese Mental Hospital." *American Journal of Psychiatry* 124 (1967): 23-28.

Cox, Harvey, ed. *The Situation Ethics Debate.* Philadelphia: Westminster Press, 1968.

Cox, J. M. *A Critical Analysis of the Roman Catholic Medico-Moral Principle of Totality and Its Applicability to Sterilizing Mutilations.* Doctoral dissertation, Claremont Graduate School, 1972.

Crabb, Lawrence, Jr. *Basic Principles of Biblical Counseling.* Grand Rapids: Zondervan, 1975.

Crane, Diana. *The Sanctity of Social Life: Physicians' Treatment of Critically Ill Patients.* New York: Russell Sage Foundation, 1975.

Creusen, S.J., I. "L'onanisme Conjugal." *Nouvelle Revuse Theologique* 59 (1932): 132-142.

CRM. *Abnormal Psychology: Current Perspectives.* Del Mar, Calif.: CRM Books, 1972, pp. 257, 267.

Cronin, Daniel A. *The Moral Law in Regard to the Ordinary and Extraordinary Means of Conserving Life.* Doctoral dissertation, Gregorian University, Rome, 1938.

Cronkhite, Leonard W., Jr. The Medical and Scientific Community and Big Government, Chairman's Address, Association of American Medical Colleges, San Francisco, November 14, 1976. *Journal of Medical Education* 52 (1977): 19-24.

Croog, Sydney H. "Interpersonal Relations in Medical Settings." In *Handbook of Medical Sociology*, edited by Howard E. Freeman, Sol Levine, and Leo G. Reeder. Englewood Cliffs, N.J.: Prentice-Hall, 1963, pp. 241-272.

Crotty, N. "Conscience and Conflict." *Theological Studies* 32 (1971): 208-232.

Cunningham, C.M., Bert. *The Morality of Organic Transplantation.* Washington, D.C.: Catholic University of America Press, 1944.

Cunningham, R. L. *Situationism and the New Morality.* New York: Appleton-Century-Crofts, 1970, pp. 35-87.

Curran, Charles E.
    1968. *A New Look at Catholic Morality.* Notre Dame, Ind.: Fides Publishers.
    1969. "Natural Law and Contemporary Moral Theology." In *Contraception: Authority and Dissent*, edited by Charles E. Curran. New York: Herder & Herder, pp. 151-175.
    1970a. *Medicine and Morals.* Washington, D.C.: Corpus Books.
    1970b. "Theology and Genetics: A Multi-Faceted Dialogue." *Journal of Ecumenical Studies* 7:61-89.
    1972. *Catholic Moral Theology in Dialogue.* Notre Dame, Ind.: Fides Publishers.
    1973a. *Politics, Medicine, and Christian Ethics: A Dialogue with Paul Ramsey.* Philadelphia: Fortress Press.
    1973b. "Sterilization: Roman Catholic Theory and Practice." *Linacre Quarterly* 40:97-108.
    1974. *New Perspectives in Moral Theology.* Notre Dame, Ind.: Fides Publishers.
    1975. *Ongoing Revision: Studies in Moral Theology.* Notre Dame, Ind.: Fides Publishers. On specificity of Christian ethics, pp. 1-37; theology of compromise, pp. 187-190; principle of double effect, pp. 173-209; cooperation, pp. 210-228.
    1977a. *Themes in Fundamental Moral Theology.* Notre Dame, Ind.: University of Notre Dame Press.
    1977b. *Issues in Sexual and Medical Ethics.* Notre Dame, Ind.: University of Notre Dame Press.

Curran, Charles E., and Hunt, Robert E. *Dissent in and for the Church: Theologians and "Humanae Vitae."* New York: Sheed & Ward, 1969.

Curran, W. J. "Legal and Medical Death: Kansas Takes the First Step." *New England Journal of Medicine* 284 (1971): 260-261.

————. "The Tuskegee Syphilis Study." *New England Journal of Medicine* 289 (October 4, 1973): 730-731.

————. "The Questionable Virtues of Genetic Screening Laws." *American Journal of Public Health* 64 (1974): 1003-1004.

————, and Shapiro, Donald E. *Law, Medicine, and Forensic Science*, 2nd ed. Boston: Little, Brown, 1974.

Curtin, Leah. *The Mask of Euthanasia* (pamphlet). Cincinnati: Nurses Concerned for Life, 1975.

Cutler, Donald R., ed. *Updating Life and Death: Essays in Ethics and Medicine.* Boston: Beacon Press, 1969.

Dalbiez, Roland. *Psychoanalytic Method and the Doctrine of Freud*, 2 vols. London: Longmans, 1941.

Dalrymple, Willard. *Foundations of Health.* Boston: Allyn & Bacon, 1959, pp. 9-30.

Danielli, James F. "Industry, Society and Genetic Engineering." *Hastings Center Report* 12 (1972): 5-7.

Danto, Arthur C. "Persons." In *Encyclopedia of Philosophy,* edited by Paul Edwards. New York: Macmillan, and The Free Press, 1967. Vol. 6, pp. 110-114.

D'Arcy, Eric. *Human Acts: An Essay on Their Moral Evaluation.* Oxford: Oxford University Press, 1963.

D'Arcy, Martin. *The Pain of the World and the Providence of God.* London: Longmans, 1936.

Daube, David. "Moral Problems in the Use of Borrowed Organs." *Annals of Internal Medicine* 60 (1964): pp. 312ff.

_____. "Limitations of Self-Sacrifice in Jewish Law and Tradition." *Theology* 72 (1969): 291-304.

Davidson, Glen W. *Living with Dying.* Minneapolis: Augsburg, 1975.

Davidson, Henry A. "Professional Secrecy." In *Ethical Issues in Medicine,* edited by Fuller E. Torrey. Boston: Little, Brown, 1968, pp. 190-194.

Davies, Edmund. "The Patient's Right to Know the Truth." *Proceedings of Royal Society of Medicine* 66 (1973): 533-536.

Davis, Bernard D. "Prospects for Genetic Intervention in Man." *Science* 170 (1970): 1279-1283.

DeArment, Daniel C. "Prayer and the Dying Patient: Intimacy Without Exposure." In *Death and Ministry: Pastoral Care of the Dying and Bereaved,* edited by Donald J. Bane et al. New York: Seabury Press, 1975, pp. 53-58.

"Debate over Psychosurgery." *Journal of American Medical Association* 225 (1973): 913-920.

"Declaration du Centre de liaison d'équipes de recerches (CLER), *Documentation Catholiques* 65 (1 September, 1968): 1469-1470.

Dedek, John F. *Human Life: Some Moral Issues.* New York: Sheed & Ward, 1972.

_____. *Contemporary Medical Ethics.* New York: Sheed & Ward, 1975.

De Koninck, Charles. *De la primauté du bien commun contre les personalistes.* Montreal: Université Laval, 1943.

De La Chapelle, Philippe. "The Origins of the Universal Declaration." *Lumen Vitae* 24 (1969): 31-49.

Delgado, Jose. *Physical Control of the Mind: Toward a Psychocivilized Society.* New York: Harper & Row, 1969.

Delhaye, Phillipe. *"Fecondite et Paternite Responsable."* *Esprit et Vie* 85 (1975): 337-344.

_____. *"La Masturbation."* *Esprit et Vie* 86 (1976): 230-254.

_____, et al. *A Symposium on Humanae Vitae and Natural Law.* *Louvain Studies* 2 (Spring 1969): 211-253.

_____; Grootaers, Jan, and Thils, Gustave, eds. *Pour relire Humanae Vitae.* Declarations episcopales du monde entier, with commentaries by eds. Paris: Duculot, 1970.

DeMarchai, Jacques E. "The Quebec Health Care System: Its Implications for Medical Education." *Journal of Medical Education* 50 (1975): 779-787.

De Marco, D. "The Philosophical Roots in Western Culture for the Pro-Abortion Stand." *Linacre Quarterly* 41 (1974): 87-99.

Denes, Magda. In *Necessity and Sorrow: Life and Death in an Abortion Hospital.* New York: Basic Books, 1976.

Denzinger, Henricus, and Schönmetzer, S.J., Adolfus. *Enchirdion Symbolorum: Definitionum et declarationum de rebus fidei et morum.* 22nd ed. Barcelona: Herder, 1963, n. 829; cf. nn. 865-875.

Deploige, Simon. *The Conflict Between Ethics and Sociology.* St. Louis: B. Herder Book Co., 1938.

"Developments in the Law — Civil Commitment of the Mentally Ill." *Harvard Law Review* 87 (1974): 1190-1406.

Devereux, George. *A Study of Abortion in Primitive Societies.* New York: Julian Press, 1955.

Devlin, Patrick. *The Enforcement of Morals.* Oxford: Oxford University Press, 1959.

Dewey, John. *Reconstruction in Philosophy.* Boston: Beacon Press, 1948 [1920], chap. 7.

_____. *Art as Experience.* New York: Putnam, Capricorn Books, 1959 [1934].

Diamond, Eugene F. "The Willowbrook Experiments." *Linacre Quarterly* 40 (1973): 133-137.

Diamond, James J. "Abortion, Animation, and Biological Hominization." *Theological Studies* 36 (1975): 305-324.

Dillon, Valerie Vance. *Life in Our Hands.* Washington, D.C.: United States Catholic Conference, Family Life Bureau, 1973.

Dinello, Daniel. "On Killing and Letting Die." *Analysis* 31 (1971): 83-86.

Dobzhansky, Theodore. *The Biological Basis of Human Freedom.* New York: Columbia University Press, 1956, pp. 118-122.

Dognin, P. D. *Initiation à Karl Marx.* Paris: Editions du Cerf., 1970.

Dolan, J. V. *"Humanae Vitae and Nature." Thought* 44 (1969): 357-358.

Doms, Herbert. *The Meaning of Marriage.* New York: Sheed & Ward, 1939.

Donceel, S.J., Joseph F. "Immediate Animation and Delayed Hominization." *Theological Studies* 31 (1970): 76-105. (a)

_____. "A Liberal Catholic View." In *Abortion in a Changing World*, edited by Robert E. Hall. 2 vols. New York: Columbia University Press, 1970. Vol. 1, pp. 39-45. (b)

_____. "Why Is Abortion Wrong?" *America* 133 (1975): 65-67.

Dorszynski, J. A. *Catholic Teaching About the Morality of Falsehood.* Washington, D.C.: Catholic University of America Press, 1949.

Douglas, Jack D. *The Social Meaning of Suicide.* Princeton, N.J.: Princeton University Press, 1967.

_____. *Deviance and Respectability: The Social Construction of Moral Meanings.* New York: Basic Books, 1970.

Downie, R. S., and Telfer, Elizabeth. *Respect for Persons.* New York: Schocken Books, 1970.

Downing, A. B. *Euthanasia and the Right to Die.* New York: Humanities Press, 1970.

Drinan, S.J., Robert F. "Catholic Moral Teaching and Abortion Laws in America." *Proceedings of Catholic Theological Society of America* 23 (1968): 118-130.

_____. "Abortion and the Law." In *Who Shall Live?* edited by Kenneth Vaux. Philadelphia: Fortress Press, 1970, pp. 51-68. (a)

_____. "The Jurisprudential Options on Abortion." *Theological Studies* 31 (1970): 149-169. (b)

Dubos, René. *Mirage of Health: Utopias, Progress, and Biological Change.* New York: Harper, 1959.

_____. "Determinants in Health and Disease." In *Britannica Perspectives.* Chicago: Encyclopedia Britannica, 1968. Vol. I, pp. 281-302.

_____. "Desparing Optimist: An Environmental Philosophy for our Times." *American Scholar* 45 (1976): 168-172.

_____, Pines, Maya, and editors of *Life, Health and Disease*; New York: Time, Inc., 1965, Chap. 7, "The Stress of Life," pp. 145ff.

Duff, Raymond S., and Campbell, A. G. M. "Moral and Ethical Dilemmas in the Special-Care Nursery." *New England Journal of Medicine* 289 (1973): 890-894.

Duff, Raymond S., and Hollingshead, August B. *Sickness and Society.* New York: Harper & Row, 1968.

Duffey, Felix D. *Psychiatry and Asceticism.* St. Louis: B. Herder Book Co., 1950.

Dummet, Michael. "The Documents of the Papal Commission on Birth Control." *New Blackfriars* 50 (1969): 211-250.

DuPont, Jacques. *Lés Beatitudes.* Rev. ed., 3 vols. Bruges: Abbaye de Saint André, 1958-1973.

Dupré, Louis. *Contraception and Catholics.* Baltimore: Helicon Press, 1964.

_____. "The Mystical Experience of the Self and Its Philosophical Significance." In *Psychiatry and the Humanities,* edited by Joseph H. Smith. New Haven: Yale University Press, 1976. Vol. 1, pp. 101-126.

Durkheim, E. *Suicide.* Glencoe, Ill.: Free Press, 1951.

Duska, Ronald, and Whelan, Mariellen. *Moral Development: A Guide to Piaget and Kohlberg.* New York: Paulist Press, 1975.

Duster, Troy. *The Legislation of Morality: Law, Drugs and Moral Judgment.* New York: The Free Press, 1970.

Dworkin, Gerland. "Autonomy and Behavior Control." *Hastings Center Report* 6 (1976): 23-28.

Eckhart, Walter. "Genetic Modification of Cells by Viruses." *Bioscience* 21 (1971): 171-173.

Edel, May, and Edel, Abraham. *Anthropology and Ethics.* Rev. ed. Cleveland: Case Western Reserve University Press, 1968.

Edelstein, Emma J., and Edelstein, Ludwig. *Asclepius: A Collection and Interpretation of the Testimonies.* 2 vols. Baltimore: John Hopkins University Press, 1945.

Edwards, R. G., and Fowler, Ruth E. "Human Embryos in the Laboratory." *Scientific American Offprints* 223 (December 1970). San Francisco: Freeman.

Ehrenreich, Barbara, and English, Deirdre. *Witches, Midwives and Nurses: A History of Women Healers.* New York: Feminist Press, 1973. (a)

_____. *Complaints and Disorders: The Sexual Politics of Sickness.* New York: Feminist Press, 1973. (b)

Eller, Vernard. "Let's Get Honest About Abortion." *Christian Century* 92 (1975): 16-18.

Ellis, Albert. "A Rational Sexual Morality." In *The New Sexual Revolution,* edited by L. A. Kirkendall and R. N. Whitehurst. Buffalo, N.Y.: Prometheus Books, 1971.

Ellul, Jacques. *The Technological Society*. New York: Knopf, 1965.

Ellwood, Paul M. "Models for Organizing Health Services and Implications of Legislative Proposals." In *Organizational Issues in the Delivery of Health Care Services*, edited by Irving K. Zole and John B. McKinlay. New York: Milbank Memorial Fund, 1974, pp. 67-90.

Emery, Alan E. H. "Social Effects of Genetic Counseling." *British Medical Journal* (1973): 724-726.

_____. "Genetic Counseling." *British Medical Journal* (1975): 219.

_____, et al. "A Genetic Register System (RAPID)." *Journal of Medical Genetics* 11 (1974): 145ff.

Emrich, Margaret. "Patient-Relations Representative: More Than a Hospital Hostess." *Hospital Topics* 49 (1971): 43-46.

Engelhardt, H. Tristram, Jr.
    1973a. "Beginnings of Personhood: Philosophical Considerations." *Perkins Journal of Theology* 27: 20-27.
    1973b. "Viability, Abortion, and the Difference Between a Fetus and an Infant." *American Journal of Obstetrics and Gynecology* 116: 429-434.
    1974. "The Ontology of Abortion." *Ethics* 84: 217-234.
    1975a. "The Concepts of Health and Disease." In *Philosophy and Medicine*, edited by Stuart F. Spicker and H. Tristram Engelhardt, Jr. Proceedings of the First Trans-Disciplinary Symposium on Philosophy and Medicine, Galveston, Texas, May 9-11, 1974. 3 vols. Boston: D. Reidel.
    1975b. "Bioethics and the Process of Embodiment." *Perspectives in Biology and Medicine* 18 (Summer): 486-500.

Engelhardt, H. Tristram, Jr., and Callahan, Daniel. "Science, Ethics and Medicine." In *The Foundations of Ethics and Its Relationship to Science*. Hastings-on-Hudson, N.Y.: Institute of Society, Ethics and the Life Sciences, 1976. Vol. 1.

English, Darrel S., ed. *Genetic and Reproductive Engineering*. New York: MSS Information Corp., 1974.

Ennis, Bruce. *Prisoners of Psychiatry*. New York: Harcourt Brace Jovanovich, 1972.

_____, and Siegel, Loren. *The Rights of Mental Patients*. New York: Avon Books, 1973.

Epstein, Charles J., et al. "The Center-Satellite System for the Wide-Scale Distribution of Genetic Counseling Services." *American Journal of Human Genetics* 27 (1975): 322-332.

Erickson, Eric. *Young Man Luther*. New York: Norton, 1958, pp. 40-48.

_____. *Identity: Youth and Crisis*. New York: Norton, 1968.

Ermecke, Gustav. "Das Problem der Universalitat oder Allgemeingultikeit sittlicher Normen innerweltlicker Lebengestaltung." *Muncher Theologische Zeitschrift* 24 (1973): 1-24.

Etzioni, Amitai. *Genetic Fix: The Next Technological Revolution*. New York: Harper & Row, Colophon Books, 1973.

"Euthanasia." Report of a meeting. *Proceedings of Royal Society of Medicine* 53 (1970): 659-670.

"Euthanasia." Special Issue. *Baylor Law Review* 27 (Winter 1975).

Euthanasia Educational Fund. "Euthanasia — An Annotated Bibliography." May 1970. New York: Euthanasia Educational Fund, 1970.

Evans, Lester J. *The Crisis in Medical Education.* Ann Arbor: University of Michigan Press, 1964.

Evans, Wayne, and Kline, Nathan S. *Psychotropic Drugs in the Year 2000: Use by Normal Humans.* Springfield, Ill.: Charles C Thomas, 1971.

Faber, Heije. *Pastoral Care in the Hospital.* Philadelphia: Westminster Press, 1972.

Faber, Heije, and Van der Schoot, Evel. *The Art of Pastoral Conversation.* Nashville, Tenn.: Abingdon, 1965.

Fackre, Gabriel. "Biomedical Reproduction." *Theology Today* 27 (1971): 409-421.

_____. "The Ethics of Abortion in Theological Perspective." *Andover-Newton Quarterly* 13 (January 1973): 222-226.

Fadali, A., et al. "An Assessment of Human Cardiac Transplantation." *American Heart Journal* 86 (1973): 721-732.

Fagin, Claire, McClure, Margaret, and Schlotfeldt, Rozela. "Can We Bring Order Out of the Chaos of Nursing Education." *American Journal of Nursing* 76 (1976): 98-107.

Faramelli, Norman J. "Lifeboat Ethics: The Case for Genocide by Benign Neglect." *Church and Society* 65 (March-April 1975): 36-39.

Farber, Leslie H. "Psychoanalysis and Morality." *Commentary* 40 (1965): 69-74.

Farberow, N. L., and Schneidman, E. D., eds. *The Cry for Help.* New York: McGraw-Hill, 1961.

Farraher, Joseph. "Notes on Moral Theology." *Theological Studies* 21 (1963): 69-79.

Farrer, Austin. *Love Almighty and Ills Unlimited.* New York: Doubleday, 1961.

Fazziola, Peter J. "The Mystery of the Unborn." *Bible Today* 78 (April 1975): 388-390.

Fein, Rashi. "On Achieving Access and Equity in Health Care." In *Economic Aspects of Health Care,* edited by John B. McKinlay. New York: Milbank Memorial Fund, 1973, pp. 23-56.

Feinbloom, Deborah H. *Transvestites and Transsexuals: Mixed Views.* Boston: Seymour Lawrence, Delacorte, 1976.

Feldman, David M. *Marital Relations: Birth Control and Abortion in Jewish Law.* New York: Schocken Books, 1974.

Ferrater Mora, Jose. *Being and Death.* Berkley: University of California Press, 1965.

Ferster, C. B. "Reinforcement and Punishment in the Control of Human Behavior by Social Agencies." *Psychiatric Research Reports of American Psychiatric Association* 10 (1968): 101-118.

Fisk, N. "Gender Dysphoria Syndrome." *Interdisciplinary Symposium on Transexualism.* Palo Alto: Stanford University Press, 1973.

Fitch, S.J., D. *"Humanae Vitae* and Reasonable Doubt." *Homiletic and Pastoral Review* 69 (1969): 516-523.

Fletcher, John. "Moral Problems in Genetic Counseling." *Pastoral Psychology* 23 (1972): 47-60.

_____. "Attitudes Towards Defective Newborns." *Hastings Center Studies* 2 (1974): 21-32.

_____. "Abortion, Euthanasia, and Care of Defective Newborns." *New England Journal of Medicine* 292 (1975): 75-78.

Fletcher, Joseph
　　1954.　*Morals and Medicine.*　Boston: Beacon Press.
　　1960.　"The Patient's Right to Die."　*Harpers,* October, pp. 138-143.
　　1966.　*Situation Ethics.*　Philadelphia: Westminster Press.
　　1967.　*Moral Responsibility: Situation Ethics at Work.*　Philadelphia: Westminster Press.
　　1971a.　"Ethical Aspects of Genetic Controls: Designed Genetic Changes in Man."　*New England Journal of Medicine* 285: 776-783.
　　1971b.　"Situation Ethics in a Changing Situation."　*Christian Century* 88: 1444-1446.
　　1972.　"Indicators of Humanhood: A Tentative Profile of Man."　*Hastings Center Report* 2: 1-3.
　　1973.　"An Ethics of Euthanasia."　In *To Live and To Die: When, Why and How,* edited by R. Williams. New York: Springer, 1973, pp. 88-97.
　　1974a.　"New Definitions of Death."　*Prism* 2: 13-16.
　　1974b.　"Abortion and the True Believer."　*Christian Century* 91: 1126-1127.
　　1974c.　"Four Indicators of Humanhood: The Enquiry Matures."　*Hastings Center Report* 4: 4-7. With replies in Correspondence 5: 4; 43-45.
　　1975.　"Triage and Lifeboat Ethics."　In *Triage in Medicine and Society: Inquiries into Medical Ethics,* edited by George R. Lucas, Jr. Houston: Institute of Religion and Human Development, 1975. Vol. 3, pp. 23-34.

Fletcher, Ronald.　*Instinct in Man: In the Light of Recent Works in Comparative Psychology.*　New York: Schocken Books, 1966.

Flew, Antony.　"On Not Deriving 'Ought' From 'Is'."　*Analysis* 25 (1964): 25-32.

————.　*Evolutionary Ethics.*　New York: St. Martin's Press, 1967.

Flexner, Abraham.　*Medical Education in The United States and Canada.*　Carnegie Foundation for the Advancement of Teaching, Bulletin no. 4.　Boston: Marymount Press, 1910. Reprinted Washington, D.C.: Science and Health Publications, 1960.

————.　*Medical Education: A Comparative Study.*　New York: Macmillan, 1925.

Foote, Phillipa.　"Moral Beliefs."　*Proceedings of Aristotelian Society* 59 (1958-1959): 83-104.

Ford, Amasa B.; Ort, Robert S.; Liske, Ralph E.; and Denton, John C.　*The Doctor's Perspective: Physicians View Their Patients and Their Practice.*　Cleveland: Case Western Reserve University, 1967, pp. 139ff.

Ford, S.J., John C., and Grisez, Germain.　"Contraception and the Infallibility of the Ordinary Magisterium."　*Theological Studies.*　In press.

Ford, S.J., John C., and Kelly, S.J., Gerald.　*Contemporary Moral Theology.*　2 vols.　Westminster, Md.: Newman Press, 1964.

Fordney-Settlage, Diane S., Motoshima, Masanabu, and Tredway, Donald S.　"Sperm Transport From the External Cervical Os to the Fallopian Tubes in Women: A Time and Quantitation Study."　*Fertility and Sterility* 24 (September 1973): 655-661.

Fortmann, S.J., Edmund J.　*Everlasting Life After Death.*　Staten Island, N.Y.: Alba House, 1976.

Foucault, Michael.　*The Birth of the Clinic: An archaeology of Medical Perception.*　New York: Pantheon, 1973.

Foye, Lawrence.　"Death with Dignity."　Hearing Before Committee on Aging, U.S. Senate, August 7, 1972. Washington, D.C.: U.S. Government Printing Office, 1972.

Fox, Marvin, ed.　*Modern Jewish Ethics: Theory and Practice.*　Athens, Ohio: Ohio University Press, 1975.

Fox, Reneé C., and Swazey, Judith P. *The Courage to Fail: A Social View of Organ Transplants and Dialysis.* Chicago: University of Chicago Press, 1970.

Francoeur, Robert T. *Utopian Motherhood: New Trends in Human Reproduction.* New York: Barnes, 1970.

_____. *Eve's New Rib: Twenty Faces of Sex, Marriage, and Family.* New York: Harcourt, Brace Jovanovich, 1972. (a)

_____. "We Can — We Must: Reflections on the Technological Imperative." *Theological Studies* 33 (1972): 428-439. (b)

Frankel, Charles. "The Spector of Eugenics." *Commentary* 57 (1974): 25-33.

Frankena, William. *Ethics.* 2nd ed. Englewood Cliffs, N.J.: Prentice-Hall, 1973.

Frankl, Victor E. *The Doctor and the Soul: An Introduction to Logotherapy.* New York: Knopf, 1955.

Fraser, F. C. "Genetic Counseling." *American Journal of Human Genetics* 26 (1974): 636-659.

Freeman, Harrop A. *Counseling in the United States.* San Francisco: Jossey-Bass, 1967.

Freeman, John M., and Cooke, Robert E. "Is There a Right to Die — Quickly?" *Journal of Pediatrics* 80 (1972): 904-908.

Freese, Arthur S. *Managing Your Doctor: How to Get the Best Possible Care.* New York: Stein & Day, 1975.

Freidmann, Theodore, and Roblin, Richard O. "Gene Therapy for Human Genetic Disease?" *Science* 175 (1972): 949-955.

Freidson, Eliot. *Professional Dominance: The Social Structure of Medical Care.* New York: Atherton Press, 1970.

_____. *Profession of Medicine: A Study of the Sociology of Applied Knowledge.* New York: Dodd, Mead, 1971.

_____, ed. *The Hospital in Modern Society.* New York: Free Press, 1963.

Freireich, Emil J. "The Best Medical Care for the 'Hopeless' Patient." *Medical Opinion.* February 1972, pp. 51-55.

_____. "Medical Perspective." In *Responsible Stewardship of Human Life,* edited by Donald McCarthy. St. Louis: Catholic Hospital Association, 1976.

Fremantle, Anne. *The Social Teachings of the Church.* New York: New American Library, Mentor Books, 1963.

Freud, Sigmund. *Beyond the Pleasure Principle.* In *Complete Works.* London: Hogarth and Institute of Psychoanalysis, 1958 [1920]. Vol. 18.

_____. *Civilization and Its Discontents.* London: Hogarth, 1930.

_____. *An Outline of Psychoanalysis.* In *Complete Works.* London: Hogarth, 1964 [1940], pp. 41ff.

Freund, Paul A. "The Legal Profession." In *The Professions in America,* edited by Kenneth S. Lynn. Boston: Houghton Mifflin, Daedulus, 1965, pp. 35-46.

Freymann, John Gordon. *The American Health Care System: Its Genesis and Trajectory.* New York: Medcom, 1974.

Friedberg, John. "Electroshock Therapy: Let's Stop Blasting the Brain." *Psychology Today,* August 1975, pp. 18ff.

Fromm, Erich. *The Revolution of Hope: Toward a Humanized Technology.* New York: Bantam Books, 1968.

_____. *Crisis of Psychoanalysis.* New York: Fawcett World Library, 1975.

Fry, Charlotte, and Miller, Hilary. "Patient Advocate — A Natural Role for the Volunteer." *The Volunteer Leader.* Fall 1975, pp. 20-31.

Fuchs, Josef. *Natural Law: A Theological Investigation.* New York: Sheed & Ward, 1963.

_____. "The Absoluteness of Moral Terms." *Gregorianum* 52 (1971): 415-458.

Furnish, Victor P. *The Love Command in the New Testament.* Nashville, Tenn.: Abingdon, 1972.

Futrell, S.J., John Carroll. "Trust in God for Future of Catholic Hospitals." *Hospital Progress,* February 1977, pp. 66-69.

Gaffney, Edward McGlynn. "Law and Theology: A Dialogue on the Abortion Decisions." *Jurist* 32 (Spring 1973): 134-152.

Gaffney, James. *Moral Questions.* New York: Paulist Press, 1974.

Gaffney, L. "Psychological Reflections on Marital Love and Contraception." *Journal of Religion and Health* 10 (1971): 11-23.

Gallon, Michael. *"Humanae Vitae:* A Pastoral Priest's Viewpoint." *Clergy Review* 53 (1968): 874-878.

Gannon, Timothy J. *Emotional Development and Spiritual Growth.* Chicago: Franciscan Herald, 1975.

Gardner, C. Q. "Deliberate Efforts to Control Human Behavior and Modify Personality." *Daedalus* 96 (1967): 347ff.

Gardner, R. F. R. "Christian Choices in a Liberal Abortion Climate." *Christianity Today* 14 (1970): 766-768.

Garrison, Fielding H. *An Introduction to the History of Medicine.* Reprinted fourth ed. Philadelphia: Saunders, 1960 [1929].

Gatch, Milton M. *Death: Meaning and Mortality in Christian Thought and Contemporary Culture.* New York: Seabury Press, 1969.

Gaylin, Willard. "Psychiatry and the Law: Partners in Crime." *Columbia Forum* 65 (Spring 1965): 23-27.

_____. "What's Normal?" *New York Magazine,* April 1, 1973, pp. 14ff. (a)

_____. "Skinner Redux." *Harpers,* October 1973, pp. 48-56. (b)

_____, and Blatte, Helen. "Behavior Modification in Prisons." *American Criminal Law Review* 13 (Summer 1975): 11-35.

_____, and Callahan, Daniel. "The Psychiatrist as Double Agent." *Hastings Center Report* 4 (1974): 11-14.

_____, Meister, Joel S., and Neville, Robert C. *Operating on the Mind.* New York: Basic Books, 1975.

Gaylin, William. "Genetic Screening: The Ethics of Knowing." *New England Journal of Medicine* 286 (1972): 1361-1362.

Geiger, H. Jack. Review of "Ivan Illich, Medical Nemesis." *New York Times Book Review,* May 2, 1976.

Gelin, Albert. *The Poor of Yahweh.* Collegeville, Minn.: Liturgical Press, 1964.

Genetic Engineering: Its Applications and Limitations. Proceedings of Symposium held in Davos, Ruschlikon-Zurich: Gottlieb Duttweiler Institute for Economic and Social Studies, 1974.

Ghoos, J. "L'Acte a Double Effet: Etude de Theologie Positive." *Ephemerides Theologiae Lovaniensis* 27 (1951): 30-52.

Giannini, Margaret, and Goodman, Lawrence. "Counseling Families During the Crisis Reaction to Mongolism." *American Journal of Mental Deficiency* 67 (1963): 740-747.

Gilbert, Sarita. "Artificial Insemination." *American Journal of Nursing* 76 (1976): 259-260.

Gilchrist, Francis G. *A Survey of Embryology.* Englewood Cliffs, N.J.: Prentice-Hall, 1968.

Gilder, George F. *Sexual Studies.* New York: Bantam Books, 1975.

Gilleman, S.J., Gerard. *The Primacy of Charity in Moral Theology.* Westminster, Md.: Newman Press, 1961.

Glaser, William A. *Paying the Doctor: Systems of Remuneration and Their Effects.* Baltimore: John Hopkins University Press, 1970. (a)

_____. *Social Settings and Medical Organization: A Cross-National Study of the Hospital.* New York: Atherton, 1970. (b)

Glass, Bentley. "Human Heredity and Ethical Problems." *Perspective in Biology and Medicine* 15 (Winter 1972): 237-253.

_____. *Human Heredity and Ethical Problems.* Philadelphia: Philadelphia Society for Health and Human Values, 1975.

Glasser, William. *Reality Therapy: A New Approach to Psychiatry.* New York: Harper & Row, 1965.

Gleason, Robert W. *Contemporary Spirituality.* New York: Macmillan, 1968.

_____, and Hagmaier, George. *Counseling the Catholic.* Mission, Kan.: Sheed, Andrews & McMeel, 1959.

Godden, B. "How Wrong Is Contraception." *Clergy Review* 53 (1968): 816-817.

Goergen, Donald. *The Sexual Celibate.* New York: Seabury Press, 1975.

Goffman, Erving. *Asylums: Essays on the Social Situation of Mental Patients and Other Inmates.* Chicago: Aldine, 1962.

Goldbrunner, Joseph. *Holiness Is Wholeness.* New York: Pantheon, 1955.

_____. *Individuation: A Study of the Depth Psychology of Carl Gustav Jung.* Notre Dame, Ind.: Notre Dame University Press, 1964.

_____. *Realization: The Anthropolony of Pastoral Care.* Notre Dame, Ind.: University of Notre Dame Press, 1966.

Goldstein, Kurt. "Health as a Value." In *New Knowledge in Human Values*, edited by Abraham M. Maslow. New York: Harper & Row, 1959, pp. 178-188.

Goode, William J. "The Theoretical Limits of Professionalization." In *The Semi-Professions and Their Organization*, edited by Amitai Etzioni. New York: The Free Press, 1969, pp. 266-313.

Gordon, H. "Genetic Counseling: Considerations for Talking to Parents and Prospective Parents." *Journal of American Medical Association* 217 (1971): 1215-1225.

Gorovitz, Samuel, et al., eds. *Moral Problems in Medicine.* Englewood Cliffs, N.J.: Prentice-Hall, 1976.

Gould, Jonathan, and Craigmyle, Lord, eds. *Your Death Warrant? The Implications of Euthanasia: A Medical, Legal, and Ethical Study.* New York: Arlington House, 1973.

Granfield, David. "The Legal Impact of the *Roe* and *Doe* Decisions." *Jurist* 32 (Spring 1973): 113-122.

Grastyán, Endré. "Emotion." In *New Encyclopedia Britannica.* 15th ed. Vol. 6, pp. 286-291.

Gray, Bradford. *Human Subjects in Medical Experimentation: A Sociological Study of the Conduct and Regulation of Clinical Research.* New York: Wiley, 1975.

Greeley, Andrew
    1972-   "The Sexual Revolution Among Catholic Clergy."
    1973.   *Review for Religious Research* 14: 91-101.
    1974.   *Ecstasy: A Way of Knowing.* Englewood Cliffs, N.J.: Prentice-Hall.
    1976a.   "Are We a Nation of Mystics?" In *Death and Beyond.* Chicago: Thomas More Press, pp. 89-111.
    1976b.   "Council or Encyclical." *Review of Religious Research* 18 (Fall): 3-24.

Green, Harold P. "Genetic Technology: Law and Policy for the Brave New World." *Indiana Law Journal* 48 (Summer 1973): 559-580.

Green, Norman N. *Jean-Paul Sartre: The Existentialist Ethic.* Ann Arbor: University of Michigan Press, 1966, pp. 44-59.

Green, Richard. "Persons Seeking Sex Change: Psychiatric Management of Special Problems." *American Journal of Psychology* 126 (1970): 1596-1603.

————. "A Research Strategy." *International Journal of Psychiatry* 9 (1970-1971): 269-273.

————. *Sexual Identity in Children and Adults.* New York: Basic Books, 1974.

Green, Ronald M. "Conferred Rights and the Fetus." *Journal of Religious Ethics* 2 (Spring 1974): 55-83. Reply by Childress, James. "A Response." *J. Relig. Ethics* 2 (Spring 1974): 77-84.

Greenberg, Roget P., et al. "The Psychological Evaluation of Patients for a Kidney Transplant and Hemodialysis Program." *American Journal of Psychiatry* 130 (1973): 247-277.

Greenberg, Selig. *The Troubled Calling: Crisis in the Medical Establishment.* New York: Macmillan, 1965.

Greene, B. L. *A Clinical Approach to Marital Problems.* Springfield, Ill.: Charles C Thomas, 1976.

Greenwood, Ernest. "The Elements of Professionalization." In *Professionalization,* edited by Howard M. Vollmer and Donald L. Mills. Englewood Cliffs, N.J.: Prentice-Hall, 1966.

Grelot, Pierre. *Man and Wife in Scripture.* New York: Herder, 1964.

Gremillion, Joseph. *The Gospel of Peace and Justice: Catholic Social Teaching Since Pope John.* Maryknoll, N.Y.: Orbis Books, 1976.

Grene, Marjorie. *Approaches to a Philosophical Biology.* New York: Basic Books, 1968, pp. 93-95.

Griese, Orville N. *The Morality of Periodic Continence.* Washington, D.C.: Catholic University Press, 1943.

Grisez, Germain G.
  1964.   *Contraception and the Natural Law.* Milwaukee: Bruce.
  1970a. *Abortion: The Myths, the Realities, the Arguments.* Washington, D.C.:
          Corpus Books.
  1970b. "Toward a Consistent Natural-Law Ethics of Killing." *American Journal
          of Jurisprudence* 15: 65-96.
  1977.   "Sucide and Euthanasia." In *Death, Dying and Euthanasia,* edited by Dennis
          J. Horan and David Mall. Washington, D.C.: University Publications, pp.
          742-818.

Grisez, Germain G., and Shaw, Russell. *Beyond the New Morality: The Responsibilities
    of Freedom.* Notre Dame, Ind.: University of Notre Dame Press, 1974.

Groat, H. T., Neal, A. G., and Kinsely, E. "Contraceptive Nonconformity Among Catholics."
    Journal for Scientific Study of Religion 14 (1975): 367-377.

Grollman, Earl A., ed. *Rabbinical Counseling.* New York: Bloch Publishing, 1967.

Gruman, Gerald J. "An Historical Introduction to Ideas about Voluntary Euthanasia: With
    a Bibliographic Survey and Guides for Interdisciplinary Studies." *Omega* 4 (Summer
    1973): 87-138.

Guerrero, Rodrigo. "Possible Effects of the Periodic Abstinence Method." In *Proceedings
    of a Research Conference on Natural Family Planning,* edited by W. A. Uricchio.
    Washington, D.C.: Human Life Foundation, 1973, pp. 84-96.

Gurney, Edward J. "Is There a Right to Die? A Study of the Law of Euthanasia." *Cumber-
    land Samford Law Review* 3 (Summer 1972): 235-261.

Gustafson, James M.
  1965.   "The Clergy in the United States." In *The Professions in America,* edited
          by Kenneth S. Lynn. Boston: Houghton Mifflin, Daedalus, pp. 70-90.
  1973a. "Genetic Engineering and the Normative View of the Human." In *Ethical
          Issues in Biology and Medicine,* edited by Preston N. Williams. Cambridge,
          Mass.: Schenkman.
  1973b. "Mongolism, Parental Desires and the Right to Life." *Perspectives in Biology
          and Medicine* 16 (Summer): 529-557.
  1974.   *Theology and Christian Ethics.* Philadelphia: United Church Press, 1974.
          "What Is Normatively Human," 229-244; "Basic Ethical Issues in the Bio-
          medical Fields," 245-272; "Genetic Engineering and the Normative View of
          the Human," 272-286.
  1975a. *Can Ethics be Christian?* Chicago: University of Chicago Press.
  1975b. *The Contributions of Theology to Medical Ethics.* Pere Marquette Theology
          Lecture. Milwaukee: Marquette University, 1975.
  1976.   *Christ and the Moral Life* (1968). Reissue. Chicago: University of Chicago
          Press, 1976.

Gustafson, James M., and Pizzulli, Francis C., commentators. "Case Studies in Bioethics:
    'Ain't Nobody Gonna Cut on My Head'." *Hastings Center Report* 5 (1975): 49-51.

Guthrie, Donald. *A History of Medicine.* Philadelphia: Lippincott, 1946, pp. 29-32; 84-110.

Gutierrez, Gustavo. *A Theology of Liberation.* Maryknoll, N.Y.: Orbis Books, 1973.

Haag, Herbut. *Is Original Sin in Scripture?* New York: Sheed & Ward, 1969.

Haigherty, Leo, ed. *Pius XII and Technology.* Milwaukee: Bruce, 1962.

Halacy, D. S., Jr. *Genetic Revolution: Shaping Life for Tomorrow.* New York: New
    American Library, Mentor Books, 1974.

Halberstam, Michael J., Stevens, Carl M., and Outka, Eugene. "Care Settings and Values." In *Ethics of Health Care*, edited by Laurence T. Tancredi. Washington, D.C.: National Academy of Medicine, 1974, pp. 231-280.

Hall, Calvin S., and Lindzey, Gardner. *Theories of Personality*. 2nd ed. New York: Wiley, 1970, pp. 7-9.

Halleck, Seymour L. *The Politics of Therapy*. New York: Science House, 1971.

_____. "Legal and Ethical Aspects of Behavioral Control." *American Journal of Psychiatry* 131 (1974): 381-385.

Halley, M. M., and Harvey, W. F. "Medical vs. Legal Definitions of Death." *Journal of American Medical Association* 204 (1968): 423-435. (a)

_____. "Law — Medicine Comment: The Definitional Dilemma of Death." *Journal of Bar Association of State of Kansas* 37 (Fall 1968): 179. (b)

_____, et al. "Definition of Death." *New England Journal of Medicine* 279 (1968): 834.

Halligan, Nicholas. "The Church as Teacher: Prologue to *Humanae Vitae*." *Thomist* 33 (1969): 675-717.

Haman, J. "Therapeutic Donor Insemination." *California Medical Journal* 90 (1973): 130-133.

Hamilton, Michael, ed. *The New Genetics and the Future of Man*. Grand Rapids, Mich.: Eerdmans, 1972.

Handy, Rollo. *The Measurement of Values*. St. Louis: Warren H. Green, 1970, pp. 181-188.

Haney, C. Allen. "Issues and Considerations in Requesting an Anatomical Gift." *Social Science and Medicine* 7 (1973): 635-642.

Hanock, Roger N. *Twentieth Century Ethics*. New York: Columbia University Press, 1974.

Hardin, Garrett. "Living on a Lifeboat." *Bioscience* 24 (1974): 561-568.

Hare, R. M. *Language of Morals*. Oxford: Oxford University Press, 1952.

Häring, C.S.S.R., Bernard.
  1961,   *The Law of Chirst*, 3 vols. Philadelphia: Westminster Press.
  1963,
  1966.
  1968a.   *Christian Renewal in a Changing World.* Garden City, N.Y.: Doubleday, Image Books.
  1968b.   *The Christian Existentialist: The Philosophy and Theology of Self-Fulfillment in Modern Society.* New York: New York University Press.
  1969.   "The Inseparability of the Unitive-Procreative Functions in the Marital Act." In *Contraception: Authority and Dissent*, edited by Charles E. Curran. New York: Herder & Herder.
  1973.   *Medical Ethics.* Notre Dame, Ind.: Fides Publishers.
  1975.   *Ethics of Manipulation: Issues in Medicine, Behavior Control and Genetics.* New York: Seabury Press.
  1976.   "New Dimensions of Responsible Parenthood." *Theological Studies* 37: 120-132.

Harman, Gilbert. *The Nature of Morality: An Introduction to Ethics*. New York: Oxford University Press, 1977.

Harmon, Nolan B. *Ministerial Ethics and Etiquette*. Nashville, Tenn.: Abingdon, 1958.

Harolds, Louis R., and Block, Melvin, eds. *Medical Malpractice — The ATL Seminar.* Rochester, N.Y.: Lawyers Cooperative Publishing Co., 1966.

Harper, Robert A. *Psychoanalysis and Psychotherapy: 36 Systems.* Englewood Cliffs, N.J.: Prentice-Hall, 1959, pp. 152-155.

Harrington, Msgr., Paul V. "The Catholic Doctor, the Catholic Hospital and Contraception." Pamphlet. Boston: Daughters of St. Paul, 1973.

Hart, H. L. A. *Law, Liberty and Morality.* New York: Random House, Vintage Books, 1963.

Hart, S.J., Thomas N. "Sin in the Concept of the Fundamental Option." *Homiletic and Pastoral Review* 71 (1970): 47-50.

Hartman, H. *Psychoanalysis and Moral Values.* New York: International Universities Press, 1960.

Harvard Medical School. "A Definition of Irreversible Coma." Ad Hoc Committee of Harvard Medical School to Examine the Definition of Brain Death. *Journal of American Medical Association* 205 (1968): 85.

Hauerwas, Stanley. *Vision and Virtue: Essays in Christian Ethical Relfection.* Notre Dame, Ind.: Fides Publishers, 1974.

Havinghurst, Clark. "Role of Competition in Cost Containment." Paper delivered at Federal Trade Commission Conference on Competition in the Health Care Sector. Washington, D.C.: June 1977.

Hayman, Howard. "An Ecological View of Health and Health Education." In *Science and Theory of Health: A Book of Readings,* edited by Herbert L. Jones, et al. Dubuque, Iowa: Brown Co., 1966, pp. 3-9.

Healy, S.J., Edwin. *Medical Ethics.* Chicago: Loyola University Press, 1956. On cooperation, pp. 102-108.

Heidgerken, Loretta E. *Teaching and Learning in the Schools of Nursing.* 3rd ed. Philadelphia: Lippincott, 1965.

Heifetz, Milton D., with Mangel, Charles. *The Right to Die: A Neurosurgeon Speaks with Candor.* New York: Putnam, 1975.

Heilbroner, Robert L. *An Inquiry into the Human Prospect.* New York: Norton, 1974.

Hemphill, Michael. "Pretesting for Huntington's Disease: An Overview." *Hastings Center Report* 6 (1973): 12-13.

Henry, Carl. *Christian Personal Ethics.* Grand Rapids, Mich.: Eerdmans, 1957.

Henry, William E., Sims, John J., and Spray, S. Lee. *The Fifth Profession: Becoming a Psychotherapist.* San Francisco: Jossey-Bass, 1971.

Hering, O.P., H. M. "De Tempore Animationis Foetus Humani." *Angelicum* 28 (1951): 18-29.

Hershey, Nathan, and Miller, Robert D. *Human Experimentation and the Law.* Germantown, Md.: Aspen Systems Corp., 1976.

Hertell, Bradley, Hendershot, G. H., and Grimm, J. W. "Religion and Attitudes Toward Abortion: A Study of Nurses and Social Workers." *Journal for Scientific Study of Religion* 13 (1974): 23-39.

Heston, L. L. "Genetics of Schizophrenic and Schizoid Disease." *Science* 167 (1970): 249-256.

Heydebrand, Wolf V. *Hospital Bureaucracy: A Comparative Study of Organizations.* New York: Dunellen, 1973.

Heymann, Philip B., and Holtz, Sara. "The Severely Defective Newborn: The Dilemma and the Decision Process." *Public Policy* 23 (Fall 1975): 381-418.

Hiatt, Howard H. "The Responsibilities of the Physician as a Member of Society: The Invisible Line." *Journal of Medical Education* 51 (1976): 30-39.

Hick, John. *Evil and the God of Love.* New York: Harper, 1966.

Hilgard, E. R., and Bower, G. H. *Theories of Learning.* 4th ed. New York: Appleton-Century-Crofts, 1974.

Hilgers, Thomas W. "The Intrauterine Device: Contraceptives or Abortifacient?" *Marriage and Family Newsletter*, January-March, 1974.

_____. "Human Reproduction: Three Issues." *Theological Studies* 38 (1977): 136-152.

_____, and Horan, Dennis J. *Abortion and Social Justice.* New York: Sheed & Ward, 1972.

Hillman, James. *Suicide and the Soul.* New York: Harper & Row, 1964.

Hiltner, Seward. *Preface to Pastoral Theology.* Nashville, Tenn.: Abingdon, 1958.

_____. *Pastoral Counseling.* Nashville, Tenn.: Abindgon, 1969. (a)

_____. *Ferment in the Ministry.* Nashville, Tenn.: Abingdon, 1969. (b)

Hilton, Bruce; Callahan, Daniel; Harris, Maureen; Condliffe, Peter; and Berkley, Bruce. *Ethical Issues in Human Genetics: Genetic Counseling and the Use of Genetic Knowledge.* New York: Plenum, 1973.

Himes, Norman E. *Medical History of Contraception.* New York: Gamut Press, 1963.

Himmelstein, Jack, and Michels, Robert. "Case Studies in Bioethics: The Right to Refuse Psychoactive Drugs." *Hastings Center Report* 3 (June 1973): 8-11.

Hinds, Stuart W. "Triage in Medicine." In *Triage in Medicine and Society: Inquiries into Medical Ethics.* Houston: Institute of Religion and Human Development, 1975. Vol. 3, pp. 6-22.

Hinnebusch, Paul. *Friendship in the Lord.* Notre Dame, Ind.: Ave Maria Press, 1974.

Hocking, William Ernest. *The Coming World Civilization.* New York: Harper, 1956.

Hoffer, William. "The Legal Limbo of AID." *Modern Medicine* 43 (1975): pp. 19ff.

Holck, Frederick H., ed. *Death and Eastern Thought.* Nashville, Tenn.: Abingdon, 1974.

Holden, J. M., Itil, T. M., and Hofstatter, L. "Prefrontal Lobotomy: Steppingstone or Pitfall?" *American Journal of Psychiatry* 127 (1970): 591-598.

Holst, Lawrence E., and Kurtz, H. *Creative Chaplaincy.* Springfield, Ill.: Charles C Thomas, 1973.

Horan, Dennis J., et al. In *Abortion and Social Justice*, edited by Thomas W. Hilgers and Dennis J. Horan. New York: Sheed & Ward, 1972. "The Legal Case for the Unborn Child," pp. 105-142; "Abortion and the Supreme Court: Death Becomes a Way of Life," pp. 301-328.

Horan, Dennis J., and Mall, David. *Death, Dying and Euthanasia.* Washington, D.C.: University Publications of America, 1977.

Horgan, J. *"Humanae Vitae" and the Bishops.* London: Irish University Press, 1972.

Horton, Paul C. "Normality — Toward a Meaningful Construct." *Comprehensive Psychiatry* 12 (1971): 54-66.

Hostie, S.J., Raymond. *Pastoral Counseling.* New York: Sheed & Ward, 1966.

Howe, Ruel J. *The Miracle of Dialogue.* New York: Seabury Press, 1963.

Hoyt, Robert, ed. *The Birth Control Debate: Interim History from the Pages of the National Catholic Reporter.* Kansas City: National Catholic Reporter, 1969.

Hudson, W. D. *Ethical Intuition.* New York: St. Martin's, 1967.

————. *Modern Moral Philosophy.* Garden City, N.Y.: Doubleday, 1970.

Hulme, William E. *Counseling and Theology.* Philadelphia: Fortress Press, 1967.

————. *Two Ways of Caring: A Biblical Design for Balanced Ministry.* Minneapolis: Augsburg, 1973.

The Human Body: Papal Teachings. Selected and arranged by the Monks of Solesmes. Boston: St. Paul Editions, 1960.

"Humanist Manifesto." *The New Humanist* 6 (May-June 1933). Reprinted in *The Humanist* 33 (January-February 1973): 13-14.

"Humanist Manifesto II." *The Humanist* 33 (September-October 1973): 4-9.

Humber, J. M. "The Case Against Abortion." *Thomist* 39 (1975): 65-84.

————, and Almeder, Robert F. *Biomedical Ethics and the Law.* New York: Plenum, 1976.

Hume, David. *An Enquiry Concerning the Principles of Morals* [1738], edited by P. H. Nidditch. New York: Oxford University Press, 1975.

Huser, Roger J. *The Crime of Abortion in Canon Law: A Historical Synopsis and Commentary.* Washington, D.C.: Catholic University Press, 1942.

Illich, Ivan D.
    1971.   *Schooling Society.* New York: Harper & Row, pp. 52ff.
    1972a. *Celebration of Awareness: A Call for Institutional Revolution.* New York: Doubleday, Anchor Books.
    1972b. "Technology and Conviviality." In *To Create A Different Future: Religious Hope and Technology*, edited by Kenneth Vaux. New York: Friendship Press, pp. 40-66.
    1976a. *Medical Nemesis: The Expropriation of Health.* New York: Pantheon.
    1976b. "Medicine Is a Major Threat to Health." Interview with Sam Keen. *Psychology Today*, May, pp. 66-77.

Ingelfinger, Franz J. "Bedside Ethics for the Hopeless Case." *New England Journal of Medicine* 289 (1973): 914-915.

————. "The Poor." In *Experiments and Research with Humans: Values in Conflict.* Washington, D.C.: National Academy of Sciences, 1975, pp. 150-170.

Ingersoll, Ralph W. "Myths of Medical Education." *Journal of Medical Education* 51 (1976): 688.

"Innovation in Science." Special Issue. *Scientific American*, September 1958.

Institute of Society, Ethics and the Life Sciences. Research Group on Ethical, Social, and Legal Issues in Genetic Counseling and Genetic Engineering. "Ethical and Social Issues in Screening for Genetic Diseases." *New England Journal of Medicine* 286 (1972): 1129-1132. (a)

————. Task Force on Death and Dying. "Refinements in Criteria for the Determination of Death." *Journal of American Medical Association* 221 (1972): 48-53. (b)

Institute for Theological Encounter with Science and Technology. *The Population Issue.* Conference, October 4-7, 1973, St. Louis University, St. Louis, Missouri.

_____. *Brain Research — Human Consciousness.* Conference on Fabricated Man III, October 10-12, 1975. St. Louis University, St. Louis, Missouri.

In The Matter of Karen Quinlan: The Complete Legal Briefs, Court Proceedings, and Decision in the Supreme Court of New Jersey. Arlington, Va.: University Publications of America, 1975.

Irion, Paul E. "The Agnostic and the Religious: Their Coping with Death." In *Death and Ministry: Pastoral Care of the Dying and Bereaved,* edited by Donald J. Bane, et al. New York: Seabury Press, 1975, pp. 205-216.

Isabel, Damien. *The Spiritual Director.* Synthesis Series. Chicago: Franciscan Herald Press, 1976.

Jacobi, Jolande. *The Way of Individuation.* New York: Harcourt Brace, 1967.

Jacobs, William. *The Pastor and the Patient: An Informal Guide to New Directions in Medical Ethics.* New York: Paulist Press, 1973.

Jakobovits, Immanuel. *Jewish Medical Ethics: A Comparative and Historical Study of the Jewish Religious Attitude to Medicine and Its Practice,* new ed. New York: Bloch Publishing, 1975.

Janssen, L. H., ed. *Population Problems and Catholic Responsibility.* Tilburg, The Netherlands: Tilburg University Press, 1975.

Janssens, Louis. "Moral Problems Involved in Responsible Parenthood." *Louvain Studies* 1 (Fall 1966): 3-18.

_____. "Ontic Evil and Moral Evil." *Louvain Studies* 4 (1972): 115-156.

Jaspers, Karl. *Nietzche and Christianity.* Chicago: Regnery, 1963 [1938].

Joannes, F. V., ed. *The Bitter Pill: Worldwide Reaction to the Encyclical "Humanae Vitae."* Philadelphia: Pilgrim Press, 1970.

Johann, Robert O. *Building the Human.* New York: Herder & Herder, 1968.

John XXIII. *Mater et Magistra.* May 15, 1961, National Catholic Welfare Conference, Washington, D.C.

Johnson, Vernon. *I'll Quit Tomorrow.* New York: Harper & Row, 1973.

Johnston, William. *Still Point: Reflections on Zen and Christian Mysticism.* New York: Harper & Row, 1971.

Jones, E. "Free Will and Determinism." *Essays in Applied Psychoanalysis* 7 (1964): 178-189.

Jones, W. T.; Sontag, F.; Becker, M. O.; and Fogeline, R. J. *Approaches to Ethics.* 2nd ed. New York: McGraw-Hill, 1969.

Jonsen, S.J., A. R. *Responsibility in Modern Religious Ethics.* Washington, D.C.: Corpus Books, 1968.

Jonsen, A. R.; Phibbs, R. H.; Tooley, W. H.; and Garland, M. J. "Critical Issues in Newborn Intensive Care: A Conference Report and Policy Proposal." *Pediatrics* 55 (1975): 756-768.

"Judaism and the Management of Birth, Life and Death." *Judaism* 24 (Spring 1975): 134-167.

Jung, Carl G. *The Development of Personality.* Collected Works. New York: Pantheon, 1954. Vol. 17.

Jungel, Eberhard. *Death: The Riddle and the Mystery.* Philadelphia: Westminster Press, 1974.

Kalish, Richard A. "Death and Dying: A Briefly Annotated Bibliography." In *The Dying Patient,* edited by Orville G. Brim, Jr., et al. New York: Russell Sage Foundation, 1970, pp. 323-380.

Kamenka, Eugene. *The Ethical Foundations of Marxism.* 2nd ed. London: Routledge, 1972.

Kanoti, G. A. "Ethical Implications in Psychotherapy." *Journal of Religion and Health* 10 (1971): 180-191.

Kaplan, Helen Singer. *The New Sex Therapy.* New York: Brunner/Mazel, 1974.

Karp, Laurence E. *Genetic Engineering: Threat or Promise?* Chicago: Nelson-Hall, 1976.

Katz, Jay, with Capron, Alexander M., and Swift Glass, Eleanor. *Experimentation with Human Beings.* New York: Russell Sage Foundation, 1972.

Katz, Jay, and Capron, Alexander M. *Catastrophic Diseases: Who Decides What?* A Psychosocial and Legal Analysis of the Problem Posed by Hemodialysis and Organ Transplantation. New York: Russell Sage Foundation, 1975.

Katz, Jay, Goldstein, Joseph, and Dershowitz, Alan M. *Psychoanalysis, Psychiatry and Law.* New York: The Free Press, 1967.

Keefe, S.J., Donald J. "A Review and Critique of the CTSA Report." *Hospital Progress,* February 1973, pp. 57-69.

Kelly, S.J., Gerald.
  1950. "The Duty of Using Artificial Means of Preserving Life." *Theological Studies* 11: 203-220.
  1951. "The Duty to Preserve Life." *Theological Studies* 12: 550-556.
  1952. "Notes on Moral Theology." *Theological Studies* 13: 59-61.
  1955. "Pope Pius XII and the Principle of Totality." *Theological Studies* 16: 373-396.
  1956. "The Morality of Mutilation: Toward a Revision of the Treatise." *Theological Studies* 17: 322-344.
  1958. *Medico-Moral Problems.* St. Louis: Catholic Hospital Association, 1958. On cooperation, pp. 322-325.

Kelly, Kevin T. "A Positive Approach to *Humanae Vitae.*" Moral Theology Forum. *Clergy Review* 57 (1972): 108-120 (Feb.); 174-186 (Mar.); 263-275 (April); 330-349 (May).

Kelsey, Beverly. "Which Infants Shall Live? Who Should Decide?" *Hastings Center Report* 5 (1975): 5-7.

Kennedy, Ian McColl. "The Kansas Statute on Death — An Appraisal." *New England Journal of Medicine* 285 (1971): 946-950.

Kerenyi, Carl. *Asklepios: Archetypal Image of the Physician's Existence.* In *Archetypal Images of Human Existence.* Princeton, N.J.: Princeton University Press, 1959, Vol. 3.

Kerner, George C. *The Revolution in Ethical Theory.* New York: Oxford University Press, 1966.

Kesey, Ken. *One Flew Over the Cuckoo's Nest.* New York: Viking, 1962 (novel).

Kiesling, O.P., Christopher. *The Future of the Christian Sunday.* New York: Sheed & Ward, 1970.

_____. *Confirmation and Full Life in the Spirit.* Cincinnati: St. Anthony's Messenger Press, 1974.

_____. *Celibacy, Friendship and Prayer.* Staten Island, N.Y.: Alba House, 1977.

Kindregan, Charles P. *The Quality of Life: Reflections on the Moral Values of American Law.* Milwaukee: Bruce, 1969.

King, J. Charles. "The Inadequacy of Situation Ethics." *Thomist* 34 (1970): 423-427.

King, Stanley H. *Perceptions of Illness and Medical Practice.* New York: Russell Sage Foundation, 1972. On relative prestige of specialities, pp. 184-188.

Kinsey, A. C., et al. *Sexual Behavior in the Human Male.* Philadelphia: Saunders, 1948.

_____. *Sexual Behavior in the Human Female.* Philadelphia: Saunders, 1953.

Kippley, J. F.
    1970.   *Covenant, Christ and Contraception.* New York: Society of St. Paul.
    1971.   "Continued Dissent: Is It Responsible Loyalty?" *Theological Studies* 32: 48-65.
    1974.   "Catholic Sexual Ethics: The Continuing Debate on Birth Control." *Linacre Quarterly* 41: 8-25. .

Kippley, J. F., and Kippley, Sheila. *The Art of Family Planning.* Cincinnati: International, Inc., Couple-to-Couple League, 1975.

Kittrie, Nicholas N. *The Right to be Different: Deviance and Enforced Therapy.* Baltimore: John Hopkins University Press, 1971.

Kleber, Karl Heinz. *De Parvitate Materiae in Sexto.* Regensburg: F. Pustet, 1971.

Klein, D. B. *A History of Scientific Psychology.* New York: Basic Books, 1970, pp. 319-360.

Klerman, Gerald L. "Drugs and Social Values." *International Journal of Addictions* 5 (May 1970): 2-19.

_____. "Psychotropic Drugs as Therapeutic Agents." *Hastings Center Studies* 2 (January 1974): 81-93.

Kline, Nathan S., and Gordon, Milton. "Case Studies in Bioethics: Amphetamine Quotas and Medical Freedom." *Hastings Center Report* 3 (1973): 8-10.

Kluge, Eike-Henner W. *The Practice of Death.* New Haven: Yale University Press, 1975.

Knauer, Peter. "The Hermeneutic Function of the Principle of Double Effect." *Natural Law Forum* 12 (1967): 132-162.

Kneller, George F. *The Art and Science of Creativity.* New York: Holt, 1965.

Knight, James. *A Psychiatrist Looks at Religion and Health.* New York: Abingdon, 1964.

_____. *Medical Student: Doctor in the Making.* New York: Appleton-Century-Crofts, 1973.

Knight, R. P. "The Comparative Clinical Status of Conditioning Theories and Psychoanalysis." In *The Conditioning Theories,* edited by Joseph Wolpe, Andrew Slater, and L. J. Reyna. New York: Holt, 1966, pp. 3-20.

Koestler, Arthur.
    1964.   *The Act of Creation.* New York: Macmillan.
    1968.   *The Ghost in the Machine.* New York: Macmillan, pp. 230ff.
    1969a. "Beyond Atomism and Holism — The Concept of the Holon." In *Beyond Reductionism: The Alpbach Symposium,* edited by Arthur Koestler and J. R. Smythies. Boston: Beacon Press, pp. 192-232.
    1969b. *Drinkers of Infinity.* New York: Macmillan.

Kohl, Marvin, ed. *Beneficent Euthanasia.* Buffalo, N.Y.: Prometheus Books, 1975.

Kohlberg, Lawrence. "Indoctrination versus Relativity in Value Education." *Theology Digest* 21 (Summer 1973): 113-119. Reprinted from *Zygon* 6 (1971): 285-310.

Kohn, Robert, and White, Kerr L., eds. *Health Care: An International Study.* Report of the WHO Collaborative Study of Medical Care Utilization. New York: Oxford University Press, 1976.

Konold, Donald E. *A History of American Medical Ethics, 1847-1912.* Madison, Wis.: State Historical Society of Wisconsin, 1962.

Kopelman, Loretta. "On Disease: Theories of Disease and Ascriptions of Disease." In *Philosophy and Medicine,* edited by Stuart F. Spicker and H. Tristram Engelhardt, Jr. Proceedings of First Trans-Disciplinary Symposium on Philosophy and Medicine, Galveston, Texas, May 9-11, 1974. 3 vols. Boston: R. Reidel, 1975.

Korein, J., et al. "On the Diagnosis of Cerebral Death: A Prospective Study." *Electroencephalography and Clinical Neurophysiology* 27 (1969): 700.

Kosnick, Anthony R. "The Present Status of the Ethical and Religious Directives for Catholic Health Facilities." *Linacre Quarterly* 40 (1973): 81-90.

_____, chairperson; with Carroll, William; Cunningham, Agnes; Modras, Ronald; and Schulte, James. *Human Sexuality: New Directions in American Catholic Thought.* New York: Paulist Press, 1977.

Kravitz, Liebe. "Patient Care Conferences." *Hospitals* 48 (1974): 55-62.

Kress, Robert. "The Church as *Communio*: Trinity and Incarnation as the Foundation of Ecclesiology." *Jurist* 36 (1976): 127-158.

Kris, Ernst. *Psychoanalytic Explorations in Art.* New York: Schocken Books, 1964.

Kron, Samuel D. "Euthanasia: A Physician's View." *Journal of Religion and Health* 7 (1968): 333-341.

Krutch, Joseph W. *Human Nature and the Human Condition.* New York: Random House, 1959, pp. 75-96.

Kübler-Ross, Elisabeth. *On Death and Dying.* New York: Macmillan, 1969.

_____. *Questions and Answers on Death and Dying.* New York: Macmillan, 1974.

Küng, Hans, ed. *The Plurality of Ministries.* In *Concilium.* New York: Seabury, 1972. Vol. 74.

Kurtz, Paul. "What Is Humanism?" In *Moral Problems in Contemporary Society,* edited by Paul E. Kurtz. Englewood Cliffs, N.J.: Prentice-Hall, 1969, pp. 1-16.

Kushnick, Theodore. "When to Refer to the Geneticist." *Journal of American Medical Association* 235 (1976): 623-625.

Kutscher, A. *Bibliography of Books on Death, Bereavement, Loss and Grief — 1955-1968.* New York: Health Sciences, 1969.

Ladd, John, ed. *Ethical Relativism.* Belmont, Calif.: Wadsworth, 1973.

Lader, Lawrence. *Abortion II: Making the Revolution.* Boston: Beacon Press, 1973.

Laetz, Ernest C. "The Rise of the Patients Representative." *Hospital Financial Management* 23 (1969): 17-21.

Laing, R. D. *The Politics of Experience.* New York: Ballantine Books, 1976.

Lamerton, Richard. *Care of the Dying.* London: Priory Press, 1973.

Landau, Richard, ed. *Regulating New Drugs.* Chicago: University of Chicago Press, 1974.

LaPlace, Jean. *Preparing for Spiritual Direction.* Chicago: Franciscan Herald Press, 1975.

_____. *Experience in the Spirit.* Chicago: Franciscan Herald Press, 1976.

Lappé, Marc.
    1971.   "The Genetic Counselor: Responsible to Whom?" *Hastings Center Report* 1: 6-11.
    1972a. "Moral Obligations and the Fallacies of 'Genetic Control'." *Theological Studies* 33: 411-427.
    1972b. "Risk-Taking for the Unborn: Ethics of In-Vitro Fertilization." *Hastings Center Report* 2, no. 1: 1-3.
    1973.   "Allegiances of Human Geneticists: A Preliminary Typology." *Hastings Center Studies* 1: 63-78.
    1975.   "Human Uses of Molecular Genetics." *Federation Proceedings* 34: 67.

Lappé, Marc, and Brody, J. A. "Genetic Counseling: A Psychotherapeutic Approach to Autonomy in Decision Making." In *Birth Defects.* Original Articles Series, XII, no. 4, edited by Daniel Bergsma, Lissy Jarvik, and Michael Sperber. New York: Basic Books, 1977.

_____, and Morison, Robert S., eds. "Ethical and Scientific Issues Posed by Human Uses of Molecular Genetics." *Annals of New York Academy of Sciences* 265 (1976): 1-208.

_____, Roblin, Richard O., and Gustafson, James M. "Ethical, Social, and Legal Dimensions of Screening for Human Genetic Disease." In *Birth Defects.* Original Articles Series, x, edited by Daniel Bergsma. Miami, Fla.: Symposia Specialists, 1974. (a)

_____, and Steinfels, Peter. "Choosing the Sex of Our Children." *Hastings Center Report* 4 (1974): 1-4. (b)

Lapsley, James N. *Salvation and Health: The Interlocking Processes of Life.* Philadelphia: Westminster Press, 1972.

Lavely, John H. "Personalism." In *The Encyclopedia of Philosophy*, edited by Paul Edwards. New York: Macmillan and The Free Press, 1967. Vol. 6, pp. 107-110.

Leach, Gerald. *The Biocrats.* Baltimore: Penguin, 1972.

Lebacqz, Karen. "Commentary 'On Natural Death' " (Californian Natural Death Act). *Hastings Center Report* 7 (1977): 14.

_____, and Engelhardt, H. Tristram, Jr. "Suicide." In *Death, Dying and Euthanasia*, edited by Dennis J. Horan and David Mall. Washington, D.C.: University Publications of America, 1977, pp. 669-741.

Lebel, S.J., Robert Roger. "Genetic Decision Making: Parental Responsibility." *Catholic Medical Quarterly* 28 (1977): 167-179.

Leclercq, Jacques. "The Universal Declaration and the Gospel." *Lumen Vitae* 55 (1969): 49-62.

Lederberg, Joshua. "A Geneticist Looks at Contraception and Abortion." *Annals of Internal Medicine* 67 (1967): 26-27.

_____. "DNA Splicing: Will Fear Rob Us of Its Benefits?" *Prism*, November 1975, pp. 33-37.

Leeman, J. S. "Euthanasia: A Man's Right to Die." *Journal of Religion and Health* 7 (1968): 342-349.

Leff, David N. "Genes, Gender, and Genital Reversal." *Medical World News*, April 18, 1977, pp. 45-58.

Leijen, A. J. "De Legende van het King: Orde van het Spreken en de Abortus" (The Legend of the Child: The Order of Speaking and Abortion). *Tijdschrift Voor Theologie* 10 (1970): 259-273.

Lejeune, Jerome. "On the Nature of Man." Lecture at American Society of Human Genetics, October 2-4, 1969.

Leo XIII. *Rerum Novarum* (1891). In *Social Wellsprings: Eighteen Encyclicals of Social Reconstruction*, edited by Joseph Husslein. 2 vols. Milwaukee: Bruce, 1949. Vol. 1.

Leonard, R. C. "The Impact of Social Trends on the Professionalization of Patient Care." In *A Sociological Framework for Patient Care*, edited by Jeannette R. Folta and Edith S. Deck. New York: Wiley, 1966, pp. 71-82.

Lepp, Ignace. *The Depths of the Soul: A Christian Approach to Psychoanalysis.* Staten Island, N.Y.: Alba House, 1965.

————. *Health of Mind and Soul.* Staten Island, N.Y.: Alba House, 1966, pp. 171-181.

————. *Death and Its Mysteries.* New York: Macmillan, 1968.

Leslie, Robert C. *Jesus and Logotherapy.* Nashville, Tenn.: Abingdon, 1965.

Lester, Andrew D. "The Abortion Dilemma." *Review and Expositor* 68 (1971): 227-244.

Lester, Gene, and Lester, David. *Suicide: The Gamble with Death.* Englewood Cliffs, N.J.: Prentice-Hall, 1971.

Levin, Arthur. *Talk Back to Your Doctor: How to Demand (and Recognize) High Quality Health Care.* Garden City, N.Y.: Doubleday, 1975.

Levin, Max. "Sexual Fulfillment in the Couple Practicing Rhythm." *Child and Family* 8 (Winter 1969): 5-13.

Levine, Myra A., et al. Special supplement. *American Journal of Nursing* 77 (May 1977): 845-876.

Lewis, C. S. *The Problem of Pain.* New York: Macmillan, 1943.

Lewis, I. M. *Ecstatic Religion: An Anthropological Study of Spirit Possession and Shamanism.* Harmondsworth, Eng.: Pelican, 1971.

Lewis, John, ed. *Beyond Chance and Necessity: A Critical Inquiry into Prof. Jacques Monod's Chance and Necessity.* Atlantic Highlands, N.J.: Humanities Press, 1974.

Ligneuel, André. *Teilhard and Personalism.* New York: Paulist Press, 1968.

Lindesmith, Alfred, and Gagnon, John. "Anomie and Drug Addiction." In *Anomic and Deviant Behavior: Discussion and Critique*, edited by Marshall Clinard. New York: Free Press, 1964.

Ling, Richard. *The Rite of Anointing the Sick and Their Pastoral Care: A Pastoral, Theological and Liturgical Commentary.* New York Clergy Conference, Yonkers, N.Y., 1973.

Lippard, Vernon W. *A Half-Century of American Medical Education.* New York: Josiah Macy, Jr. Foundation, 1975.

Lobo, S.J., George. *Current Problems in Medical Ethics.* Allahabad, India: St. Paul Editions, 1974.

Lockerby, Florence K. "Representative Personalizes Care." *Hospitals* 47 (1973): 51-53.

London, Perry. *The Modes and Morals of Psychotherapy.* New York: Holt, 1964.

————. *Behavior Control.* New York: Harper & Row, 1969.

_____. "The Psychotherapy Boom: From the Long Couch for the Sick to the Push Button for the Bored." *Psychology Today*, June 1974, pp. 62-68.

Long, Edward Leroy. *A Survey of Christian Ethics.* New York: Harper & Row, 1963.

Longo, C.F.A., Brother Warren. *Toward a Theology of Health and Healing.* Doctoral dissertation, Mundelein College, Chicago, 1973.

Longwood, Merle. "Ethics and the Taking of Life." *Linacre Quarterly* 26 (1974): 64-76.

Lorber, John. "Selective Treatment of Myelomeningocele: To Treat or Not to Treat." *Pediatrics* 53 (1974): 307-308.

Lorentz, Konrad Z. *On Aggression.* New York: Harcourt Brace, 1966.

Louisell, David D., and Noonan, John T., Jr. "Constitutional Balance." In *The Morality of Abortion: Legal and Historical Perspectives*, edited by John T. Noonan, Jr. Cambridge, Mass.: Harvard University Press, 1970, pp. 220-262.

Lucas, George R., Jr. "Famine and Global Policy: An Interview with Joseph Fletcher." *Christian Century* (1975): 753-758. (a)

_____. "Triage." In *Inquiries Into Medical Ethics*, edited by Donald G. McCarthy. Houston, Texas: Institute of Religion and Human Development, 1975. Vol. 3: *Medicine and Society.* (b)

Luft, L. L., et al. "Effects of Peer Review on Outpatient Therapy." *American Journal of Psychiatry* 133 (1976): 891-895.

Lynch, H. T. "Subjective Perspective of a Family with Huntington's Chorea: Implications for Genetic Counseling." *Archives of General Psychiatry* 27 (1972): 67-72.

Lynn, Kenneth S., ed. *The Professions in America.* Boston: Houghton Mifflin, Daedalus, 1965.

Lyonnet, Stanislaus. *Sin, Redemption and Sacrifice.* Rome: Biblical Institute, 1970.

Lyons, Catherine. *Organ Transplants: The Moral Issues.* Philadelphia: Westminster Press, 1970.

Mabe, Alan R., ed. "New Technologies and Strategies for Social Control: Ethical and Practical Limits." Special number. *American Behavioral Scientist* 18 (May-June 1975).

McAuliffe, Robert M., and Bosen, Mary. *The Essentials of Chemical Dependency.* Minneapolis: Chemical Dependency Services, 1972.

McCabe, O.P., Herbert. *What Is Ethics All About?* Washington, D.C.: Corpus Books, 1969.

McCarthy, Donald G.
    1973.   (ed.) *Inquiries into Medical Ethics.* Houston, Tex.: Institute of Religion and Human Development. Vol. 1: *Beginnings of Personhood.*
    1975a. "The Use and Abuse of Cardiopulmonary Resuscitation." *Hospital Progress,* April, pp. 64-72.
    1975b. (ed.) *Inquiries into Medical Ethics.* St. Louis: Catholic Hospital Association. Vol. 2: *Responsible Stewardship of Human Life.*
    1977.   "Medication to Prevent Pregnancy after Rape." *Linacre Quarterly* 44: 210-222.

McCarthy, Donald G., and Moraczewski, O.P., Albert. *An Ethical Evaluation of Fetal Experimentation: An Interdisciplinary Study.* St. Louis: Pope John XXIII Medical-Moral Research and Education Center, 1976.

McClearn, G. E., and DeFries, J. C. *Introduction to Behavioral Genetics.* San Francisco: Freeman, 1973, pp. 272ff.

McClendon, James. *Biography as Theology*. Nashville, Tenn.: Abingdon, 1974.

McCormick, S.J., Richard A.
    1968.   "Past Church Teaching on Abortion." *Proceedings of Catholic Theological Society of America* 23: 133-137.
    1969.   "HV: A Round of Reactions." *Theological Studies* 30: 635-644.
    1971.   "Vasectomy and Sterilization." Reply to letter of L. L. deVeber, M.D. *Linacre Quarterly* 38: 7; 9-10.
    1972.   "The New Directives and Institutional Medico-Moral Responsibility." *Chicago Studies* 11 (Fall): 305-311.
    1973a.   *Ambiguity in Moral Choice*. 1973 Pere Marquette Theology Lecture. Milwaukee, Wis.: Marquette University.
    1973b.   "Notes on Moral Theology." *Theological Studies* 34: 53-102.
    1973c.   "The Silence Since HV." *America* 21: 30-33.
    1974a.   "To Save or Let Die: The Dilemma of Modern Medicine." *Journal of American Medical Association* 229: 172-176.
    1974b.   "Proxy Consent in the Experimentation Situation." *Perspectives in Biology and Medicine* 118 (Autumn): 2-20.
    1975.   "Notes on Moral Theology." *Theological Studies* 36: 77-129.
    1976a.   "The Preservation of Life." *Linacre Quarterly* 43: 94-100.
    1976b.   "Experimentation in Children: Sharing in Sociality." *Hastings Center Report* 6: 41-46.
    1976c.   "Notes on Moral Theology." *Theological Studies* 37: 70-119.
    1977.   "Notes on Moral Theology." *Theological Studies* 38: 57-114.
    1978.   "Notes on Moral Theology." *Theological Studies* 39: 76-138.

McDermott, S.J., Brian O. "Original Sin: Recent Developments." *Theological Studies* 38 (1977): 478-572.

McDonagh, Enda. *Invitation and Response: Essays in Christian Moral Theology*. Dublin: Gill and Macmillan, 1972.

————. *Gift and Call: Towards a Christian Theology of Morals*. St. Meinrad, Ind.: Abbey Press, 1975.

MacDonald, S. "The Meaning of Abortion." *American Ecclesiastical Review* 169 (1975): 219-236.

McEllhenney, John Galen. *Cutting the Monkey Rope*. Valley Forge, Pa.: Judson Press, 1973.

McFadden, O.S.A., Charles J. *Medical Ethics*. 6th ed. Philadelphia: Davis, 1967. On co-operation, pp. 357-372; truthfulness and professional secrecy, pp. 389-414.

————. *The Dignity of Life: Moral Values in a Changing Society*. Huntington, Ind.: Our Sunday Visitor, 1976, pp. 186ff.

McGinnis, J. Michael. "The Rising Costs of Hospital Care: Mandate for Academic Intro-spection." *Journal of Medical Education* 51 (1976): 602-604.

McGlothlin, William H., issue ed. "Chemical Comforts of Man: The Future." Special issue. *Journal of Social Issues* 27, no. 3 (1971).

McGrath, Patrick. *The Nature of Moral Judgment*. Notre Dame, Ind.: University of Notre Dame, 1969.

Machan, Tibor R. *The Pseudo-Science of B. F. Skinner*. New York: Arlington House, 1974.

McHugh, James T., ed. *Death, Dying and the Law*. Bishops' Committee for Pro-Life Activ-ities, NCCB. Hungtington, Ind.: Our Sunday Visitor, 1976.

Mack, Arien. *Death in American Experience*. New York: Schocken Books, 1973.

McKegney, F. P., and Lange, P. "The Decision to No Longer Live on Chronic Hemodialysis." *American Journal of Psychiatry* 128 (1971): 267-274.

McKusick, Victor A. "The Growth and Development of Human Genetics as a Clinical Discipline." *American Journal of Human Genetics* 27 (1975): 261-273.

McLemore, S. Dale, and Hill, Richard J. "Role Change and Socialization in Nursing." *Pacific Sociological Review* 8 (1965): 21-27.

MacMurray, John. *The Self as Agent.* London: Faber & Faber, 1957.

_____. *Persons in Relation.* London: Faber & Faber, 1961.

McNeill, S.J., John J. *The Church and the Homosexual.* Mission, Kans.: Sheed, Andrews & McMeel, 1976.

McNeill, John T. *A History of the Care of Souls.* New York: Harper & Row, 1951.

MacNutt, O.P., Francis. *Healing.* Notre Dame, Ind.: Ave Maria Press, 1974. Paperback edition. Bantam Books, 1977.

_____. *Healing Through Prayer.* New York: Bantam Books, 1977.

MacQuarrie, John. *Three Ethical Issues.* New York: Harper & Row, 1970, chap. 4, "Rethinking the Natural Law," pp. 82-110.

McQuillan, Florence L. "Patients Present Their Bill of Rights." *Nursing Home Administrator* 19 (January-February 1965): 53-54.

McReavy, L. L. "The Essential Doctrine of HV." *Clergy Review* 53 (1968): 861-867.

McSorley, Harry J. "Some Ecclesiological Reflections on *Humanae Vitae.*" *Bijdragen* 30 (1969): 3-8.

Maguire, Daniel.
    1972.   "The Freedom to Die." *Commonweal* 96 (August): 423-427.
    1974a. *Death by Choice.* Garden City, N.Y.: Doubleday.
    1974b. "Death, Legal and Illegal." *Atlantic Monthly*, February, pp. 72-85.
    1974c. "Ethical Meaning and the Problem of Death." *Anglican Theological Review* 56: 258-279.

Mainelli, Vincent P., ed. *Social Justice: The Catholic Position.* Washington, D.C.: Consortium Press, 1975.

Malone, Robert J. "Is There a Right to a Natural Death?" *New England Law Review* 9 (Winter 1974): 293-310.

Mangan, J. "An Historical Analysis of the Principle of Double Effect." *Theological Studies* 10 (1949): 40-61.

_____. "The Wonder of Myself: Ethical-Theological Aspects of Direct Abortion." *Theological Studies* 31 (1970): 125-148.

Mann, Kenneth W. *Deadline for Survival: A Survey of Moral Issues in Science and Medicine.* New York: Seabury Press, 1970.

Mannes, Marya. "A Woman's View of Abortion." In *The Case for Legalized Abortion*, edited by A. F. Guttmacher. Berkely, Calif.: Diabolo Press, 1967, pp. 59ff.

_____. *Last Rights.* New York: Morrow, 1974.

Manning, Francis V. "The Human Meaning of Sexual Pleasure and the Morality of Premarital Intercourse." *American Ecclesiastical Review* 165 (1971): 18-28.

_____. "The Human Meaning of Sexual Pleasure . . . ." *American Ecclesiastical Review* 166 (1972): 3-21; 302-319.

Marcuse, Herbert. *One-Dimensional Man: Studies in the Ideology of Advanced Industrial Society.* Boston: Beacon Press, 1964.

_____. *Eros and Civilization.* Boston: Beacon Press, 1974.

Maritain, Jacques. *Three Reformers: Luther, Descartes, Rousseau,* rev. ed. London: Sheed & Ward, 1929, pp. 54ff.

_____. *Creative Intuition in Art and Poetry.* Bollingen Series. New York: Pantheon, 1953.

Mark, Vernon H. "Brain Surgery in Aggressive Epileptics." *Hastings Center Report* 3 (1973): 1-5.

_____, and Ervin, Frank R. *Violence and the Brain.* New York: Harper & Row, 1970.

Markland, Colin. "Transexual Surgery." *Obstetrics & Gynecology Annual* 4 (1975): 309-330.

Marshall, Donald S., and Suggs, Robert C., eds. *Human Sexual Behavior: Variations Across the Ethnographic Spectrum.* New York: Basic Books, 1971.

Marshall, John, and Rowe, Beverly. "Psychologic Aspects of the Basal Body Temperature Method of Regulating Births." In *Proceedings of a Research Conference on Natural Family Planning,* edited by W. A. Uricchio. Washington, D.C.: Human Life Foundation, 1973.

Martelet, Gustave. *L'existence humaine et l'amour, pour mieux comprendre L'encyclicque Humanae Vitae.* Paris: Desclee, 1969.

Marx, Karl. *The Economic and Philosophic Manuscripts of 1844.* Introduction by D. J. Struik. Translated by Martin Milligan. New York: International Publishers, 1964, pp. 179ff.

Marx, O.S.B., Paul. *Death Without Dignity: Killing for Mercy.* Collegeville, Minn.: Liturgical Press, 1975.

Maslow, Abraham H. *Religion: Values and Peak Experiences.* Columbus, Ohio: Ohio State University Press, 1964.

_____. *Motivation and Personality.* 2nd ed. New York: Harper & Row, 1970.

Masters, William H., and Johnson, Virginia.
    1966. *Human Sexual Response.* Boston: Little, Brown.
    1970. *Human Sexual Inadequacy.* Boston: Little, Brown.
    1976. *The Pleasure Bond.* New York: Bantam Books. Paperback edition.
    1977. *Ethical Issues in Sex Research and Therapy.* Boston: Little, Brown.

May, Rollo. *Love and Will.* New York: Norton, 1969.

May, Rollo, et al., eds. *Existence: A New Dimension of Psychology.* New York: Basic Books, 1958.

May, William E.
    1975. *Becoming Human: An Invitation to Christian Ethics.* Dayton, Ohio: Pflaum Press.
    1976a. "Proxy Consent to Human Experimentation." *Linacre Quarterly* 43: 73-84.
    1976b. *The Nature and Meaning of Chastity.* Synthesis series. Chicago: Franciscan Herald Press.
    1977a. "Situationism and Contemporary Roman Catholic Moral Theology." Unpublished paper. Courtesy of author.
    1977b. "Sterlization: Catholic Teaching and Catholic Practice." *Homiletic and Pastoral Review* 77 (August-September): 9-22.

Mays, Lowell H. "The Right of Suicide." *Dialogue* 12 (1973): 289-292.

Mead, Margaret. "Rights to Life." *Christianity and Crisis* 32 (1973): 288-292.

Meadows, Donella H.; Meadows, Dennis L.; Randers, Jorgen; and Behrens, William W. *The Limits to Growth.* New York: Universe Books, 1972.

Mechanic, David. *Medical Sociology: A Selective View.* New York: Free Press, 1968.

_____. *Politics, Medicine, and Social Science.* New York: Wiley, 1974.

Medvedev, Roy A., and Medvedev, Zhores A. *A Question of Madness.* New York: Knopf, 1971.

Meerlo, J. "Change of Sex and Collaboration with the Psychosis." *American Journal of Psychiatry* 124 (1967): 263.

Mehl, Roger. *Catholic Ethics and Protestant Ethics.* Philadelphia: Westminster Press, 1971.

Meier, Anton Meinrad. *Das peccatum mortale ex toto genere suo.* Regensurg: Pustet, 1966.

Mendelsohn, Everett, Swazey, Judith P., and Taviss, Irene, eds. *Human Aspects of Biomedical Innovation.* Cambridge, Mass.: Harvard University Press, 1971.

Menninger, Karl.
    1938. *Man Against Himself.* New York: Harcourt Brace.
    1942. *Love Against Hate.* New York: Harcourt Brace.
    1958. *Theory of Psychoanalytic Technique.* New York: Basic Books. On transference, pp. 77-98.
    1963. *The Vital Balance.* New York: Viking, pp. 401-417.
    1968. *Crime of Punishment.* New York: Viking.
    1973. *Whatever Became of Sin?* New York: Hawthorn.

"Mental Illness: A Suspect Classification." *Yale Law Journal* 83 (1974): 1237-1271.

Merkelbach, O.P., Benedictus. *Summa Theologiae Moralis.* 10th ed. 3 vols. Burge, Belgium: Desclee de Brouwer, 1959. Vol. 1: On cooperation, nn. 487-492.

Merleau-Ponty, Maurice. *Phenomenology of Perception.* New York: Humanities Press, 1962.

Merton, Robert K. *Some Thoughts on the Professions in American Society* (address). Brown University, 1960.

_____, Reader, George G., and Kendall, Patricia. *The Student Physician.* Cambridge, Mass.: Harvard University Press, 1957.

Merton, Thomas. *Contemplative Prayer.* New York: Doubleday, 1971.

_____. *The Asian Journal of Thomas Merton.* New York: New Directions, 1973.

Messner, Johannes. *Social Ethics: Natural Law in the Western World.* St. Louis: B. Herder Book Co., 1965. On subsidiarity, pp. 45ff; common good, 207ff; corporatism (functionalism), pp. 436ff; unions, pp. 834ff; 903ff; codetermination, pp. 844ff; 908; 971.

Meyer, J. K. "Psychiatric Considerations in the Sexual Reassignment of Non-Intersex Individuals." *Clinics in Plastic Surgery* 1 (1974): 275-283.

Michaels, Robert. "Ethical Issues of Psychological and Psychotherapeutic Means of Behavior Conrol." *Hastings Center Report* 3 (1973): 11-13.

Middleton, Carl L., Jr. "Principles of Life-Death Decision Making." *Linacre Quarterly* 42 (1975): 268-278.

Middleton, E. "Ovulation Control with Stilbestrol." *Obstetrics & Gynecology* 26 (1965): 253-260.

Milgram, Stanley. *Obedience to Authority.* New York: Harper & Row, 1974.

Milhaven, John. "Epistemology of the Abortion Debate." *Theological Studies* 31 (1970): 106-124.

_____. "Christian Evaluations of Sexual Pleasure." *American Society of Christian Ethics: Selected Papers*, 1976. Missoula, Mont.: University of Montana Printing Department, 1976, pp. 63-74.

Mill, John Stuart. *Utilitarianism and Other Writings.* Cleveland: New American Library, Meridian Books, 1962. Originally published in 1863.

Mills, C. Wright. *The Power Elite.* New York: Oxford University Press, 1956.

Mills, Don Harper. "The Kansas Death Statute — Bold and Innovative." *New England Journal of Medicine* 285 (1971): 968-969.

Milunsky, Aubrey, ed. "The Prevention of Genetic Disease and Mental Retardation." Philadelphia: Saunders, 1975.

_____, and Annas, A. J. *Genetics and the Law.* New York: Plenum, 1975.

Mitchell, Kenneth R. *Hospital Chaplain.* Philadelphia: Westminster Press, 1966.

Mitford, Jessica. *The American Way of Death.* 2nd ed. New York: Simon & Schuster, 1975.

Modell, Walter. "The Will to Live." *New England Journal of Medicine* 290 (1974): 907-908.

Modesta, R.S.M., Sister Mary. "Patient Relations Representatives Bridge Communications Gap." *Hospital Progress*, September 1970, pp. 30-32.

Moltmann, Jurgen. *Theology of Hope.* New York: Harper & Row, 1967.

Money, J., and Gaskin, R. "Sex Reassignment." *International Journal of Psychiatry* 9 (1970-1971): 249-269.

Monod, Jacques. *Chance and Necessity: An Essay on the Natural Philosophy of Modern Biology.* New York: Knopf, 1971.

Montange, Charles H. "Informed Consent and the Dying Patient." *Yale Law Journal* 83 (1974): 1632-1664.

Moody, Howard. "Abortion: Woman's Right and Legal Problem." *Christianity and Crisis* 31 (1971): 27-32.

Moody, Raymond A., Jr. *Life After Life.* New York: Bantam Books, 1975.

Moore, Charles A. *The Status of the Individual in East and West.* Honolulu: University of Hawaii Press, 1967.

Moore, F. D. "Medical Responsibility for the Prolongation of Life." *Journal of American Medical Association* 206 (1968): 384-386.

Moore, G. E. *Principia Ethica.* London: Cambridge University Press, 1903.

Moore, Wilbert E., and Rosenblum, Gerald W. *The Professions: Roles and Rules.* New York: Russell Sage Foundation, 1970, pp. 51-65; 174-186.

Moraczewski, O.P., Albert S. "Theological Pharmacology: A Study of Drugs and Values." *Linacre Quarterly* 40 (1973): 205-212.

Moreno, O.P., Antonio. *Jung, Gods and Modern Man.* Notre Dame, Ind.: University of Notre Dame Press, 1970.

Morison, Robert S., and Kass, Leon R. "Death: Process or Event?" *Science* 173 (1971): 694-702.

Morris, Desmond. *The Naked Ape.* New York: McGraw-Hill, 1967.

Morris, J. M. "Compounds Interfering with Ovum Implantation." *American Journal of Obstetrics & Gynecology* 96 (1966): 804-810.

Morrow, John F. "The Prospects for Gene Therapy in Humans." In *Ethical and Scientific Issues Posed by Human Uses of Molecular Genetics,* edited by Marc Lappé and Robert S. Morison. New York: New York Academy of Sciences, 1976.

Moss, Peter. *Medicine and Morality.* London: Harrap, 1974.

Motulsky, Arno G., et al. *Genetic Counseling.* New York: MSS Information Corp., 1974.

Mounier, Emmanuel. *Personalism.* London: Routledge, 1952.

Muller, Hubert J. *Uses of the Future.* Bloomington, Ind.: Indiana University Press, 1974.

Mulligan, J. J. "Confessor, Penitent and *Humanae Vitae.*" *Homiletic and Pastoral Review* 69 (1969): 507-515.

Munter, Suessmann. In *Encyclopaedia Judaica.* New York: Macmillan, 1971. Vol. 11: "Medicine," col. 1177-1195.

Murphy, Jeffree G. "Total Institutions and the Possibility of Consent to Organic Therapies." *Human Rights* 5 (Fall 1975): 25-45.

Murray, Robert F., Jr. "Problems Behind the Promise: Ethical Issues in Mass Genetic Screening." *Hastings Center Report* 2 (1972): 10-13.

_____, and Soble, Alan. "Case Studies in Bioethics: Drug Treatment or Drug Addiction?" *Hastings Center Report* 4 (1974): 11-12.

Mushkin, Selma J. "Directions for Health Services Research." In *Consumers Incentives and Health Care,* edited by Selma J. Muskin. New York: Milbank Memorial Fund, 1974, pp. 385-415.

Mussallem, H. K. "The Changing Role of the Nurse." *American Journal of Nursing* 69 (1969): 514-517.

Naegle, Kaspar D. *Health and Healing.* San Francisco: Jossey-Bass, 1970, pp. 8ff.

Nardone, Roland M. "The Nexus of Biology and the Abortion Issue." *Jurist* 33 (Spring 1973): 153-161.

Nasr, Seyyed Hassein. *The Encounter of Man and Nature: The Spiritual Crisis of Modern Man.* London: G. Allen, 1968.

National Conference of Catholic Bishops.
    1968. *Human Life in Our Day: A Pastoral Letter* (15 November) Washington, D.C.: United States Catholic Conference.
    1973. *Pastoral Guidelines for Catholic Hospitals and Health Care Personnel.* Washington, D.C.: United States Catholic Conference.
    1974. *Documentation on the Right to Life and Abortion.* Washington, D.C.: United States Catholic Conference.
    1976a. *To Live in Christ Jesus: A Pastoral Reflection on the Moral Life.* Washington, D.C.: United States Catholic Conference.
    1976b. *Respect Life.* Respect Life Committee. Washington, D.C.: United States Catholic Conference.

Navone, S.J., John J. *Personal Witness: A Biblical Spirituality.* New York: Sheed & Ward, 1967.

Neale, Robert E. *The Art of Dying.* New York: Harper & Row, 1973.

Nelson, C. Ellis, ed. *Conscience: Theological and Psychological Perspectives.* New York: Newman Press, 1964.

Nelson, J. Robert. "What Does Theology Say about Abortion." *Christian Century* 90 (1973): 124-128.

Nelson, James B. *Human Medicine: Ethical Perspectives on New Medical Issues.* Minneapolis: Augsburg, 1974.

Neumann, Erich. *The Origins and History of Consciousness.* Bollinger Series. New York: Pantheon, 1964, pp. 318-320.

Neuner, S.J., J., and Dupuis, S.J., J. *The Christian Faith in the Doctrinal Documents of the Catholic Church.* Rev. ed. Westminster, Md.: Christian Classics, 1975, pp. 550-618.

Neville, Robert C. "Where Do the Poets Fit In?" Review of *Beyond Freedom and Dignity* by B. F. Skinner. *Hastings Center Report* 1 (1971): 6-8.

————. "Ethical and Philosophical Issues of Behavior Control." Paper presented at American Association for Advancement of Science Meeting, 1973.

————, and Steinfels, Peter, commentators. "Case Studies in Bioethics: Blood Money: Should a Rich Nation Buy Plasma from the Poor?" *Hastings Center Report* 2 (1972): 8-10.

"New Technologies and Strategies for Social Control: Ethical and Practical Limits." Special issue. *American Behavioral Scientist* 18 (May-June 1975).

Niebuhr, H. Richard. *The Responsible Self.* New York: Harper & Row, 1963.

Nielson, Kai. *Ethics Without God.* Buffalo: Prometheus Books, 1973.

Nogar, O.P., Raymond J. *The Wisdom of Evolution.* New York: Doubleday, 1963, pp. 76ff.

Nolan, O.S.A., Martin. "The Principle of Totality in Moral Theology." In *Absolutes in Moral Theology*, edited by Charles E. Curran. Washington, D.C.: Corpus Books, 1968.

Nolen, William A. *Surgeon Under the Knife.* New York: Coward-McGann, 1976.

Nolin, O.S.B., Kieran. "Attitudes of Medical Staff to Sacramental Ministry in Public Hospitals." Unpublished paper read at Institute of Religious and Human Development, Texas Medical Center, Houston, 1972.

Noonan, John T., Jr.
 1965. *Contraception: A History of Its Treatment by the Catholic Theologians and Canonists.* New York: Harvard University Press, Belknap Press. On zero population growth, pp. 18-25; on Church's middle course in sex ethics, pp. 56-106.
 1966. "Authority, Usury and Contraception." *Dublin Review* 509: 201-229.
 1967. "Abortion and the Catholic Church: A Summary History." *Natural Law Forum* 12: 85-131.
 1970a. "An Almost Absolute Value in History." In *The Morality of Abortion: Legal and Historical Perspectives*, edited by John T. Noonan, Jr. Cambridge, Mass.: Harvard University Press, pp. 1-59.
 1970b. (ed.) *The Morality of Abortion: Legal and Historical Perspectives.* Cambridge, Mass.: Harvard University Press.
 1973. "Responding to Persons: Methods of Moral Argument in Debate Over Abortion." *Theological Digest* 21: 291-307.

Nouwen, Henri J.
 1970. *Intimacy: Pastoral Psychological Essays.* Notre Dame, Ind.: Fides Publishing.

1971. *Creative Ministry.* New York: Doubleday.
1972. *The Wounded Healer: Ministry in Contemporary Society.* New York: Doubleday.
1973. *Reaching Out: The Three Movements of Spiritual Life.* New York: Doubleday.

Novak, David. *Suicide and Morality.* New York: Scholars Press, 1971.

Noyes, R., Jr. "Seneca on Death." *Journal of Religion and Health* 12 (1973): 223-240.

Nozick, Robert. *Anarchy, State and Utopia.* New York: Basic Books, 1974.

Oates, Wayne E. *The Bible in Pastoral Care.* Philadelphia: Westminster Press, 1953.

_____. *Protestant Pastoral Counseling.* Philadelphia: Westminster Press, 1962.

_____. *Pastoral Counseling.* Philadelphia: Westminster Press, 1974.

O'Callaghan, D. F. "*Humanae Vitae* in Perspective: Survey of Recent French Writing." *Irish Theological Quarterly* 37 (1970): 309-321.

Oden, Thomas C. *Radical Obedience.* Philadelphia: Westminster Press, 1964.

_____. *Should Treatment be Terminated? Moral Guidelines for Christian Families and Pastors.* New York: Harper & Row, 1976.

O'Donnell, S.J., Thomas J. *Morals in Medicine.* Washington, D.C.: Newman Press, 1957.

_____. "The Directives: A Crisis of Faith." *Linacre Quarterly* 39 (1972): 139-146.

_____. *Medicine and Christian Morality.* Staten Island, N.Y.: Alba House, 1976.

O'Flaherty, S.J., V.M. *How to Cure Scruples.* Milwaukee: Bruce, 1966.

Oken, D. "What to Tell Cancer Patients: A Study of Medical Attitudes." *Journal of American Medical Association* 175 (1961): 1120-1128.

Olesen, Virginia, ed. *Women and Their Health: Research Implications for a New Era.* Proceedings of Conference at University of California, San Francisco, August 1-2, 1975. Washington, D.C.: U.S. Department of Health, Education, and Welfare, 1976.

Olin, Grace B., and Olin, Harry S. "Informed Consent in Voluntary Hospital Admissions." *American Journal of Psychiatry* 132 (1975): 938-941.

O'Meara, O.P., Thomas F. "Liturgy and Eschatological Life Within the Hospital." *Hospital Progress,* October 1975, pp. 68-92.

O'Neill, O.P., Colman E. *Meeting Christ in the Sacraments.* Staten Island, N.Y.: Alba House, 1964.

Oraison, Marc. *Love, Sin and Suffering.* New York: Macmillan, 1964.

Ornstein, Robert E. *The Psychology of Consciousness.* San Francisco: Freeman, 1972.

O'Rourke, O.P., Kevin D.
1974a. "Is Your Health Facility Catholic?" *Hospital Progress,* April, pp. 40-44.
1974b. "The Christian Affirmation of Life." *Hospital Progress,* July, pp. 65-72.
1975. "Fetal Experimentation: An Evaluation of the New Federal Norms." *Hospital Progress,* September, pp. 60-69.
1976. "An Analysis of the Church's Teaching on Sterilization." *Hospital Progress,* May, pp. 68-75.

Osmond, Humphry. "The Medical Model of Psychiatry: Love It or Leave It." *Medical Annals of District of Columbia* 41 (1972): 171-175.

Osmundsen, John A. "We Are All Mutants — Preventive Genetic Medicine: A Growing Clinical Field Troubled by a Confusion of Ethicists." *Medical Dimensions* 2 (1973): 5-7; 26-28.

Outka, Gene. *Norm and Context in Christian Ethics.* New York: Scribners, 1968.

————. *Agape: An Ethical Analysis.* New Haven: Yale University Press, 1972.

Outler, Albert C. "The Beginnings of Personhood: Theological Considerations." *Perkins Journal of Theology* 27 (Fall 1973): 28-34.

Owen, D. R. G. *Body and Soul: A Study of the Christian View of Man.* Philadelphia: Westminster Press, 1956.

Packard, Vance. *The People Shapers.* Boston: Little, Brown, 1977.

Pacoe, Larry V.; Naar, Roy; Guyetl, I. P. R.; and Wells, Richard. "Training Medical Students in Interpersonal Relationship Skill." *Journal of Medical Education* 51 (1976): 743-750.

Palazzini, Pietro, and Canals, Salvador. *Sin: Its Reality and Nature: A Historical Survey.* New York: Scepter, 1964.

Palmer, Paul. "Who Can Anoint the Sick?" *Worship* 48 (1974): 81-92.

Pankratz, Lorden, and Pankratz, Deanna. "Determinants in Choosing a Nursing Career." *Nursing Research* 16 (Spring 1967): 169-172.

————. "Nursing Autonomy and Patient's Rights: Development of a Nursing Attitude Scale." *Journal of Health and Social Behavior* 15 (1974): 211-215.

Paris Statement of 1966. In *A Catholic/Humanist Dialogue*, edited by Paul Kurtz and Albert Dondeyne. Buffalo: Prometheus Books, 1972, pp. 3ff.

Parnes, Sidney J., and Harding, Harold F., eds. *A Source Book for Creative Thinking.* New York: Scribner, 1962.

Parry, Hugh J., et al. "National Patterns of Psychotherapeutic Drug Use." *Archives of General Psychiatry* 28 (1973): 769-783.

Parsons, Talcott. *The Social System.* Glencoe, Ill.: Free Press, 1951.

Patterson, C. H. *Theories of Counseling and Psychotherapy*, 2nd ed. New York: Harper & Row, 1973, pp. 521-540.

Paul VI.
    1967.   March 26 *The Development of Peoples (Populorum Progressio).* Washington, D.C.: United States Catholic Conference.
    1968a. *Humanae Vitae: Encyclical Letter on the Regulation of Birth.* Washington, D.C.: United States Catholic Conference.
    1968b. July 31 Allocution. "La préparation, let but, et l'esprit de l'encyclique." *Documentation Catholique* 65 (1 September): 1458-1461.
    1971a. May 14 *A Call to Action: Apostolic Letter on Eightieth Anniversary of "Rerum Novarum."* Washington, D.C.: United States Catholic Conference.
    1971b. November 30 Issued by Synod of Bishops. *Justice in the World. The Pope Speaks* 16: 377-384.
    1972. *Apostolic Constitution on the Sacrament of Annointing the Sick.* Washington, D.C.: United States Catholic Conference.
    1973. December 10 Message to President of United Nations General. *The Pope Speaks* 18 (1974): 304-307.

Paul, J. "State Eugenic Sterilization: A Brief Overview." In *Eugenic Sterilization*, edited by Jonas Robitscher. Springfield, Ill.: Charles C Thomas, 1973, pp. 25-40.

Pearn, J. H. "Patients' Subjective Interpretation of Risks Offered in Genetic Counseling." *Journal of Medical Genetics* 10 (1973): 129-134.

Peele, Stanton, with Brodsky, Archie. *Love and Addiction.* New York: Taplinger, 1975.

Pekkanen, John. *The American Connection: Profiteering and Politicking in the "Ethical" Drug Industry.* Chicago: Follett, 1973.

Penelhuam, Terence. "Personal Identity." In *The Encyclopedia of Philosophy*, edited by Paul Edwards. New York: Macmillan, The Free Press, 1967. Vol. 6, pp. 95-106.

Perlin, Seymour. *A Handbook for the Study of Suicide.* New York: Oxford University Press, 1975.

Perrucci, Robert. *Circle of Madness: On Being Insane and Institutionalized in America.* Englewood Cliffs, N.J.: Spectrum Books, 1974.

Peterkin, E. K. *Care for the Dying.* Collegeville, Minn.: Liturgical Press, 1975.

Phillips, D. Z., and Mounce, H. O. "On Morality's Having a Point." *Philosophy* 40 (1965): 308-319.

Phipps, William E. *Was Jesus Married?* New York: Harper & Row, 1970.

_____. "Masturbation: Vice or Virtue?" *Journal of Religion and Health* 16 (1977): 183-196.

"Physical Manipulation of the Brain." Special supplement. *Hastings Center Report*, May 1973.

Piaget, Jean. *The Moral Judgement of the Child.* New York: The Free Press, 1965 [1929].

Pieper, Josef.
    1958. *Happiness and Contemplation.* New York: Pantheon.
    1964. *Leisure, the Basis of Culture.* New York: New American Library.
    1966. *Four Cardinal Virtues.* Notre Dame, Ind.: University of Notre Dame Press, pp. 3-42.
    1969. *Death and Immortality.* New York: Herder & Herder.
    1974. *About Love.* Chicago: Franciscan Herald Press.

Pierce, V. *Swan Point Cemetery.* 10 Rhode Island 227 [1872].

Pines, Maya. *The Brain Changers: Scientists and the New Mind Control.* New York: Harcourt Brace Jovanovich, 1973.

Pittenger, Norman. "Suffering and Love." *Expositor's Times* 85 (1973): 19-22.

Note: Unless otherwise noted, the following references to works of Pius XI and Pius XII are to *The Human Body: Papal Teachings* (Boston: St. Paul Editions, 1960.) (HB).

Pius XI
    1930. December 31. *Casti Connubi.* HB nn. 4-12.

Pius XII
    1944. November 12. "Allocution to the Italian Medical-Biological Union of St. Luke." HB nn. 44-67.
    1945. May 20. "Allocution to Italian Sporting Associations." HB nn. 78-94.
    1949. September 29. "Allocution to the delegates at the Fourth International Congress of Catholic Doctors." HB nn. 165-179.
    1950. August 12. *Humani Generis.* Encyclical letter. Washington, D.C.: United States Catholic Conference, 1950.
    1951. October 29. "Allocution to Italian Midwives." HB nn. 243-315.
    1952. September 14. "Allocution to the First International Congress of Histopathology." HB nn. 349-381.

1956a. May 14. "Allocution to a Group of Eye Specialists." HB nn. 637-649.

1956b. May 19. "Allocution to the Second World Congress on Fertility and Sterility." HB nn. 650-666.

1957. November 24. "Prolongation of Life: Allocution to an International Congress of Anesthesiologists." *The Pope Speaks* 4: 393-398.

1962. Pius XII and Technology. Compiled by Leo J. Hagerty. Milwaukee: Bruce.

Platt, Michael. "Commentary: On Asking to Die." *Hastings Center Report* 5 (1975): 9-12.

Plé, O.P., Albert. "Alert au Traducianisme: Apropos d l'avortement." *La Vie Spirituelle.* (Supplement) 24 (1971): 70.

Poe, William D. "Do We Need Restraint in Medicine?" *Christian Century* 90 (1973): 914-918.

Polyani, Michael. *Personal Knowledge: Toward a Post-Critical Philosophy.* New York: Harper & Row, Torchbooks, 1964.

Pontifical Commission on Peace and Justice. "Church and Human Rights." *Osservatore Romano* (Eng. ed.) 6 (1973); 6-10 (23 Oct.); 8-9 (30 Oct.); 6-8 (6 Nov.); 9-10 (13 Nov.).

Pontoppidun, Henning, et al. "Optimum Care for Hopelessly Ill Patients." *New England Journal of Medicine* 295 (1976): 362-364.

Popoff, David. In consultation with G. Ray Funkhouser. "What Are Your Feelings About Death and Dying?" Part three of a three-part survey: euthanasia, suicide, and allowing to die. *Nursing* 75 (1975): 40-50.

Popper, Karl. *The Open Society and Its Enemies.* London: Routledge, 1966.

"Population." Special issue. *Theological Studies* 35 (March 1974).

Potter, Van Rennselaer. *Bioethics: Bridge to the Future.* Englewood Cliffs, N.J.: Prentice-Hall, 1971.

Potts, Timothy C. "The Arguments of *Humanae Vitae.*" *Month* 41 (1969): 144-156.

Powell, Francis D. *Theory of Coping Systems: Change in Supportive Health Organizations.* Cambridge, Mass.: Schenkman, 1975.

Powledge, Tabitha M. "New Trends in Genetic Legislation." *Hastings Center Report* 12 (1973): 6-7.

————. "Dangerous Research and Public Obligation." *New York Times*, August 24, 1974.

————. "The Genetic Engineers Still Await Guidelines." *New York Times*, February 15, 1976.

Premack, David. "Linguistic Competence of Apes." In *Origins and Evolution of Language and Speech*, edited by Stevan R. Harnad, H. D. Steklis, and J. Lancaster. *Annals New York Academy of Science* 280 (1976): 544-611.

Presser, Harriet B. "Perfect Fertility Control: Consequences for Women and the Family." In *Toward the End of Growth: Population in America*, edited by C. F. Westoff, et al. Englewood Cliffs, N.J.: Prentice-Hall, 1973.

Pretzel, P. W. "Philosophical and Ethical Considerations of Suicide Prevention." *Bulletin of Suicidology* 4 (1968): 30-38.

Progoff, Ira. *The Symbolic and the Real.* New York: Julian Press, 1963.

Prucha, Milan. "Marxism and the Existential Problems of Man." In *Socialist Humanism: An International Symposium*, edited by Erich Fromm. Garden City, N.Y.: Doubleday, 1965, pp. 138-147.

Prümmer, O.P., Dominicüs M. *Manuale Theologiae Moralis.* 14th ed. 3 vols. Barcelona: Herder, 1960.

Prussin, Jeffrey A. "NHI Prospects: Quick Enactment Unlikely Despite Carter Election." *Hospital Progress,* February 1977, pp. 62-65.

Pruyseur, Paul W. *The Minister as Diagnostician: Personal Problems in Pastoral Perspective.* Philadelphia: Westminster Press, 1976.

Pugh, George Edgin. *The Biological Origin of Human Values.* New York: Basic Books, 1977.

Purtilo, Ruth. *The Allied Health Professional and the Patient: Techniques of Effective Interaction.* Philadelphia: Saunders, 1973.

_____. *Essays for Professional Helpers: Some Psycho-Social and Ethical Considerations.* Thorofare, N.J.: Charles B. Slack, 1975.

Quay, Paul. "Morality by Calculation of Values." *Theology Digest* 23 (1975): 347-364.

Quesnell, John Q. *The Message of Christ and the Counselor.* Synthesis Series. Chicago: Franciscan Herald Press, 1976.

Rabkin, Mitchell T., Gillerman, G., and Rice, N. R. "Orders: Not Resuscitate." *New England Journal of Medicine* 295 (1976): 364-366.

Rachel, James. "Active and Passive Euthanasia." *New England Journal of Medicine* 292 (1975): 78-80.

Rahmeier, Paul W. "Abortion and the Reverence for Life." *Christian Century* 88 (1971): 556-560.

Rahner, S.J., Karl.
1961-
1975. *Theological Investigations.* 12 vols. New York: Seabury Press. Vol. 2: "On the Question of a Formal Existential Ethics," pp. 217-234.
1963. *The Church and the Sacraments.* In *Questiones Disputatae,* no. 9. New York: Herder & Herder.
1965. *On the Theology of Death.* New York: Herder & Herder.
1968a. "On the Encyclical *Humanae Vitae.*" English translation in *National Catholic Reporter,* September 18.
1968b. *Theology of Pastoral Action.* Westminster, Md.: Christian Classics.

Rahner, Karl, et al. "Resurrection." In *Sacramentum Mundi.* New York: Herder & Herder, 1968. Vol. 5, pp. 323-342.

Ramsey, Ian T. "Biology and Personality." In *Biology and Personality,* edited by Ian T. Ramsey. Oxford: Blackwell, 1965, pp. 174-206.

Ramsey, Paul.
1962. *Christian Ethics.* Englewood Cliffs, N.J.: Prentice-Hall.
1965. *Deeds and Rules in Christian Ethics.* Edinburgh: Oliver & Boyd, pp. 144ff.
1967. "The Sanctity of Life." *Dublin Review* 241 (Spring): 3-21.
1968. "On Taking Sexual Responsibility Seriously Enough." In *Social Ethics: Issues in Ethics and Society,* edited by Gibson Winter. New York: Harper & Row, pp. 44-54. Comments on Quaker View of Sex, pp. 24-43.
1970a. *Fabricated Man: The Ethics of Genetic Control.* New Haven: Yale University Press.
1970b. *The Patient as Person.* New Haven: Yale University Press.
1972. "Genetic Therapy: A Theologian's Response." In *The New Genetics and the Future of Man,* edited by Michael P. Hamilton. Grand Rapids, Mich.: Eerdmans.

1973a. "Abortion: A Review Article." *Thomist* 37: 174-226.

1973b. "Screening: An Ethicist's View." In *Ethical Issues in Human Genetics*, edited by Bruce Hilton. New York: Plenum.

1975. *The Ethics of Fetal Research.* New Haven: Yale University Press.

1976. "The Enforcement of Morals: Non-Therapeutic Research on Children." *Hastings Center Report* 6: 21-30.

1977. *Ethics at the Edges of Life.* New Haven: Yale University Press.

Rand, Ayn. *The Virtue of Selfishness: A New Concept of Egoism.* New York: New American Library, Signet Books, 1964.

Rapaport, Felix T., ed. *A Second Look at Life.* New York: Grune & Stratton, 1973.

_____, et al. "Recent Advances in Clinical and Experimental Transplantation." *Journal of American Medical Association* 237 (1977): 2835-2840.

Ratner, Herbert. "Periodic Abstinence: An Editorial." *Child and Family* 7 (Fall 1968): 290-295.

Ravich, Ruth, and Rehr, Helen. "Ombudsman Program Provides Feedback." *Hospitals* 48 (1974): 62-67.

Rawls, John. *A Theory of Justice.* Cambridge, Mass.: Harvard University Press, 1971.

Read, David H. C. "Dying Patient's Concept of God." In *Death and Ministry: Pastoral Care of the Dying and Bereaved*, edited by Donald J. Bane. New York: Seabury, 1975, pp. 59-63.

Reader, W. J. *Professional Men.* New York: Basic Books, 1966, p. 2.

Reed, George. "Congress and State Legislatures Pass Conscience Clause Legislation." *Hospital Progress*, July 1973, pp. 18-20.

Reich, Warren T., and Smith, Harmon, commentators. "Case Studies in Bioethics: On the Birth of a Severely Handicapped Infant." *Hastings Center Report* 3 (1973): 10-12.

Reid, Keith. *Nature's Network: The Story of Ecology.* Garden City, N.Y.: Natural History Press, 1970.

Reidlich, Fritz, and Mollica, Richard F. "Overview: Ethical Issues in Contemporary Psychiatry." *American Journal of Psychiatry* 133 (1976): 125-135.

Reiser, Stanley J., Dyck, Arthur J., and Curran, William J. *Ethics in Medicine: Historical Perspectives and Contemporary Problems.* Cambridge, Mass.: M.I.T. Press, 1977.

Reisman, L. E., and Matheny, A. P., Jr. *Genetics and Counseling in Medical Practice.* St. Louis: Mosby, 1969.

Rescher, Nicholas. *Introduction to Value Theory.* Englewood Cliffs, N.J.: Prentice-Hall, 1969, pp. 1-19.

Resnick, H. L. P., ed. *Suicidal Behaviors.* Boston: Little, Brown, 1968.

Restak, Richard M. *Pre-Meditated Man: Bioethics and the Control of Future Human Life.* New York: Viking, 1975.

Richardson, Cyril C. "A Christian Approach to Ecology." *Religion in Life* 41 (Winter 1972): 462-479.

Richardson, Herbert W. *Nun, Witch, Playmate.* New York: Harper & Row, 1971.

Rieff, Philip. *The Triumph of the Therapeutic: Uses of Faith After Freud.* New York: Harper & Row, Torchbooks, 1968.

Riese, Walter. *The Conception of Disease: Its History, Its Versions, Its Nature.* New York: Philosophical Library, 1953.

Rigali, S.J., Norbert J. "On Christian Ethics." *Chicago Studies* 10 (1971): 227-247.

"The Right of a Patient to Refuse Blood Transfusions: A Dilemma of Conscience and Law for Patient and Hospital." *University of San Fernando Valley Law Review* 3 (1974): 91-104.

Rite of Baptism for Children. Washington, D.C.: United States Catholic Conference, 1971. On importance of infant baptism, n. 8.

Rite of Christian Initiation of Adults (provisional text). Washington, D.C.: United States Catholic Conference, 1974.

Rite of Penance (study edition). Washington, D.C.: United States Catholic Conference, 1975.

Rizzo, Robert, and Yonder, Paul. "Definition and Criteria of Clinical Death." *Linacre Quarterly* 40 (1973): 223-233.

Robertson, John A. "Involuntary Euthanasia of Defective Newborns: A Legal Analysis." *Stanford Law Review* 27 (1975): 213-267.

Robinson, Norman H. G. *The Groundwork of Christian Ethics.* Grand Rapids, Mich.: Eerdmans, 1972.

Robitscher, Jonas.
    1966. *Pursuit of Agreement: Psychiatry and the Law.* Philadelphia: Lippincott.
    1972a. "Courts, State Hospitals and the Right to Treatment." *American Journal of Psychiatry* 129: 298-304.
    1972b. "The Right to Die." *Hastings Center Report* 2: 11-14.
    1972c. "The Right to Psychiatric Treatment: A Social-Legal Approach to the Plight of the State Hospital Patient." *Villanova Law Review* 18: 11-36.
    1975. "The Impact of New Legal Standards on Psychiatry or Who are David Bazelon and Thomas Szasz and Why are they Saying Such Terrible Things About Us? Or Authoritarianism Versus Nihilism in Legal Psychiatry." *Journal of Psychiatry and Law* 37: 11-36.

Rogers, Carl R. *Client-Centered Therapy.* Boston: Houghton Mifflin, 1951.

Rogers, Cornish. "Biomedics, Psychosurgery and Laissez-Faire." *Christian Century* 90 (1973): 1076-1078.

Rokeach, Milton. *The Open and Closed Mind.* New York: Basic Books, 1962.

_____. *The Nature of Human Values.* New York: The Free Press, 1973.

Rondet, Henri. *Original Sin: The Patristic and Theological Background.* Staten Island, N.Y.: Alba House, 1972.

Rordorf, Willy. *Sunday: The History of the Day of Rest and Worship in the Earliest Centuries of the Christian Church.* Philadelphia: Westminster Press, 1968.

Rorvik, David. *Brave New Baby: Promise and Peril of Biological Revolution.* Garden City, N.Y.: Doubleday, 1969.

Rose, Steven. *The Conscious Brain.* New York: Knopf, 1973.

Rosengren, William R., and Lefton, Mark. *Hospitals and Patients.* New York: Atherton Press, 1969.

Rosenham, D. L. "On Being Sane in Insane Places." *Science* 179 (1973): 250-258.

Rosenthal, David. "Changes in Moral Values Following Psychotherapy." *Journal of Consulting Psychology* 19 (1955): 431-436.

_____. *Genetics of Psychopathology.* New York: McGraw-Hill, 1971.

Rosner, Fred. *Modern Medicine and Jewish Law.* New York: Yeshiva University Press, 1972.

Rosoff, S. D., et al. "The EEG in Establishing Brain Death: A 10-Year Report with Criteria and Legal Safeguards in the 50 States." *Electroencephalography and Clinical Neurophysiology* 24 (1968): 283-284.

Ross, W. D. *Foundations of Ethics.* New York: Oxford University Press, 1939.

_____. *The Right and the Good.* New York: Oxford University Press, 1965.

Roszak, Betty, and Roszak, Theodore. *Masculine/Feminine: Readings in Sexual Mythology and the Liberation of Women.* New York: Harper & Row, 1964.

Roszak, Theodore. *The Making of a Counterculture: Reflections on the Technocratic Society and Its Youthful Opponents.* Garden City, N.Y.: Doubleday, 1969.

_____. *Where the Wasteland Ends: Politics and Transcendance in Postindustrial Society.* Garden City, N.Y.: Doubleday, 1972, pp. 3-27.

Rothman, David J. *The Discovery of the Asylum.* Boston: Little, Brown, 1971.

_____. "Behavior Modification in Total Institutions." *Hastings Center Report* 5 (1975): 17-24.

Rouse, Lara L., Hood, Wanda, and Allen, Louis T. "Patient Council." *American Journal of Public Health* 61 (1971): 2383-2386.

Rousseau, Jeans-Jacques. *Discourse Upon the Origin and Foundations of Inequality Among Mankind in Social Contract and Discourses.* [1753]. New York: Dutton, 1976.

Roy, Rustum, and Bube, Richard H. "Is There a Christian Basis for a Sexual Revolution?" *Journal of American Scientific Affiliation* 26 (1974): 70-81.

Royce, James E. *Man and His Nature: A Philosophical Psychology.* New York: McGraw-Hill, 1961.

Rubin, Isadore. "What Areas of Agreement on Sexual Ethics Are There for the Religionist and the Humanist?" *Pastoral Psychology* 21 (1970): 10-18.

Rudel, Harry, and Kincl, Fred. "The Biology of Anti-Fertility Steroids." *Acta Endocrinologica* 51 (1966): 21-25.

Rudin, Josef. "A Catholic View of Conscience." In *Conscience: Theological and Psychological Perspectives*, edited by C. Ellis Nelson. Westminster, Md.: Newman Press, 1964.

_____. *Psychotherapy and Religion.* Notre Dame, Ind.: University of Notre Dame Press, 1968, 57-90; 173-202.

Rudkovsky, David. *The Rights of Prisoners.* New York: Avon Books, 1973.

Ruesch, Jurgen, and Bateson, Gregory. *Communication: The Social Matrix of Psychiatry.* New York: Norton, 1951, pp. 50-93.

Ruff, S.J., Wilfried. "Das embryonale Werder des Individuums." *Stimmen der Zeit* 181 (1968): 107-119.

_____. "Individualitat und Personalitat in embryonalen Werden." *Theologie und Philosophie* 45 (1970): 24-59.

Rugg, Harold. *Imagination.* New York: Harper & Row, 1963.

Russell, J. L. "Contraception and the Natural Law." *Heythrop Journal* 10 (1969): 121-134.

Russell, O. Ruth. *Freedom to Die: Moral and Legal Aspects of Euthanasia.* New York: Human Sciences Press, 1975. Paperback edition, Dell, 1976.

Russo, S.J., Biagio. *Humanae Vitae: Commento ai commenti.* Naples: Edizioni Dehoniane, 1969.

Sadler, Alfred, et al. "The Uniform Anatomical Gift Act." *Journal American Medical Association* 206 (1968): 2501-2506.

Sagov, Stanley E., and Brodsky, Archie. *The Active Patient's Guide to Better Medical Care.* New York: McKay, 1976.

Sahuc, Louis J. *La morale catholique est-elle humaine?* Paris: Bloud et Gay, 1970.

St. John-Stevas, Norman. *Life, Death and the Law: Law and Christian Morals in England and the United States.* Bloomington, Ind.: Indiana University Press, 1961.

_____. *The Agonising Choice: Birth Control, Religion and the Law.* Bloomington, Ind.: Indiana University Press, 1971.

"The Sale of Human Body Parts." *Michigan Law Review* 72 (1974): 1182-1264.

Saltman, Jules, and Zimering, Stanley. *Abortion Today.* Springfield, Ill.: Charles C Thomas, 1973.

Sanford, Agnes. *The Healing Gifts of the Spirit.* New York: Pillar Books, 1976.

Sapp, Stephen. *Sexuality, the Bible, and Science.* Philadelphia: Fortress Press, 1977. On biological and cultural bases of sexual identity, pp. 79-106.

Sarvis, Betty, and Rodman, Hyman. *The Abortion Controversy.* New York: Columbia University Press, 1973.

"Scarce Medical Resources." *Columbia Law Review* 69 (1969): 620-692.

Schaefer, John. "The Morality of Breath." *Journal of Pastoral Counseling* 25 (1971): 112-176.

Schall, S.J., J. V. "The Long-Range Significance of the Encyclical HV." *Month* 40 (1968): 245-251.

Schillebeeckx, O.P., Edward. *Christ: The Sacrament of the Encounter with God.* New York: Sheed & Ward, 1963.

_____. *Marriage: Human Reality and Saving Mystery.* New York: Herder, 1964.

_____. *Revelation and Theology,* 2 vols., Vol. 1. New York: Sheed & Ward, 1968, pp. 3-24.

Schnackenburg, Rudolf. *The Moral Teaching of the New Testament.* New York: Herder & Herder, 1965.

Schneiderman, Lawrence J., et al. "Birth Control, Sterilization and Abortion." *Western Journal of Medicine* 120 (1974): 174-179.

Schneidman, Edwin S., ed. *Essays in Self-Destruction.* New York: Science House, 1967.

_____, ed. *On the Nature of Suicide.* San Francisco: Jossey-Bass, 1969.

_____, and Farberow, Norman L. *Clues to Suicide.* New York: McGraw-Hill, 1959.

_____, and Litman, Robert E. *The Psychology of Suicide.* New York: Science House, 1970.

Schoeck, Helmut, and Wiggins, James W., eds. *Relativism and the Study of Man.* Princeton, N.J.: Van Nostrand, 1961.

Schroeder, H. H. "Some Misinterpretations of the Kantian Ethics." *Philosophical Review* 49 (1940): 424-426.

Schubert-Soldern, Rainer. *Mechanism and Vitalism.* Notre Dame, Ind.: University of Notre Dame Press, 1962.

Schüller, Bruno. *Die Begründung sittlicher Urteile: Typen ethischer Argumentation in der katholischen Moraltheologie.* Düsseldorf: Patmos Verlag, 1973.

————. "Neuere Beiträge zum Thema 'Begründung sittlicher Normen'." *Theologische Berichte*, no. 4. Zurich: Benziger, 1974, pp. 109-182.

Schur, E. M., ed. *The Family and the Sexual Revolution.* London: G. Allen, 1966.

Schwartz, Harry. *The Case for American Medicine: A Realistic Look at Our Health Care System.* New York: McKay, 1972.

Schwartz, Richard. "Psychiatry's Drift Away from Medicine." *American Journal of Psychiatry* 131 (1974): 129-134.

Schwitzgebel, Robert L., and Schwitzgebel, Ralph K., eds. *Psychotechnology: Electronic Control of Mind and Behavior.* New York: Holt, 1973.

Scott, Byron T. "Doctors and Dying: Is Euthanasia Now Becoming Accepted?" *Medical Opinion* 10 (1974): 31-34.

Scott, Graham D. "Abortion and the Incarnation." *Journal of Evangelical Theological Society* 17 (1974): 29-44.

Sedgwick, Peter. "Illness — Mental and Otherwise." *Hastings Center Studies* 1, no. 3 (1973): 19-40.

Sellers, James. *Theological Ethics.* New York: Macmillan, 1966.

Senate Judiciary Committee. "Draft Legislation on Euthanasia and Refusal of Treatment." February 22, 1973.

Shakow, David. "Ethics for a Scientific Age: Some Moral Aspects of Psychoanalysis." *Psychoanalytic Review* 52 (Fall 1965): 5-18.

Shannon, Thomas A., ed. *Bioethics: Basic Writings on the Key Ethical Questions that Surround the Major Modern Biological Possibilities and Problems.* New York: Paulist Press, 1976.

Shannon, William H. *The Lively Debate: Response to "Humanae Vitae."* New York: Sheed & Ward, 1970.

Shapiro, Michael H. "Who Merits Merit? Problems in Distributive Justice and Utility Posed by the New Biology." *Southern California Law Review* 48 (1974): 318-370.

Shaw, Margery W. "Genetic Counseling." *Science* 184 (1974): 751.

Shaw, Russell. *Abortion on Trial.* Dayton: Pflaum Press, 1968.

Shehan, Lawrence Cardinal. *"Humanae Vitae: 1968-1973."* *Homiletic and Pastoral Review* 74 (1973): 14-32 (Nov.); 20-32 (Dec.).

Sheps, Cecil G. "The Influence of Consumer Sponsorship on Medical Services." In *Organizational Issues in the Delivery of Health Services*, edited by Irving K. Zola and John B. McKinlay. New York: Milbank Memorial Fund, 1974, pp. 365-392.

Shibutani, Tamotsu. *Society and Personality.* Englewood Cliffs, N.J.: Prentice-Hall, 1961.

Shinn, Roger L. "Personal Decisions and Social Policies in a Pluralist Society." *Perkins Journal of Theology* 27 (Fall 1973): 58-63.

Shinsheimer, Robert L. "Prospects for Future Scientific Developments: Ambush or Opportunity." In *Ethical Issues in Human Genetics*, edited by Bruce Hilton, et al. New York: Plenum, 1973.

Shirer, William. *The Rise and Fall of the Third Reich*. New York: Simon & Shuster, 1960. On the medical experiments, pp. 1274-1289.

Shor, Joel. "The Ethics of Freud's Psycho-Analysis." *International Journal of Psycho-Analysis* 152 (1961): 116-122.

Shore, Milton E., and Golann, Stuart E., eds. *Current Ethical Issues in Mental Health*. Rockville, Md.: National Institute of Mental Health, 1973.

Shriver, Donald W., Jr. "Lifeboat Ethics: The Case for the Mainlanders." *American Society of Christian Ethics*. Selected Papers, 1976, pp. 17-32.

Siegel, Seymour. "A Bias for Life." *Hastings Center Report* 5 (1975): 23-25.

Siegler, Miriam, and Osmond, Humphrey. *Models of Madness, Models of Medicine*. New York: Macmillan, 1974.

_____, and Mann, Harriet. "Laing's Models of Madness." In *R. D. Laing and Anti-Psychiatry*, edited by R. Boyers and R. Orrill. New York: Harper & Row, 1972.

Sieverts, Steven. *Health Planning Issues and Public Law 93-641*. Chicago: American Hospital Association, 1977.

Sigerist, Henry E. *A History of Medicine*. New York: Oxford University Press, 1951.

_____. In *Henry E. Sigerist on Medicine*, edited by Milton E. Roemer and James M. MacKintosh. New York: MD Publishers, 1960. "An Outline of the Development of the Hospital," pp. 319-326; "The Special Position of the Sick," pp. 9-22.

Silverman, Daniel; Saunders, Michael G.; Schwab, Robert S.; and Masland, Richard L. "Cerebral Death and the Electroencephalogram: Report of the Ad Hoc Committee of the American Electroencephalographic Society on the EEG Criteria for Determination of Brain Death." *Journal of American Medical Association* 209 (1969): 1505-1510.

Silverman, Daniel, et al. "Irreversible Coma Associated with Electrocerebral Silence." *Neurology* 20 (1970): 525-533.

Silverman, Milton, and Lee, Phillip R. *Pills, Profits and Politics*. Berkeley: University of California Press, 1974.

Silving, Helen. "Euthanasia: A Study in Comparative Criminal Law." *University of Pennsylvania Law Review* 103 (1954): 350-389.

Simmons, R., and Fulton, J. "Ethical Issues in Kidney Transplant." In *Is It Moral to Modify Man?*, edited by Claude A. Frazier. Springfield, Ill.: Charles C Thomas, 1973.

Simon, Lawrence. "The Ethics of Triage." *Christian Century* 92 (1975): 12-15.

Simon, Yves. *The Tradition of Natural Law*. New York: Fordham University Press, 1965.

Singer, Daniel M. "Impact of the Law on Genetic Counseling." *Birth Defects*. Original Articles Series, IX (April 1974). White Plains, N.Y.: National Foundation March of Dimes, 1974, pp. 34-38.

Singer, Peter. *Animal Liberation: A New Ethics for Our Treatment of Animals*. New York: New York Review, 1975.

Skinner, B. F.
1953.   *Science and Human Behavior*. New York: Macmillan.
1964.   "Behaviorism at Fifty." In *Behaviorism and Phenomenology*, edited by T. W. Wann. Chicago: University of Chicago Press.

1971. *Beyond Freedom and Dignity.* New York: Knopf.

1974. *About Behaviorism.* New York: Random House.

Slater, Robert L. *World Religions and World Community.* New York: Columbia University Press, 1963.

Sloan, Frank, and Feldman, Roger. "Monopolistic Elements in the Market for Physicians' Services." Paper delivered at the Federal Trade Commission Conference on Competition in the Health Care Sector, June 1977.

Sloane, Robert M., and LeRoy, Betty. *A Guide to Health Facilities,* 2nd ed. St. Louis: Mosby, 1977.

Small, Leonard. *The Briefer Psychotherapies.* New York: Brunner/Mazel, 1971.

Smart, J. J., and Williams, B. *Utilitarianism: For and Against.* London: Cambridge University Press, 1973.

Smart, Ninian. *The Religious Experience of Mankind,* 2nd ed. New York: Scribner, 1976, pp. 390-441; 517-556.

Smith, Charles, et al. "Individuals at Risk in Families with Genetic Disease." *Journal of Medical Genetics* 8 (1971): 453-459.

Smith, David B., and Kaluzny, Arnold D. *The White Labyrinth: Understanding the Organization of Health Care.* Berkeley, Calif.: McCutchan, 1975.

Smith, David T., ed. *Abortion and the Law.* Cleveland: Western Reserve University Press, 1967.

Smith, G., and Smith, E. D. "Selection for Treatment in Spina Bifida Cystica." *British Medical Journal* 4 (1973): 189-197.

Smith, Harmon L. *Ethics and the New Medicine.* Nashville, Tenn.: Abingdon, 1970.

————. "The Minister as Consultant to the Medical Team." *Journal of Religion and Health* 14 (1975): 7-13.

Smith, Luke M. "The System Barriers to Quality Nursing." In *A Sociological Framework for Patient Care,* edited by Jeanette R. Folta and Edith S. Deck. New York: Wiley, 1966, pp. 134-155.

Smith, Raymond K. "Training and Certification for Pastoral Care: Is It A Success." *Hospital Progress,* February 1977, pp. 74-75.

Smith, William B. "Catholic Hospitals and Sterilization." *Linacre Quarterly* 44 (1977): 107-116.

Smythies, J. R., ed. *Brain and Mind: Modern Concepts of the Nature of Mind.* London: Routledge, 1965.

Snyder, Solomon. *Madness and the Brain.* New York: McGraw-Hill, 1973.

Søe, Niels Hansen. In *The Encyclopedia of the Lutheran Church,* edited by Julius Bodensieck. Minneapolis: Augsburg, 1965, Vol. 1: *Ethics,* pp. 810-813.

Somers, Herman M., and Somers, Anne R. "The Changing Doctor-Patient Relationship." From *Doctors, Patients and Health Insurance.* Washington, D.C.: Brookings Institute, 1961.

Sottocornola, S.J., F. *A Look at the New Rite of Penance.* Washington, D.C.: United States Catholic Conference, 1975.

Soukup, O.P., Jacques W. "Human Experimentation — Reasonably Free and Adequately Informed Consent: A Personal Partnership in Moral Decision-Making." Masters thesis, Aquinas Institute of Theology, Dubuque, Iowa, 1976.

Soulen, Richard N. *Care for the Dying.* Atlanta, Ga.: John Knox Press, 1975.

Spector, William. "Health, Human." *New Encyclopedia Britannica,* 15th ed. 1975. Vol. 8, pp. 687-884.

Spicq, O.P., Ceslaus. *Agape in the New Testament.* 3 vols. St. Louis: B. Herder Book Co., 1963.

Spitzer, W. O., and Saylor, C. L. *Birth Control and the Christian: A Protestant Symposium on the Control of Human Reproduction.* Wheaton, Ill.: Tyndale House, 1969. Appendix I: Protestant official statements, pp. 415-464.

Spivak, Jonathan. Conference summary. In *Controls of Medicine.* Washington, D.C.: National Academy of Sciences, 1975, pp. 175-180.

Spoonhour, J. M. "Psychosurgery and Informed Consent." *University of Florida Law Review* 26 (Spring 1974): 432-452.

Sprague, Ruth L. "Abortion: The Right to be Wanted." *Christianity and Crisis* 27 (1967): 220-222.

Spring, Charles M. "The Other Side of the Situation Ethics Debate." *Religion and Life* 39 (1970): 221-228.

Stark, Werner. *The Sociology of Religion.* 5 vols. London: Routledge, 1966. Vol. 1.

Stedman's Medical Dictionary. 23rd ed. Baltimore: Williams & Wilkins, 1976.

Stein, Edward V. *Guilt: Theory and Therapy.* Philadelphia: Westminster Press, 1968.

Stein, Leonard I. "The Doctor-Nurse Game." *Archives of General Psychiatry* 16 (1967): 699-703.

Steinfels, Peter. "Confronting the Other Drug Problem." *Hastings Center Report* 2 (1972): 4-6.

Steppacher, Robert C., and Mauser, Judith S. "Suicide in Male and Female Physicians." *Journal of American Medical Association* 228 (1974): 323-328.

Stern, Curt. *Principles of Human Genetics.* 3rd ed. San Francisco: Freeman, 1973, 690ff.

Stevens, Robert, and Stevens, Rosemary. *Welfare Medicine in America: A Case Study of Medicaid.* New York: The Free Press, 1974.

Stevens, Rosemary. *American Medicine and the Public Interest.* New Haven: Yale University Press, 1971.

Stevenson, Charles L. *Ethics and Language.* New Haven: Yale University Press, 1944.

Stinson, Charles. "Theology and the Baron Frankenstein: Cloning and Beyond." *Christian Century* 89 (1972): 60-63.

Stone, Alan A. "Psychiatry and the Law." *Psychiatric Annals* 1 (1971): 18-44.

_____. "The Right to Treatment and the Psychiatric Establishment." *Psychiatric Annals* 4 (1974): 21ff.

_____. "Overview: The Right to Treatment — Comments on the Law and Its Impact." *American Journal of Psychiatry* 132 (1975): 1125-1134.

Stott, John R. W. "Reverence for Human Life." *Christianity Today* 16 (1972): 852-856.

Strauss, Anselm L., Glaser, Barney, and Quint, Jeanne. "The Nonaccountability of Terminal Care." *Hospitals* 38 (1964): 73-87.

Strawson, P. F. *Individuals: An Essay in Descriptive Metaphysics.* London: Methuen, 1959, pp. 87-116.

Strickler, Ronald C., Keller, P. W., and Warren, J. C. "Artificial Insemination with Fresh Donor Semen." *New England Journal of Medicine* 289 (1975): 848-852.

Suchman, Edward A. "The Addictive Diseases as Socio-Environmental Health Problems." In *Handbook of Medical Sociology*, edited by Howard E. Freeman, Sol Levine, and Leo G. Reeder. Englewood, Cliffs, N.J.: Prentice-Hall, 1963, pp. 123-144.

Sullivan, Frank W. "Peer Review and Professional Ethics." *American Journal of Psychiatry* 134 (1977): 186-188.

Sullivan, Joseph V. *The Morality of Mercy Killing.* Westminster, Md.: Newman Press, 1952.

Sullivan, Michael T. "The Dying Person — His Plight and His Right." *New England Law Review* 8 (1973): 197-216.

Sumner, Charles Graham. *Folkways.* New York: Ginn, 1934 [1906].

Supreme Court of New Jersey. "In the Matter of Karen Quinlan: An Alleged Incompetent." *355 Atlantic Reporter*, 2d, 647. (1976).

Sweet, William H. "Treatment of Medically Intractable Mental Disease by Limited Frontol Leucotomy." *New England Journal of Medicine* 289 (1973): 1117-1125.

Swift, Francis W. "An Analysis of the American Theological Reaction to Janssens' Stand on 'The Pill'." *Louvain Studies* 1 (Fall 1966): 19-53.

Symington, J. W. with Kramer, Thomas R. "Does Peer Review Work?" *American Scientist* 65 (1977): 17-20.

"Symposium on Psychosurgery." *Boston University Law Review* 54 (March 1974): 215-353.

Szasz, Thomas.
    1961.   *The Myth of Mental Illness.* New York: Hoeber-Harper.
    1968a. *Ethics of Psychoanalysis.* New York: Dell. Paperback edition.
    1968b. "Problems Facing Psychiatry: The Psychiatrist as Party to Conflict." In *Ethical Issues in Medicine*, edited by E. Fuller Torrey. Boston: Little, Brown.
    1970.   *The Manufacture of Madness: A Comparative Study of the Inquisition and the Mental Health Movement.* New York: Harper & Row.
    1971a. "The Ethics of Suicide." *Antioch Review* 31 (Spring): 7-17.
    1971b. "The Ethics of Addiction." *American Journal of Psychiatry* 128: 541-546.
    1974a. *Ceremonial Chemistry: The Ritual Persecution of Drugs, Addicts, and Pushers.* New York: Doubleday.
    1974b. *The Myth of Mental Illness.* Rev. ed. New York: Harper & Row.
    1977a. "A Different Dose for Different Folks." *Sceptic* (January-February): 46-49.
    1977b. *The Theology of Medicine: The Political-Philosophical Foundations of Medical Ethics.* New York: Harper & Row.

Szasz, Thomas, and Hollender, Marc H. "The Basic Models of the Doctor-Patient Relationship." *American Medical Association Archives of Internal Medicine* 97 (1956): 585-592.

Szebenyi, A. L. "Reflections of A Biologist." *Theological Studies* 33 (1972): 450-456.

Tachibana, S. *The Ethics of Buddhism.* London: Oxford University Press, 1926.

Talbot, John A. "Radical Psychiatry: Examination of the Issues." *American Journal of Psychiatry* 131 (1974): 121-128.

Tancredi, Laurence R., ed. *Ethics of Health Care.* Papers of the Conference on Health Care and Changing Values, November 27-29, 1973. Washington, D.C.: Institute of Medicine, National Academy of Medicine, 1974.

Tavard, George H. "Ecumenism in Ethics." *Journal of Ecumenical Studies* 10 (Summer 1973): 575-576.

_____. "Ethical Ghettos in the Ecumenical Age." *Worldview* March 1974, pp. 10-12.

Taylor, Lee. *Occupational Sociology.* New York: Oxford University Press, 1968, p. 476.

Taylor, S.J., Michael J., ed. *The Mystery of Suffering and Death.* Staten Island, N.Y.: Alba House, 1973.

Teale, A. E. *Kantian Ethics.* Westport, Conn.: Greenwood Press, 1975.

Teilhard de Chardin, Pierre. *The Future of Man.* New York: Harper & Row, 1964.

Temkin, Owsei. "The Scientific Approach to Disease: Specific Entity and Individual Sickness." In *Scientific Change,* edited by A. C. Crombie. London: Heinemann, 1963, pp. 629-660.

_____. "Health and Disease." In *Dictionary of the History of Ideas,* edited by Philip P. Weiner. New York: Scribners, 1973. Vol. 2, pp. 395-407.

Thielicke, Helmut. *The Ethics of Sex.* New York: Harper & Row, 1964.

_____. *Theological Ethics.* 2 vols. Philadelphia: Fortress Press, 1969. Vol. 1: "Moral Dilemmas," pp. 609-668.

Thils, Gustave. *L'infallibilité pontificiale: sources, conditions, limits.* Paris: Duculot, 1968. On criteria of infallibility, pp. 179-185; on infallibility on moral matters, pp. 207-211.

Thomson, Judith Jarvis. "The Right to Privacy." *Philosophy and Public Affairs* 4 (Summer 1975): 295-314.

Thornton, Edward E. *Theology and Pastoral Counseling.* Englewood Cliffs, N.J.: Prentice-Hall, 1964.

Tietze, Christopher. "Ranking of Contraceptive Methods by Levels of Effectiveness." Report to American Association of Planned Parenthood Physicians, Boston, April 9-10, 1970. In *Advances in Planned Parenthood.* Vol. 6, pp. 117-126. *Excerpta Medica* International Congress Series. New York: Excerpta Medica, 1971.

Tillich, Paul.
  1955.   "Moralisms and Morality from the Point of View of the Ethicist." In *Ministry and Medicine in Human Relations,* edited by Iago Galdston. New York: International Universities Press, pp. 125-140.
  1961.   "The Meaning of Health." *Perspectives in Biology and Medicine* 5: 92-100.
  1963.   *Christianity and the Encounter of the World Religions.* New York: Columbia University Press.
  1967a.   "The Meaning of Health." In *Religion and Medicine,* edited by David Belgum. Ames, Iowa: Iowa State University Press, pp. 3-12.
  1967b.   *Systematic Theology.* 3 vols. Chicago: University of Chicago Press. Vol. 1, 85ff; pp. 147ff.

Titmus, Richard. *The Gift Relationship: From Human Blood to Social Policy.* New York: Pantheon, 1971. Penguin ed., 1973.

Toffler, Alvin. *Future Shock.* New York: Random House, 1970.

Tooley, Michael. "A Defense of Abortion and Infanticide." *Philosophy and Public Affairs* 2 (1972): 37-65.

Torrey, E. Fuller. *The Mind Game: Witchdoctors and Psychiatrists.* New York: Bantam Books, 1972.

_____. *The Death of Psychiatry.* Radnor, Pa.: Chilton, 1974.

Toulmin, Stephen. *An Examination of the Place of Reason in Ethics.* New York: Cambridge University Press, 1950.

Touraine, Alain. *The Post-Industrial Society.* New York: Random House, 1971.

Tournier, Paul. *The Meaning of Persons.* London: SMC Press, 1957, pp. 128ff.

_____, ed. *Medicine of the Whole Person.* Waco, Texas: Word Books, 1973.

"Toward a Definition of Fetal Life: Ethical and Legal. Options and Their Implications for Biologists and Physicians." Symposium. *Clinical Research* 23 (1975): 211-244.

Travis, Terry A., Noyes, Russell, Jr., and Brightwell, Dennis R. "The Attitudes of Physicians Toward Prolonging Life." *International Journal of Psychiatry in Medicine* 5 (1974): 17-26.

Treffert, Darold A. "The Practical Limits of Patients' Rights." *Psychiatric Annals* 5 (1975): 91-96.

Trendler, Moshe. *Medical Ethics: A Compendium of Jewish Moral, Ethical and Religious Principles in Medical Practice.* New York: Committee on Religious Affairs of the Federation of Jewish Philanthropies of New York, 1975.

Triche, Charles, III, and Triche, Diane Samson. *The Euthanasia Controversy 1812-1974.* Bibliography with select annotations. Troy, N.Y.: Whitson, 1975.

Trowell, Hugh. *The Unfinished Debate on Euthanasia.* London: SCM Press, 1973.

Trubo, Richard. *An Act of Mercy: Euthanasia Today.* Plainview, N.Y.: Nash Publishing, 1973.

Uhr, Leonard Merrick, and Miller, James G. *Drugs and Behavior.* New York: Wiley, 1960.

Ulanov, Ann, and Ulanov, Barry. *Religion and the Unconscious.* Philadelphia: Westminster Press, 1975.

Ulich, Robert. "On Education of Teachers." In *Intellectual Foundations of American Education,* edited by Harold J. Carter. New York: Pitman, 1968, pp. 577-583.

Ulrich, Roger, Stachik, Thomas, and Mabry, John. *Control of Human Behavior.* 3 vols. Glenview, Ill.: Scott, Foresman, 1974.

Underwood, Kenneth. *The Church, the University, and Social Policy.* 2 vols. Middletown, Conn.: Wesleyan University Press, 1972. Vol. 1, pp. 422-436.

United Church of Christ Eighth General Synod. "Freedom of Choice Concerning Abortion." *Social Action* 38 (1971): 9-12.

United Nations. *Universal Declaration of Human Rights.* New York: United Nations Publications, 1948.

Uricchio, W. A., ed. *Proceedings of a Research Conference on Natural Family Planning.* Washington, D.C.: Human Life Foundation, 1973.

Urmson, J. O. *Emotive Theory of Ethics.* New York: Oxford University Press, 1969.

United States Catholic Conference. *Ethical and Religious Directives for Catholic Health Facilities.* Approved by National Conference of Catholic Bishops and the United States Catholic Conference November 1971 as "the national code, subject to the approval of the bishop for use in the diocese." Washington, D.C.: U.S. Catholic Conference, 1971.

_____. *Selected Documentation from the New Sacramentary.* Washington, D.C.: U.S. Catholic Conference, 1974.

_____. "Guidelines for the Determination of Brain Death." *Hospital Progress,* December 1975, p. 26.

U.S. Department of Health, Education, and Welfare. Public Health Service. National Institutes of Health, National Institute of Neurological Diseases and Stroke, Applied Neurologic Research Branch. *Brain Death: A Bibliography with Key-Word and Author Indexes* edited by Andrew J. K. Smith and J. Kiffin Penry. DHEW Publication No. (NIH) 73-347. Washington, D.C.: Government Printing Office, 1972.

_____. *Report of the Secretary's Commission on Medical Malpractice*, January 16, 1973, Washington, D.C.

_____. *Protection of Human Subjects: Fetuses, Pregnant Women, and "in Vitro" Fertilization*, August 8, 1975, Washington, D.C.

Valenstein, Eliot S. *Brain Control: A Critical Examination of Brain Stimulation and Psychosurgery.* New York: Wiley, 1973.

Valsecchi, Ambrogio. *Controversy: The Birth Control Debate, 1958-1968.* Washington, D. C.: Corpus Books, 1968.

_____. *Regulation des Naissances.* Gembloux: J. Duculot, 1970.

Van Allen, Rogers. "Artificial Insemination (AIH): A Content Re-Analysis." *Homiletic and Pastoral Review* 70 (1970): 363-372.

Van den Haag, Ernest. *Punishing Criminals: Concerning a Very Old and Painful Question.* New York: Basic Books, 1975.

Van der Poel, Cornelius J. "The Principle of Double Effect." In *Absolutes in Moral Theology*, edited by Charles E. Curran. Washington, D.C.: Corpus Books, 1968, pp. 186-210.

Van Hoose, William H., and Kottler, Jeffrey A. *Ethical and Legal Issues in Counseling and Psychotherapy.* San Francisco: Jossy-Bass, 1977.

Van Kaam, Adrian. *The Addictive Personality.* Synthesis series. Chicago: Franciscan Herald Press, 1966.

Van Roo, S.J., W. A. "Infants Dying Without Baptism: A Survey of Recent Literature and a Determination of the State of the Question." *Gregorianum* 35 (1954): 406-473.

Vatican II Documents.
    Quotations and citations are from Flannery, O.P., Austin, ed. *Vatican II: The Conciliar and Post Conciliar Documents.* Collegeville, Minn.: Liturgical Press, 1975. Cf. also Abbott, S.J., Walter M., ed. *The Documents of Vatican II.* New York: Association Press, 1966.
    1964a. *Dogmatic Constitution on the Church. (Lumen Gentium*, 21 November), pp. 350-426.
    1964b. *Decree on Ecumenism (Unitatis Redintegratio*, 21 November), pp. 452-470.
    1965a. *Declaration on the Relation of the Church to Non-Christian Religions (Nostra Aetate*, 28 October), pp. 738-742.
    1965b. *Declaration on Religious Liberty (Dignitatis Humanae*, 7 December), pp. 799-812.
    1965c. *Pastoral Constitution on the Church in the Modern World (Gaudium et Spes*, 7 December), pp. 903-1001.

Vaux, Kenneth. *Biomedical Ethics: Morality for the New Medicine.* New York: Harper & Row, 1974.

Veatch, Henry. *Rational Man: A Modern Introduction to Aristotle's Ethics.* Bloomington, Ind.: Indiana University Press, 1962.

_____. *For an Ontology of Morals: A Critique of Contemporary Ethical Theory.* Evanston, Ill.: Northwestern University Press, 1971.

Veatch, Robert M.
    1972a. "The Unexpected Chromosome: The Counselor's Dilemma." *Hastings Center Report* 2, no. 1: 8-9.
    1972b. "Brain Death: Welcome Definition or Dangerous Judgment?" *Hastings Center Report* 2: 10-13.
    1972c. "Medical Ethics: Professional or Universal." *Harvard Theological Review* 65: 531-539.
    1973a. "Does Ethics Have an Empirical Basis?" *Hastings Center Studies* 1, no. 1: 50-65.
    1973b. "The Medical Model: Its Nature and Problems." *Hastings Center Studies* 1, no. 3: 59-76.
    1974. "Drugs and Competing Drug Ethics." *Hastings Center Studies* 2: 68-80.
    1975. "The Whole-Brain-Oriented Concept of Death: An Outmoded Philosophical Formulation." *Journal of Thanatology* 3, no. 1: 13-30.
    1976. *Death, Dying, and the Biological Revolution: Our Last Quest for Responsibility.* New Haven: Yale University Press.

Veatch, Robert M., and Branson, Roy. *Ethics and Health Policy.* Cambridge, Mass.: Ballinger, 1976.

_____, Gaylin, Willard, and Councilman, Morgan, eds. *The Teaching of Medical Ethics.* Hastings-on-the-Hudson, N.Y.: Institute of Society, Ethics and the Life Sciences, 1973.

Vereecke, Louis. "Preface a l'histoire de la theologie morale moderne." In *Studia Moralia.* Rome: Edicion Ancora, 1962. Vol. 1: Academia Alfonsiana, pp. 87-129.

Verwoerdt, Adriaan. *Communications with the Fatally Ill.* Springfield, Ill.: Charles C Thomas, 1966.

Viederman, Milton, and Burke, Daniel. "Saying 'No' to Hemodialysis." *Hastings Center Report* 4 (1974): 8-10.

Virginia Department of Health. *Holland v. Sisters of St. Joseph,* 1974.

Visscher, Maurice B. *Humanistic Perspectives in Medical Ethics.* Buffalo: Prometheus Books, 1972.

Vodiga, Bruce. "Euthanasia and the Right to Die — Moral, Ethical and Legal Perspectives." *Chicago-Kent Law Review* 51 (Summer 1974): 1-40.

Volpe, E. Peter. *Human Heredity and Birth Defects.* Indianapolis: Bobbs-Merrill, Pegasus, 1971.

Von Hildebrand, Dietrich. *The Encyclical "Humanae Vitae": A Sign of Contradiction.* Chicago: Franciscan Herald Press, 1969.

Vonier, Anscar. *A Key to the Doctrine of the Eucharist.* London: Burns Oates, 1931.

Wade, Francis C. "Potentiality in the Abortion Discussion." *Review of Metaphysics* 22 (1975): 239-255.

Wahlberg, Rachel Conrad. "The Woman and the Fetus: 'One Flesh'?" *Christian Century* 88 (1971): 1045-1048.

_____. "Abortion: Decisions to Live With." *Christian Century* 90 (1973): 691-693.

Walkefield, John C. *Artful Childmaking: Artificial Insemination and Catholic Teaching.* St. Louis: Pope John XXIII Institute for Medical Moral Research and Education, in press.

Walgrave, O.P., John H. *Person and Society: A Christian View.* Pittsburgh: Duquesne University Press, 1965, pp. 94-116.

Walker, Earl, et al. "An Appraisal of the Criteria of Cerebral Death." *Journal of American Medical Association* 237 (1977): 982-986.

Wallenmaier, Thomas E. "A Philosopher Looks at Medical Ethics." *Journal of Medical Education* 50 (1975): 99-100.

Walters, L. "Technology Assessment and Genetics." *Theological Studies* 33 (1972): 666-683.

Wardwell, Walter I. "Limited, Marginal, and Quasi Practioneers." In *Handbook of Medical Sociology*, edited by Howard E. Freeman, Sol Levine, and Leo G. Reeder. Englewood Cliffs, N.J.: Prentice-Hall, 1963, pp. 212-240.

Warnock, Mary. *Ethics Since 1900*. London: Oxford University Press, 1960.

Warwick, Donald. Review of Ivan Illich, *Medical Nemesis*. *Commonweal* 103 (1976): 570-572.

Wasmuth, Carl E., Jr. "The Concept of Death." *Ohio State Law Journal* 30 (1969): 32-60.

Wasserstrom, Richard. "The Status of the Fetus." *Hastings Center Report* (1975): 18-22.

Wassmer, S.J., Thomas A. "Contemporary Attitudes of the Roman Catholic Church Toward Abortion." *Journal of Religion and Health* 7 (1968): 311-323.

Watson, James D. "Moving Toward the Clonal Man: Is This What We Want?" *The Atlantic*. May 1971, pp. 50-53.

Weber, Leonard J. *Who Shall Live? The Dilemma of Severely Handicapped Children and Its Meaning for Other Moral Questions*. New York: Paulist Press, 1976.

Weinberg, George H. *Society and the Healthy Homosexual*. New York: St. Martin's Press, 1972.

Weinberg, Martin. *Sex Research: Studies from the Kinsey Institute*. New York: Oxford University Press, 1976.

Wells, William W. "Drug Control of School Children: The Child's Right to Choose." *Southern California Law Review* 46 (1973): 585-616.

Wender, Paul H. "The Case of MBD." *Hastings Center Studies* 2, no. 1 (January 1974): 94-102.

————. *The Hyperactive Child*. New York: Crown, 1973.

Wertham, Frederic. *A Sign for Cain*. New York: Paperback Library, 1969.

Wertz, Richard W. *Readings on Ethical and Social Issues in Biomedicine*. Englewood Cliffs, N.J.: Prentice-Hall, 1973.

West, Louis Jolyon. "Psychiatry, 'Brainwashing,' and the American Character." *American Journal of Psychiatry* 120 (1964): 842-850.

————. "Ethical Psychiatry and Biosocial Humanism." *American Journal of Psychiatry* 126 (1969): 226-239.

————. "Hallucinogenic Drugs: Perils and Possibilities." *Hastings Center Studies* 2, no. 1 (January 1974): 103-112.

Westberg, Granger E. *Good Grief: A Constructive Approach to the Problem of Loss*. Rock Island, Ill.: Augustana Press, 1971.

Westley, Richard J. "Some Reflections on Birth-Control." *Listening* 12 (Spring 1977): 43-61.

Westoff, Charles F., and Rindfuss, Ronald R. "Sex Preselection in the United States: Some Implications." *Science* 184 (1974): 633-636.

Wheeler, Harvey. *Operant Conditioning: Social and Political Aspects.* San Francisco: Freeman, 1973, pp. 22-56.

White, Andrew Dickson. *A History of the Warfare of Science with Theology in Christendom* [1896]. New York: Dover, 1960. Vol. 2, pp. 55-63.

White, John, ed. *The Highest State of Consciousness.* Garden City, N.Y.: Doubleday, Anchor Books, 1972.

White, Robert B., and Engelhardt, H. Tristram, Jr. "Case Studies in Bioethics: A Demand to Die." *Hastings Center Report* 5 (1975): 9ff.

White, Victor. *God and the Unconscious.* London: Harvill Press, 1952.

Whitehead, Alfred North. *Process and Reality* [1929]. New York: Macmillan and The Free Press, 1957.

"Why You Do What You Do: Sociobiology: A New Theory of Behavior." *Time Magazine,* 1 August 1977, pp. 54-63.

Wilensky, Harold L. "The Professionalization of Everyone?" *American Journal of Sociology* 70 (1964): 137-158.

Wilke, J. C., and Wilke, Barbara. *Handbook on Abortion.* Cincinnati: Hayes Publishing, 1975.

Wilkins, Leslie T. "Putting 'Treatment' on Trial." *Hastings Center Report* 5 (1975): 35-37.

Williams, Cornelius. "The Hedonism of Acquinas." *Thomist* 38 (1974): 257-290.

Williams, G. H. "Religious Residues and Presuppositions in the American Debate on Abortion." *Theological Studies* 31 (1970): 10-75.

Williams, Glarville L. *The Sanctity of Life and Criminal Law.* New York: Knopf, 1968.

Williams, Mary Kay. *Abortion: A Collision of Rights.* Washington, D.C.: National Catholic News Service, 1972.

Williams, Preston, et al. *Ethical Issues in Biology and Medicine.* Cambridge, Mass.: Schenkman, 1973.

Wilson, Edward O. *Sociobiology: The New Synthesis.* Cambridge, Mass.: Harvard University Press, 1975. (a)

_____. *Sociobiology: The New Synthesis.* Cambridge, Mass.: Harvard University Press, Belknap Press, 1975. (b)

Wilson, Jerry B. *Death by Decision: The Medical, Moral and Legal Dilemmas of Euthanasia.* Philadelphia: Westminster Press, 1975.

Wilson, Miriam G. "Genetic Counseling." *Current Problems in Pediatrics* 5 (1975): 1-51.

Wilson, Robert N. "Patient-Practitioner Relationships." In *Handbook of Medical Sociology,* edited by Howard E. Freeman, Sol Levine, and Leo G. Reeder. Englewood Cliffs, N.J.: Prentice-Hall, 1963, pp. 273-295.

Winter, Arthur. *Surgical Control of Behavior.* Springfield, Ill.: Charles C Thomas, 1971.

Winter, Gibson, ed. *Social Ethics: Issues in Ethics and Society.* New York: Harper & Row, 1968.

Wise, Carroll A. *Pastoral Counseling: Its Theory and Practice.* New York: Harper, 1951.

_____. *The Meaning of Pastoral Care.* New York: Harper & Row, 1966.

Wittlin, Alma S. "The Teacher." In *The Professions in America,* edited by Kenneth S. Lynn. Boston: Houghton Mifflin, 1965, pp. 91-109.

Wolpe, Joseph. "The Comparative Clinical Status of Conditioning Theories and Psychoanalysis." In *The Conditioning Therapies: The Challenge of Psychiatry*, edited by Joseph Wolpe, Andrew Slater, and L. J. Reyna. New York: Holt, 1966, pp. 3-20.

_____. *The Practice of Behavior Therapy*. New York: Pergamon Press, 1973.

Wolstenholme, G. E. W., and O'Connor, Maeve. *Ethics in Medical Progress: With Special Reference to Transplantation*. Boston: Little, Brown, 1966.

Worden, J. William. "The Right to Die." *Pastoral Psychology* 23 (1972): 9-14.

Working Party of the Newcastle Regional Hospital Board. "Ethics of Selective Treatment of Spina Bifida." *Lancet* 1 (1975): 85-88.

World Health Organization. *First Ten Years of WHO*. Geneva: World Health Organization, 1958, p. 459.

Wygant, W. E., Jr. "A Protestant Minister's View of Abortion." *Journal of Religion and Health* 11 (1972): 269-277.

Wylie, Charles M. "The Definition and Measurement of Health and Disease." *Public Health Reports* 85 (1970): 100-104.

Young, James Harvey. "Social History of American Drugs Legislation." In *Drugs in Our Society*, edited by Paul Talalay. Baltimore: John Hopkins University Press, 1964.

Zaehner, R. C. *Concordant Discord*. London: Oxford University Press, 1970.

Zumbro Valley Medical Society. *Religious Aspects of Medical Care: A Handbook of Religious Practices of all Faiths*. Medicine and Religion Committee. St. Louis: Catholic Hospital Association, 1975.

INDEX

AUTHORS CITED FREQUENTLY